WORKBOOK

Bob Elling • J. David Bergeron

EMERGENCY CARE

Ninth Edition

■ DANIEL LIMMER

■ MICHAEL F. O'KEEFE

■ HARVEY D. GRANT

■ ROBERT H. MURRAY, JR.

■ J. DAVID BERGERON

Contributors

BETH LOTHROP ADAMS
BOB ELLING
DAVID M. HABBEN
FITZGERALD PETERSEN

Medical Editor

EDWARD T. DICKINSON, M.D., FACEP

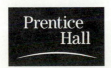

Prentice Hall

BRADY/PRENTICE HALL HEALTH
Upper Saddle River, New Jersey 07458

Dedicated to my two beautiful daughters: Laura and Caitlin. And to my lovely wife Kirsten.
May you always maintain humility as your accomplishments meet the stars!

B.E.

NOTICE ON CARE PROCEDURES

This workbook reflects current EMS practices based on the 1994 U.S. Department of Transportation's EMT-Basic National Standard Curriculum. It is the intent of the authors and publisher that this workbook be used as part of a formal Emergency Medical Technician education program taught by qualified instructors and supervised by a licensed physician. The procedures described in this workbook are based upon consultation with EMS and medical authorities. The authors and publisher have taken care to make certain that these procedures reflect currently accepted clinical practice; however, they cannot be considered absolute recommendations.

The material in this workbook contains the most current information available at the time of publication. However, federal, state, and local guidelines concerning clinical practices, including, without limitation, those governing infection control and universal precautions, change rapidly. The reader should note, therefore, that new regulations may require changes in some procedures.

It is the responsibility of the reader to familiarize himself or herself with the policies and procedures set by federal, state, and local agencies as well as the institution or agency where the reader may be employed. The author and the publisher of this workbook disclaim any liability, loss, or risk resulting directly or indirectly from the suggested procedures and theory, from any undetected errors, or from the reader's misunderstanding of the text. It is the reader's responsibility to stay informed of any new changes or recommendations made by any federal, state, and local agency as well as by his or her employing institution or agency.

If when reading this workbook you find an error, have an idea for how to improve it, or simply want to share your comments with us, please send your letter to one of the following addresses below.

Brady Marketing Department
Prentice Hall
One Lake Street
Upper Saddle River, New Jersey 07458

bobelling@usa.net

NOTICE ON BCLS PROCEDURES

The national standards for BCLS are reviewed and revised on a regular basis and may change slightly after this book is printed. It is important that you know the most current procedures for CPR, both for the classroom and your patients. The most current information may always be downloaded from www.bradybooks.com or obtained from your instructor.

Prentice-Hall International (UK) Limited, *London*
Prentice-Hall of Australia Pty. Limited, *Sydney*
Prentice-Hall Canada Inc., *Toronto*
Prentice-Hall Hispanoamericana, S.A., *Mexico*
Prentice-Hall of India Private Limited, *New Delhi*
Prentice-Hall of Japan, Inc., *Tokyo*
Prentice-Hall Singapore Pte. Ltd.
Editora Prentice-Hall do Brasil, Ltda., *Rio de Janeiro*

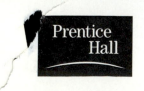

10 9 8 7 6 5

ISBN 0-13-031951-1

Contents

Introduction

▶ OVERVIEW

This workbook is designed to accompany the textbook *Emergency Care,* Ninth Edition. The workbook covers the course knowledge and U.S. Department of Transportation (DOT) skill objectives to which all standardized testing instruments are referenced. It is neither meant to replace the text nor is it meant to be a substitute for a well-designed course in emergency care.

This is a self-instructional workbook. It has been designed to allow you to work at your own pace and evaluate your own progress. To benefit from this workbook, follow the procedures in this introduction. Thousands of EMT-B students before you have used prior editions of this workbook as part of their emergency medical training. The system works, having helped them to learn and excel on state and national certification and registration examinations. By doing your best on each chapter, you, as well as those patients to whom you deliver emergency care, will benefit.

This edition continues the emphasis of the 1994 DOT curriculum on patient assessment. In addition, there are a number of updated sections and new features in this workbook. Additional Case Studies have been added and the EMT-Basic Performance Checklists have been updated. Two new features have been added to the workbook: Virtual Street Scenes and Web Simulations, which are both described below.

▶ FEATURES

Each chapter in the workbook contains these specific elements:

- **Match Terminology/Definitions**—In this section, you are asked to match chapter terminology with appropriate definitions, which are included in the chapter's running text, appear in the chapter glossary, or both. The terms have been placed in alphabetical order so that after reading the definitions you can quickly select the appropriate term.
- **Multiple-Choice Review**—This section provides some 25 to 45 questions (on average). Emphasis is placed on multiple-choice questions, since this is the format of state and national exams used for certification or registration. Practice in answering multiple-choice questions can help improve your understanding of the material as well as your course grades. These multiple-choice questions generally appear in the sequential order that the topics appear in the textbook, enabling you to build on prior knowledge. When similar questions appear in the three Interim Exams, the order is scrambled, as is done on state and national exams.
- **Complete the Following**—This section focuses on your recalling and listing specific information on chapter objectives, such as the signs and symptoms of shock or the five stages of grief.
- **Label the Diagram/Photograph and Complete the Chart**—In some chapters, you are asked to study a visual and to identify its content or to complete a partially filled-in chart. These diagrams, photographs, and charts correspond to those in the textbook.
- **Virtual Street Scenes**—Each chapter of the textbook has a section called Street Scenes. They are designed to apply what you have learned in the chapter to a situation that could easily be found in your work as an EMT-B. In the workbook, you are asked to reread the Street Scenes and then use your imagination and the knowledge you have obtained thus far in your course to answer a few more questions.
- **Web Simulations**—Using the Internet, a number of cases have been designed to complement the topics in the textbook and workbook. These are referred to in the workbook, and the internal (URL) is listed.
- **Case Study**—After every few chapters, a case study requires you to synthesize information that you have learned up to that particular point in the course and to apply this knowledge to a real-life situation. As each step of the case is presented, you are asked a series of questions that build on the facts of the case.
- **Answer Key**—The Answer Key at the back of the workbook provides answers for all of the above-mentioned workbook elements. For the Virtual Street Scenes questions, rationales appear for each answer. For the Multiple-Choice Review questions, rationales are provided where appropriate along with the textbook page reference where each topic is discussed.
- **EMT-Basic Skills Performance Checklists**—Most workbook chapters include a listing of the EMT-B skills that incorporate national

standards or the DOT EMT-B curriculum description of a method of doing each skill. These checklists are from the *Pocket Reference for the EMT-B and First Responder*. This handy pocket-size reference contains not only all of the steps of each of the EMT-B skills, but also many of the medical terms, abbreviations, anatomical charts, and reference tools used in the field.

▶ STEPS FOR SUCCESS

To get the most out of this workbook, you should complete the following eight steps:

Step 1—Learn the Course Objectives

Each chapter of the textbook begins with objectives—objectives that were developed as a part of the U.S. Department of Transportation's EMT-B 1994 training curriculum. Most state and national certifying examinations are based on these course objectives. To score well on those exams, you must learn the objectives of the course. Use the objectives in the textbook in the following way:

1. Read them over.
2. Read the text.
3. Reread the objective in the form of a question.
4. Write down your answer to each question on a blank piece of paper.
5. Perform a self-assessment or ask your instructor to assess how well you understand the material in the chapter.

Step 2—Learn the Language of the EMT-Basic

Emergency Medical Services (EMS) is clearly a medical field and as such it is necessary for the EMT-Basic to learn and understand the language of medicine. This will help you communicate with the other members of the health-care team in a clear, concise, and accurate manner. In addition, learning the language of medicine will facilitate your understanding of medical and trade journal articles as you work to keep current in the constantly changing EMS field.

First, review the medical terminology in the text and then put aside the text. Next, test your understanding of the terminology by completing the Match Terminology/Definitions exercise in each workbook chapter. Complete the entire matching exercise before checking your answers against the Answer Key. For those terms you were unable to match, write down the word on

one side of a 3" × 5" card and write the definition on the other side of the card. Carry these cards in your pocket and refer to them frequently to help you learn the terms.

Step 3—Learn the Structure of the Body

The language of medicine also includes learning the names and locations of the structures of the human body. Imagine being unable to control serious bleeding because you could not find the pressure point in the arm! To help you learn the structures of the body, in workbook chapters in which it is appropriate, anatomical drawings and diagrams are provided. For example, the drawing of the respiratory system in the workbook has blank numbered lines that point to each of the system's different structures. Label each structure as requested and check your answers in the back of the workbook. For those you miss, go to the textbook page suggested and study the body structure again.

Step 4—Answer the Multiple-Choice Questions

For each Multiple-Choice Review, complete the entire exercise at one sitting. Read each question and all the answer choices before you mark your answer. If you jump to a conclusion without fully reading the question, you could answer incorrectly. Also, watch out for questions with negative expressions or the word "except." You will notice that the author has minimized the use of "all of the above" as an answer to questions in this edition. This was done to ensure that exam items mirror those used in standardized tests. Once you have completed the exercise, refer to the Answer Key to check your performance. A textbook page reference has been provided for the theory or principle tested in each question. Many answers have an "author's comment" whenever it is appropriate to clarify the answer to a question.

You will need to practice reading, and not reading into, multiple-choice questions. If it has been many years since you took a standardized test, leave extra time to review this section of each workbook chapter. If you notice any trends in your performance on these questions, you may wish to consult your instructor for "test-taking assistance."

Step 5—Utilize the Virtual Street Scenes and Web Simulations in this workbook and on the Internet.

Step 6—Review the EMT-Basic Skill Performance Checklists

Whenever a skill is introduced in the chapter, a checklist has been included in the workbook. Work in pairs and use these checklists to test each other.

Step 7—Take the Interim Exams

Once you have completed each individual workbook chapter, move on to the next chapter and repeat steps one to five. Interim Exams appear after Modules 2, 4, and 7 and are similar to the interim exams your instructor may give in the EMT-Basic course. Each exam covers material in the chapters that precede it. Therefore, when you have completed all of the material preceding an exam, it's time to take the Interim Exam.

Also be sure to review the extra materials in the Appendix sections that appear at the end of the workbook.

Step 8—Pay Close Attention to the Case Studies

The case studies integrated in the workbook help you synthesize your knowledge and apply it to real-life situations. They actually put you at a scene and require you to think quickly and accurately. Answers at the back of the workbook will help you sort out any problems you confront.

So that's it in eight simple steps. It will take your time and commitment to work through each of the steps. Since this is a self-instructional workbook, it will be up to you to reward yourself for doing well on chapters. At the same time, you need to be honest with yourself. If you are having difficulty with a chapter, let your instructor know immediately so he or she can offer additional assistance.

It is the hope of the *Emergency Care* authors and development team that using this workbook as an integral part of your EMT-Basic training package will help you improve your understanding of the material and enhance your performance in the field. After all, isn't quality patient care what EMS is all about? See you in the streets!

▶ ACKNOWLEDGMENTS

The authors of the *Emergency Care Workbook*, Ninth Edition would like to thank the publishing team led by Julie Alexander, Laura Edwards, and Lois Berlowitz for all their hard work and support on the *Emergency Care* series. Appreciation is extended to Dan Limmer and Mike O'Keefe for their friendship and confidence and the opportunity to partake in this important project. Gratitude is extended to Terse Stamos and Jo Cepeda for excellent manuscript editing. And last, but not least, a special thanks to J. David Bergeron.

▶ ABOUT THE NINTH EDITION WORKBOOK AUTHOR

Bob Elling, MPA, REMT-P, has been involved in EMS since 1975. He is an active paramedic with the Town of Colonie (NY) EMS Department, and National Faculty for the AHA. Regional Faculty for the NYS Bureau of EMS. Bob also is a Professor of EMS for the American College of Prehospital Medicine. He has served as a paramedic and lieutenant for NYC EMS, Program Director for the Hudson Valley Community College's Institute of Prehospital Emergency Medicine in Troy, New York, Associate Director of the NYS EMS Program, the Education Coordinator for PULSE: Emergency Medical Update, and is on the JEMS editorial review board. He is the author of the *Pocket Reference for the EMT-B and First Responder*, *MedReview for the EMT-B*, coauthor of *Essentials of Emergency Care*, *PARAMEDIC CARE:Principles & Practice Workbook Volume 5*, and of *First Responder: Exam Preparation and Review*. You can reach him at his e:mail address: bobelling@USA.net

Chapter One
INTRODUCTION TO EMERGENCY MEDICAL CARE

MATCH TERMINOLOGY/DEFINITIONS

A. State laws that allow an EMS system to exist

B. An all out effort by EMS personnel to improve the service provided from the moment of contact to the moment of delivery to the most appropriate medical facility and personnel

C. The provision for physician input and direction of patient care, training, and quality assurance of an emergency medical service or system

D. A system designed to get trained personnel to the patient as quickly as possible and to provide emergency care on the scene, en route to the hospital, and in the hospital

E. Policy or protocol issued by a Medical Director that authorizes EMT-Bs or others to perform particular skills in certain situations

F. Lists of steps, such as assessment and interventions, to be taken in different situations that are developed by the Medical Director of an EMS system

G. A communications system that has the capability of automatically identifying the caller's phone number and location

H. A system for telephone access to report emergencies in which a dispatcher answers the call, takes the information, and alerts EMS or the fire or police departments as needed

I. An EMT-B or other person authorized by a Medical Director to give medications and provide emergency care

J. A physician who assumes the ultimate responsibility for the patient care aspects of the EMS system

_____ **1.** Designated agent

_____ **2.** EMS system

_____ **3.** Enabling legislation

_____ **4.** Enhanced 9-1-1

_____ **5.** Medical direction

_____ **6.** Medical Director

_____ **7.** 9-1-1 system

_____ **8.** Protocols

_____ **9.** Quality improvement

_____ **10.** Standing order

_____ **1.** The earliest documented emergency medical service was in
- **A.** England in the 1890s.
- **B.** France in the 1790s.
- **C.** Seattle in the 1970s.
- **D.** Miami in the 1960s.

_____ **2.** In 1966, the _____ charged the United States _____ with developing EMS standards.
- **A.** Uniform Traffic Act : Department of Transportation
- **B.** President : Fire Academy
- **C.** National Highway Safety Act : Department of Transportation
- **D.** American Medical Association : Department of Health & Human Services

_____ **3.** Of the following, which is <u>not</u> a major component in the National Highway Traffic Safety Administration's EMS system assessment standards?
- **A.** transportation
- **B.** computerization
- **C.** communications
- **D.** evaluation

_____ **4.** An example of a "specialty" hospital in the EMS system is a(n)
- **A.** emergency department.
- **B.** correctional facility.
- **C.** poison control center.
- **D.** primary care center.

_____ **5.** National levels of EMS training include all of the following <u>except</u>
- **A.** advanced first aid.
- **B.** First Responder.
- **C.** EMT-Intermediate.
- **D.** EMT-Paramedic.

_____ **6.** The major emphasis of the curriculum for the EMT-B deals with _____ of the ill or injured patient in the prehospital setting.
- **A.** immediate life-threatening care
- **B.** interpretation of electrocardiograms
- **C.** assessment and care
- **D.** techniques of advanced airway care

_____ **7.** Patient care provided by the EMT-B should be
- **A.** delayed until transportation.
- **B.** based on assessment findings.
- **C.** guided by the service's attorney.
- **D.** based upon your diagnosis of the patient.

_____ **8.** An example of assuring continuity during the transfer of care of the patient would be
- **A.** providing pertinent patient information to the hospital staff.
- **B.** performing more hospital procedures in the field.
- **C.** only giving a report directly to a physician.
- **D.** none of the above.

_____ **9.** Patient advocacy is
- **A.** assessing your patient.
- **B.** abandoning your patient.
- **C.** executing your primary responsibility as an EMT-B.
- **D.** speaking up for your patient.

_____ **10.** Good personality traits are very important to the EMT-B. You should be
- **A.** cooperative and resourceful.
- **B.** cunning and inventive.
- **C.** respectful and condescending.
- **D.** emotionally stable and shy.

_____ **11.** If an EMT-B is <u>not</u> in control of personal habits, he/she might
- **A.** contaminate the patient's wounds.
- **B.** make inappropriate decisions.
- **C.** render improper care.
- **D.** do all of the above.

_____ **12.** To prevent violating patient confidentiality, the EMT-B should
- **A.** communicate with medical direction.
- **B.** perform an accurate interview.
- **C.** avoid inappropriate conversation.
- **D.** develop the ability to listen to others.

_____ **13.** Way(s) in which an EMT-B may further his/her EMS education include
- **A.** re-reading the EMT-B textbook.
- **C.** attending EMS conferences.
- **B.** repeating the EMT-B course.
- **D.** all of the above.

_____ **14.** A system of continuous self-review of all aspects of an EMS system for the purpose of identifying and correcting aspects of the system that require improvement is called
- **A.** off-line medical direction.
- **C.** quality improvement.
- **B.** patient advocacy.
- **D.** continuing education.

_____ **15.** Obtaining feedback from patients and the hospital staff is a means of
- **A.** obtaining on-line medical direction.
- **B.** providing quality improvement.
- **C.** determining what is wrong with patients.
- **D.** avoiding charges of negligence.

_____ **16.** Participation in continuing education and keeping carefully written documentation are examples of the EMT-B's role in
- **A.** patient advocacy.
- **C.** quality improvement.
- **B.** medical direction.
- **D.** transfer of care.

_____ **17.** Every EMS system should have a
- **A.** minimum of three EMT-Bs on each vehicle.
- **B.** call review on a monthly basis.
- **C.** contract with the local hospital.
- **D.** Medical Director.

_____ **18.** An EMT-B is operating as the Medical Director's
- **A.** employee.
- **C.** designated agent.
- **B.** replacement.
- **D.** peer.

_____ **19.** The difference between on-line (direct) and off-line (indirect) medical direction is that
- **A.** off-line does not need protocols.
- **B.** off-line orders are given by the on-duty physician, usually over the radio or phone.
- **C.** on-line uses standing orders.
- **D.** on-line orders are given by the on-duty physician, usually over the radio or phone.

_____ **20.** An example of a medication carried by EMT-Bs that may require a physician consult to administer is
- **A.** lidocaine.
- **C.** oxygen.
- **B.** activated charcoal.
- **D.** aspirin.

COMPLETE THE FOLLOWING

1. List at least six of the categories and standards of an EMS system as established by the National Highway Traffic Safety Administration.

    A. _____

    B. _____

    C. _____

    D. _____

    E. _____

    F. _____

2. List the four types of specialty hospitals.

    A. _____

    B. _____

    C. _____

    D. _____

3. List the four levels of EMS certification.

    A. _____

    B. _____

    C. _____

    D. _____

VIRTUAL STREET SCENES

(First review the Street Scenes on pages 10–11 in the textbook. Then answer the question below.)

What responsibilities of the EMT-B are illustrated in this scenario?

WEB SIMULATION

For interactive case studies that will help you review and practice basic skills, visit the *Emergency Care 9e Companion Website* at www.bradybooks.com/emergencycare.

Chapter Two

THE WELL-BEING OF THE EMT-BASIC

Match Terminology/Definitions

A. Infection control based on the presumption that all body fluids are infectious

B. Mental health professionals and peer counselors who work as a team to provide emotional and psychological support to EMS personnel who are or have been involved in a highly stressful incident

C. The removal or cleansing of dangerous chemicals or other dangerous or infectious materials

D. Equipment such as eye wear, mask, gloves, gown, turnout gear, or helmet that protect the EMS worker from infection and/or from hazardous materials and the dangers of rescue operations

E. The organisms that cause infection, such as viruses and bacteria

F. An emergency involving multiple patients

G. When a patient mentally tries to postpone death for a short time

H. The release of a harmful substance into the environment

I. When a rescuer becomes overwhelmed by the stress of a scene

J. When a patient gets upset and questions, "Why me?"

K. Injections given to a rescuer that are designed to prevent him/her from getting a disease

L. When a patient puts off dealing with the inevitable end of the process of dying

M. A potentially infectious material

N. A high efficiency particulate air respirator or mask designed to reduce the spread of tuberculosis (TB)

O. Test that determines if a person has been exposed to TB

_____ **1.** Anger

_____ **2.** Bargaining

_____ **3.** Biohazard

_____ **4.** Body substance isolation (BSI)

_____ **5.** Critical incident stress debriefing (CISD) teams

_____ **6.** Decontamination

_____ **7.** Denial

_____ **8.** Distress

_____ **9.** Hazardous-material incident

_____ **10.** HEPA

_____ **11.** Immunizations

_____ **12.** MCI

_____ **13.** Pathogens

_____ **14.** Personal protective equipment (PPE)

_____ **15.** PPD test

_____ 1. The most important job of the EMT-B is to
  A. stay physically safe and emotionally well.
  B. immediately assess the patient and call the hospital.
  C. provide medical advice to friends and community members.
  D. check the unit at the end of each shift.

_____ 2. An organism that causes infection is referred to as a(n)
  A. airborne.   C. allergen.
  B. bloodborne.   D. pathogen.

_____ 3. Precautions the EMT-B should take when dealing with all patients are known as
  A. universal precautions.   C. body substance isolation.
  B. general isolation.   D. quarantine isolation.

_____ 4. To provide body substance isolation, the EMT-B may need to use
  A. handwashing and SCBA.
  B. HEPA mask and shoe covers.
  C. disposable gloves and eye protection.
  D. paper gown and leather gloves.

_____ 5. An EMT-B should routinely wear a mask when treating a patient with
  A. hepatitis B.   C. AIDS.
  B. potential for blood or fluid spatter.   D. all of the above.

_____ 6. When an EMT-B covers a patient's mouth and nose with a mask to prevent the spread of an airborne disease, he/she should
  A. monitor the respirations and airway closely.
  B. write "TB alert" on the patient's prehospital care report.
  C. wear a surgical mask to reduce the spread of TB.
  D. notify his/her supervisor prior to transporting the patient.

_____ 7. All of the following are ways the EMT-B can plan safety precautions in advance of the call except
  A. keeping his/her tetanus immunization current.
  B. maintaining a list of communicable patients.
  C. verifying immune status.
  D. obtaining hepatitis B vaccine.

_____ 8. It is suggested that all EMT-Bs be immunized with all of the following vaccines except
  A. tetanus.   C. purified protein derivative.
  B. hepatitis B.   D. measles.

_____ 9. A federal organization responsible for issuing guidelines for employee safety around biohazards is called the
  A. Food and Drug Administration.
  B. Federal Communications Commission.
  C. Occupational Safety and Health Administration.
  D. Public Health Service.

_____ 10. Every employer of EMT-Bs must provide free of charge
  A. a yearly physical examination.   C. a hepatitis B vaccination.
  B. a life insurance policy.   D. universal health insurance.

_____ 11. A federal act that establishes procedures by which emergency response workers can find out if they have been exposed to life-threatening infectious diseases is
A. OSHA 1910.1030.
B. Ryan White CARE Act.
C. NFPA 1207.
D. OSHA 1910.1200.

_____ 12. After contact with the blood or body fluids of a patient, an EMT-B may submit a request for a determination of exposure to his/her
A. employer.
B. Medical Director.
C. designated officer.
D. local hospital.

_____ 13. Always assume that any person with
A. a cold has a bloodborne disease.
B. a productive cough has TB.
C. a fever has typhoid.
D. dehydration and sores has AIDS.

_____ 14. Which of the following is true about treating a contaminated patient at a hazardous-material incident?
A. Take the patient to the ambulance.
B. Bring the patient to the hospital.
C. Wear a SCBA when treating the patient.
D. Delay treatment until the patient is decontaminated.

_____ 15. The EMT-B can safeguard his/her well-being by
A. understanding and dealing with job stress.
B. ensuring scene safety.
C. taking body substance isolation.
D. all of the above.

_____ 16. Each of the following is an example of a call that has a high potential for causing excess stress on EMS providers except
A. trauma to infants and children.
B. an adult cardiac arrest.
C. elder abuse.
D. death or serious injury of a coworker.

_____ 17. Some warning signs that an EMT-B is being affected by stress include
A. overeating and ringing in the ears.
B. rapid urination and sweating.
C. indecisiveness and guilt.
D. increased sexual activity and sleep.

_____ 18. All of the following are recommended life-style changes an EMT-B may take to deal with job stress except
A. develop more healthful and positive dietary habits.
B. devote time to relaxation.
C. exercise.
D. avoid talking about his/her feelings.

_____ 19. A meeting held by a team of peer counselors and mental health professionals within 24 to 72 hours after a major incident is a(n)
A. incident critique.
B. MCI.
C. critical incident stress debriefing.
D. quality circle.

_____ 20. For a CISD to be effective,
A. it must not be an investigation of the events of the call.
B. information discussed must remain confidential.
C. an EMT-B must feel open to discuss feelings, fears, and reactions.
D. all of the above.

_____ **21.** A CISD can be effective in returning personnel to work quicker because
    A. the debriefing can be combined with an incident critique.
    B. pressure from their peers is provided.
    C. it helps them suppress their feelings.
    D. it can accelerate the recovery process.

_____ **22.** When a patient finds out that he is dying, he may go through which of the following emotional stages?
    A. anger and laughter
    B. denial and empathy
    C. depression and acceptance
    D. bargaining and elation

_____ **23.** A dying patient may go through emotional stages in the following order:
    A. acceptance, rage, depression, acceptance, bargaining.
    B. denial, anger, bargaining, depression, acceptance.
    C. bargaining, acceptance, denial, anger, depression.
    D. depression, bargaining, denial, acceptance, anger.

_____ **24.** An EMT-B will occasionally need to assist the patient who has a terminal illness. Experts suggest all of the following <u>except</u>
    A. listen empathetically to the patient.
    B. tell the patient that everything will be all right.
    C. be tolerant of angry reactions from the patient or family members.
    D. try to recognize the patient's needs.

_____ **25.** All of the following are part of the three "Rs" of reacting to danger except
    A. retreat.
    B. respond.
    C. radio.
    D. reevaluate.

COMPLETE THE FOLLOWING

1. List five types of calls with a high potential of stress for EMS personnel.

    A. _____

    B. _____

    C. _____

    D. _____

    E. _____

2. List five signs and symptoms of stress.

    A. _____

    B. _____

    C. _____

    D. _____

    E. _____

3. List at least five of the critical elements of the infection control plan required by Title 29 Code of Federal Regulation 1910.1030.

A. _____

B. _____

C. _____

D. _____

E. _____

VIRTUAL STREET SCENES

(First review the Street Scenes on page 30 in the textbook. Then answer the questions below.)

1. Since the EMT-B had some open cuts on his hands and was exposed to the patient's blood from the facial laceration, what are some of the diseases he may have been exposed to?

2. Due to the potential exposure to HIV, what medication, tests, and instructions would you expect the ED physician to prescribe for the EMT-B?

3. Aside from wearing PPE, could the EMT-B have prevented contracting any of these bloodborne diseases? Explain your answer.

4. Of the diseases the EMT-B may have been exposed to, which one would he have the greatest chance of catching and how serious is the disease?

WEB SIMULATION

For interactive case studies that will help you review and practice basic skills, visit the *Emergency Care 9e Companion Website* at www.bradybooks.com/emergencycare.

EMT-BASIC SKILLS PERFORMANCE CHECKLIST

▶ HANDWASHING PROCEDURE

❑ Remove watch and rings. Roll up sleeves.

❑ Adjust water flow and temperature.

❑ Wet hands and distal forearms.

❑ Dispense soap into hands.

❑ Scrub lower arms and hands. Clean around and under the nails.

❑ Rinse thoroughly under running water to remove all soap. Do not touch the sink!

❑ Use a paper towel to shut off the faucet to avoid recontaminating hands.

NOTE: Even though you wear protective gloves with your patients, handwashing must still be performed immediately after each call.

Chapter Three

MEDICAL/LEGAL AND ETHICAL ISSUES

Match Terminology/Definitions

A. Permission to treat an unconscious patient until he becomes conscious

B. A written order given by the physician based upon a decision by a patient prior to his/her demise

C. Being held legally responsible

D. An obligation to provide emergency care to a patient

E. Permission given by adults who are of legal age and mentally competent to make a rational decision in regard to their medical well-being

F. Permission from the patient to treat him/her

G. A series of laws, varying in each state, designed to provide immunity from liability to individuals trying to help in emergencies

H. The collective medical, legal, and ethical guidelines that govern the EMT-B

I. Not providing the standard of care

J. A finding of failure to act properly in a situation in which there was a duty to act

K. A legal document, usually signed by the patient and his/her physician, to "do not resuscitate"

L. The obligation not to reveal information obtained about a patient except to other health-care professionals involved in the patient's care, or under subpoena, or in a court of law

M. Leaving a patient after care has been initiated and before the patient has been transferred to someone with equal or greater medical training

N. Child who is married or of a specific age who, in certain states, can make legal decisions

O. Subjecting a patient to unwanted care and transport may be considered this in a court of law

_____ **1.** Abandonment

_____ **2.** Advance directive

_____ **3.** Battery

_____ **4.** Breach of duty

_____ **5.** Confidentiality

_____ **6.** Consent

_____ **7.** DNR order

_____ **8.** Duty to act

_____ **9.** Emancipated minor

_____ **10.** Expressed consent

_____ **11.** Good Samaritan laws

_____ **12.** Implied consent

_____ **13.** Liability

_____ **14.** Negligence

_____ **15.** Scope of practice

_____ **1.** The collective set of regulations and ethical considerations governing the EMT-B is called
   A. duty to act.   **C.** advance directives.
   B. scope of practice.   **D.** Good Samaritan laws.

_____ **2.** Legislation that governs the skill and medical interventions that may be performed by an EMT-B is
   A. uniform throughout the country.
   B. different from state to state.
   C. uniform for regions within a state.
   D. governed by the U.S. Department of Transportation.

_____ **3.** When the EMT-B makes the physical/emotional needs of the patient a priority, this is considered a(n) _____ of the EMT-B.
   A. advance directive   **C.** ethical responsibility
   B. protocol   **D.** legal responsibility

_____ **4.** Which one of the following is not a type of consent required for any treatment or action by an EMT-B?
   A. child and mentally incompetent adult
   B. implied
   C. applied
   D. expressed

_____ **5.** When you inform the adult patient of a procedure you are about to perform and its associated risks, you are looking for
   A. expressed consent.   **C.** implied consent.
   B. negligence.   **D.** applied consent.

_____ **6.** Consent that is based on the assumption that an unconscious patient would approve the EMT-B's life-saving interventions is called
   A. expressed.   **C.** implied consent.
   B. negligence.   **D.** applied consent.

_____ **7.** Your record of a patient's refusal of medical aid or transport should include all of the following except
   A. informing the patient of the risks and consequences of refusal.
   B. documenting the steps you took.
   C. signing of the form by the Medical Director.
   D. obtaining a "release" form with the patient's witnessed signature.

_____ **8.** Forcing a competent adult patient to go to the hospital against his will may result in _____ charges against the EMT-B.
   A. abandonment   **C.** implied consent
   B. assault and battery   **D.** negligence

_____ **9.** Which one of the following is an action you should not take if a patient refuses care?
   A. Leave phone stickers with emergency numbers.
   B. Recommend that a relative call the family physician to report the incident.
   C. Tell the patient to call her family physician if the problem reoccurs.
   D. Call a relative or neighbor who can stay with the patient.

_____ **10.** Another name for a DNR order is
   A. deviated nervous response.   **C.** refusal of treatment.
   B. duty not to react.   **D.** advance directive.

_____ 11. There are varying degrees of DNR orders, expressed through a variety of detailed instructions that may be part of the order, such as
  A. allowing for CPR only if cardiac or respiratory arrest was observed.
  B. allowing comfort care measures such as intravenous feeding.
  C. disallowing the use of long-term life-support measures.
  D. specifying only five minutes of artificial respiration will be attempted.

_____ 12. In a hospital, long-term life-support and "comfort care" measures would consist of intravenous feeding and
  A. routine inoculations.
  B. the use of a respirator.
  C. infection control by the health-care providers.
  D. hourly patient documentation.

_____ 13. If an EMT-B with a duty to act fails to provide the standard of care, and if this failure causes harm or injury to the patient, the EMT-B may be accused of
  A. breach of promise.   C. abandonment.
  B. negligence.   D. assault.

_____ 14. Termination of care of the patient without assuring the continuation of care at the same level or higher is called
  A. liability infraction.   C. abandonment.
  B. battery.   D. breach of duty.

_____ 15. The EMT-B should not discuss information about a patient outside of relaying pertinent information to the physician at the Emergency Department. Information considered confidential includes
  A. patient history gained through interview.
  B. assessment findings.
  C. treatment rendered.
  D. all of the above.

_____ 16. The EMT-B can release confidential patient information in all of the following circumstances except
  A. to inform other health-care professionals who need to know information to continue care.
  B. to report incidents required by state law, such as rape or abuse.
  C. to comply with a legal subpoena.
  D. to protect the other victims of a motor vehicle collision.

_____ 17. Medical identification insignia that indicate serious patient medical conditions come in the form of all of the following except
  A. bracelets.   C. cards.
  B. necklaces.   D. patches.

_____ 18. When treating a critical patient who has an organ donor card, the EMT-B should
  A. transport without delay and document a DNR.
  B. treat the patient the same as any other patient and inform the ED physician.
  C. withhold oxygen therapy from the patient to keep the organ hypoxic.
  D. do all of the above.

_____ 19. At a crime scene, the EMT-B should
  A. avoid disturbing any evidence at the scene unless emergency care requires.
  B. immediately remove the patient from the scene.
  C. move all obstacles from around the patient to make more room to work.
  D. search the house for clues to the cause of the crime.

_____ 20. Commonly required reporting situations include all of the following except
  A. child and elder abuse.   C. sexual assault.
  B. crimes in public places.   D. domestic abuse.

COMPLETE THE FOLLOWING

1. In order for a patient to refuse care or transport, what three conditions must be fulfilled?

   A. _____

   B. _____

   C. _____

2. A finding of negligence, or failure to act properly, requires that all of the following circumstances be proven:

   A. _____

   B. _____

   C. _____

3. Four examples of conditions that may be listed on a medical identification device (such as a necklace, bracelet, or card) include:

   A. _____

   B. _____

   C. _____

   D. _____

VIRTUAL STREET SCENES

(First review the Street Scenes on page 43 in the textbook. Then answer the questions below.)

1. Suppose you observed that the patient's home was filthy. Would it be a violation of patient confidentiality to discuss the "roach house" with fellow workers? Explain.

2. Is it appropriate to write that the patient has AIDS on the prehospital care report? Explain your answer.

3. Is a patient's vomitus a hazard to your health? If so, what BSI equipment would be appropriate?

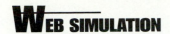

WEB SIMULATION

For interactive case studies that will help you review and practice basic skills, visit the *Emergency Care 9e Companion Website* at www.bradybooks.com/emergencycare.

EMT-BASIC SKILLS PERFORMANCE CHECKLIST

▶ PATIENT REFUSAL PROCEDURE

❏ Spend time effectively communicating with the patient (includes reasoning, persistence, and strategies to convince the patient to go to the hospital).

❏ Clearly inform the patient of the consequences of not going to the hospital.

❏ Consult with medical direction.

❏ Contact family to help convince the patient.

❏ Call law enforcement who may be able to order or "arrest" the serious patient in order to force the patient to go to the hospital.

❏ Try to determine why the patient is refusing care.

❏ Complete thorough documentation of the refusal. Have both the patient and a witness (e.g., bystander, police officer) sign the refusal release .

NOTE: Procedure may differ by state and jurisdiction. Always follow your Medical Director's advice.

CASE STUDY

▶ A WITNESSED COLLISION: FIRST ON THE SCENE

It's a summer morning and you are traveling on the interstate highway with your family to the lake. Although the speed is posted at 55 mph, traffic has been moving along at least 10 mph faster. All of a sudden, you observe the station wagon a few cars in front of you going from the center lane to the passing lane, cutting off a car, and then veering off the center of the road down a ravine and rolling over numerous times. The vehicle comes to rest on its roof.

1. If you are an off-duty EMT-B, must you legally stop to offer assistance?

2. Are you protected from a lawsuit? Explain your answer.

3. Are you protected from a liability suit provided your treatment is appropriate?

As you secure your vehicle off the shoulder and assign another helper to set out some flares, your spouse uses a cellular phone to call for emergency assistance.

4. In most communities, what is the universal emergency phone number?

5. What types of questions would you expect the dispatcher to ask about the collision?

6. What emergency response agencies would you expect to be sent?

As you carefully climb down through the brush to the car, you notice there are two patients who were ejected from the vehicle. Another citizen arrives and she identifies herself as an EMT-B. You ask her to check out the two ejected patients while you check the car for additional patients. She reports one ejected patient is dead, and the other is unconscious and has an obvious head injury.

7. As additional help arrives, how can they help with this patient?

8. What types of injuries could the patient have?

9. Do you need permission to treat the patient?

Inside the car there is a conscious male patient approximately 40 years old who appears to have been injured by the steering wheel in the left upper quadrant of his abdomen. He also has a broken upper left leg. You also notice that the car continues to leak gasoline from the dented fuel tank. After obtaining some additional help, you decide to carefully move this patient out of the car.

10. What potential injuries might this patient have?

11. How can you help minimize further injury to the leg?

12. Do you need permission to treat this patient? Explain.

Once the patient is out of the car, two ambulances arrive as well as the fire department with a paramedic engine and a heavy rescue truck. Meanwhile the police have arrived and are dealing with the traffic congestion that has developed.

13. Since there is now plenty of help, can you leave?

14. What would be the problem if you left prior to help arriving?

Chapter Four

THE HUMAN BODY

MATCH TERMINOLOGY/DEFINITIONS

▶ PART A

A. Main branch of the respiratory system that enters each of the lungs

B. Upper chambers of the heart

C. Muscle that divides the chest cavity from the abdominal cavity

D. The carotid and this pulse are considered central pulses

E. Tiny blood vessels

F. Pulse in the neck at the side of the larynx

G. Body system that transports blood throughout the body

H. Area directly posterior to the mouth

I. Pulse in the arm used to take a blood pressure

J. Area directly posterior to nose

K. Ring-shaped structure that forms the lower larynx

L. Structure that contains the vocal cords

M. Structure that closes to prevent food from going into the trachea during swallowing

N. Pulse on the top of the foot

O. Vessels that carry blood away from the heart

_____ **1.** Arteries

_____ **2.** Atria

_____ **3.** Brachial pulse

_____ **4.** Bronchi

_____ **5.** Capillaries

_____ **6.** Cardiovascular system

_____ **7.** Carotid pulse

_____ **8.** Cricoid cartilage

_____ **9.** Diaphragm

_____ **10.** Dorsalis pedis pulse

_____ **11.** Epiglottis

_____ **12.** Femoral pulse

_____ **13.** Larynx

_____ **14.** Nasopharynx

_____ **15.** Oropharynx

Part B

A. Area that includes the oropharynx and nasopharynx

B. Parts of the blood needed to form blood clots

C. Watery, salty fluid that makes up over one half of the blood's volume

D. Pulse that may be palpated on the posterior aspect of the medial malleolus

E. Structure that carries inhaled air from the larynx to the bronchi; also called the windpipe

F. Vessels that carry blood from the capillaries back to the heart

G. Blood pressure created in the arteries when the left ventricle contracts and forces blood into circulation

H. Body system that takes in oxygen and eliminates carbon dioxide

I. Socket that holds the ball of the femur

J. Lower chambers of the heart

K. Muscle type that works without the patient thinking about its operation

L. Two large veins that return blood to the heart

M. Long bone in the upper leg

N. Pulse on the thumb side of the wrist

O. Bone at the back of the lower leg

_____ 1. Acetabulum

_____ 2. Femur

_____ 3. Fibula

_____ 4. Involuntary muscle

_____ 5. Pharynx

_____ 6. Platelets

_____ 7. Plasma

_____ 8. Posterior tibial pulse

_____ 9. Radial pulse

_____ 10. Respiratory system

_____ 11. Systolic

_____ 12. Trachea

_____ 13. Veins

_____ 14. Venae cavae

_____ 15. Ventricles

Part C

A. Medial anterior portion of the pelvis

B. Vertebrae that form the back of the pelvis

C. Standing face forward with palms forward

D. Inferior most division of the spine that is referred to as the tailbone

E. Towards or closer to the midline

F. Lower jaw bone

G. Round ball of bone on the inside of the ankle

H. Wide bony ring that can be felt near the waist

I. System that consists of sensory and motor nerves

J. Round ball of bone on the outside of the ankle

K. Facial bone that surrounds each of the eyes

L. Breastbone

M. Seven vertebrae in the neck

N. Bones of the ankle

O. Medial and larger of the two bones of the lower leg

_____ 1. Anatomical position

_____ 2. Cervical spine

_____ 3. Coccyx

_____ 4. Iliac crest

_____ 5. Lateral malleolus

_____ 6. Mandible

_____ 7. Medial

_____ 8. Medial malleolus

_____ 9. Orbit

_____ 10. Peripheral nervous system

_____ 11. Pubis

_____ 12. Sacral spine

_____ 13. Sternum

_____ 14. Tarsals

_____ 15. Tibia

PART D

A. Inferior tip of the sternum

B. Upper arm bone

C. Away from the midline

D. Nerves that transmit information from the body to the spinal cord and brain

E. When two points on the extremities are compared, the point closer to the torso

F. Outermost layer of the skin

G. When two points on the extremities are compared, the point farther away from the torso

H. Nerves that carry messages from the brain to the body

I. Above or towards the head end of the torso

J. Layer of the skin in which the hair follicles, sweat glands, and oil glands are located

K. Bones in the fingers and toes

L. Joint where three bones of upper arm and forearm are connected

M. Front side of the torso

N. Heel bone

O. Back side of the torso

_____ 1. Anterior

_____ 2. Calcaneus

_____ 3. Dermis

_____ 4. Distal

_____ 5. Elbow

_____ 6. Epidermis

_____ 7. Humerus

_____ 8. Lateral

_____ 9. Motor nerves

_____ 10. Phalanges

_____ 11. Posterior

_____ 12. Proximal

_____ 13. Sensory nerves

_____ 14. Superior

_____ 15. Xiphoid process

PART E

A. Body system that regulates metabolic functions such as sugar absorption by the cells

B. Body system that governs sensations, movement, and thought

C. Lateral bone of the forearm aligned with the thumb

D. Bones that make up the hand

E. Highest portion of the shoulder

F. Medial bone of the forearm

G. Bones that make up the wrist

H. Shoulder blade

I. Bone in the front of the shoulder

J. The body less the extremities and the head

K. Lying on the back

L. An imaginary line drawn vertically from the center of the clavicle to the nipple below

M. Sitting on a stretcher with body at 45-to-60 degree angle

N. Similar on both sides of the body

O. Lying supine with the legs elevated a few inches

_____ 1. Acromion process

_____ 2. Bilaterally

_____ 3. Carpals

_____ 4. Clavicle

_____ 5. Endocrine system

_____ 6. Fowler's

_____ 7. Metacarpals

_____ 8. Mid-clavicular

_____ 9. Nervous system

_____ 10. Radius

_____ 11. Scapula

_____ 12. Supine

_____ 13. Torso

_____ 14. Trendelenburg

_____ 15. Ulna

PART F

A. Muscle under conscious control of the brain

B. Four divisions of the abdomen used to pinpoint the location of pain

C. Referring to the sole of the foot

D. Blood vessels that supply the muscle of the heart

E. Referring to the back of the body

F. Upper jaw bone

G. Body system that provides protection and movement

H. Blood pressure in the arteries when the left ventricle is refilling

I. Knee cap

J. Vertebrae of the lower back

K. Rib area of the spinal column

L. Imaginary line drawn vertically through the middle of the body

M. Anatomical term for the armpit

N. Patient's left side

O. Lying on the stomach or face down

_____ 1. Abdominal quadrants

_____ 2. Axilla

_____ 3. Coronary arteries

_____ 4. Diastolic

_____ 5. Dorsal

_____ 6. Left side

_____ 7. Lumbar spine

_____ 8. Maxilla

_____ 9. Midline

_____ 10. Musculoskeletal system

_____ 11. Patella

_____ 12. Plantar

_____ 13. Prone

_____ 14. Thoracic spine

_____ 15. Voluntary muscle

MULTIPLE-CHOICE REVIEW

_____ 1. All of the following are body systems except
    A. respiratory.
    B. cardiovascular.
    C. abdominal.
    D. musculoskeletal.

_____ 2. If a patient is lying on his left side, this position is called the _____ position.
    A. Fowler's
    B. recovery
    C. left supine
    D. left prone

_____ 3. When a patient is placed in a sitting-up position on a stretcher, this position is called
    A. prone.
    B. supine.
    C. Fowler's.
    D. Trendelenburg.

_____ 4. When a patient is lying flat with head lower than legs, this position is called
    A. prone.
    B. supine.
    C. Fowler's.
    D. Trendelenburg.

_____ 5. The musculoskeletal system has three main functions. It gives the body shape, provides for body movements, and
    A. gives the body sensation.
    B. protects vital internal organs.
    C. provides for the body's outer covering.
    D. allows transport of oxygen into the cells.

_____ 6. The upper jaw is also called the
    A. mandible.
    B. orbit.
    C. maxillae.
    D. nasal bone.

_____ 7. The spinal column includes the _____ vertebrae.
A. thoracic and coccyx   C. lumbar and sternal
B. cervical and orbit   D. sacrum and pelvic

_____ 8. An injury to the spinal cord at the _____ level may be fatal because control of the muscles of breathing arise from the spinal cord at this level.
A. lumbar   C. cervical
B. sacral   D. thoracic

_____ 9. Bones in the lower extremities include the
A. femur, calcaneus, and phalanges.
B. ischium, tibia, and ulna.
C. orbit, lumbar, and shin.
D. radius, fibula, and metatarsals.

_____ 10. Bones in the upper extremities include the
A. humerus and radius.   C. phalanges and tibia.
B. humerus and calcaneus.   D. ulna and cervical.

_____ 11. The types of muscle tissue include
A. voluntary.   C. cardiac "automaticity."
B. involuntary.   D. all of the above.

_____ 12. The type of muscle that allows body movement such as walking is called
A. voluntary.   C. cardiac.
B. involuntary.   D. smooth.

_____ 13. Involuntary, or smooth, muscle is found in the
A. trachea.   C. heart.
B. walls of the blood vessels. D. quadriceps and biceps.

_____ 14. The structure in the throat that is described as the voice box is called the
A. pharynx.   C. trachea.
B. larynx.   D. sternum.

_____ 15. A leaf-shaped valve that prevents food and foreign objects from entering the trachea is called the
A. pharynx.   C. larynx.
B. epiglottis.   D. bronchi.

_____ 16. Oxygen passes from the environment to the lungs in what order?
A. nose, bronchi, larynx, trachea, lung
B. larynx, esophagus, trachea, bronchi, alveoli
C. mouth, pharynx, trachea, bronchi, alveoli
D. epiglottis, trachea, cricoid, bronchi, alveoli

_____ 17. When the diaphragm and intercostal muscles relax, the size of the chest cavity
A. increases, causing inhalation.   C. decreases, causing exhalation.
B. increases, causing exhalation.   D. decreases, causing inhalation.

_____ 18. The difference between the adult airway and the pediatric airway is that
A. the adult's tongue takes up proportionately more space in the mouth than the child's.
B. the trachea is softer and more flexible in an adult.
C. the cricoid cartilage is softer in an adult.
D. all structures are smaller and more easily obstructed in a child.

_____ 19. The right atrium
A. receives blood from the venae cavae.
B. receives blood from the pulmonary veins.
C. pumps blood to the lungs.
D. pumps blood to the body.

_____ 20. The aorta
  A. is the major artery originating from the heart.
  B. divides at the level of the nipples into the iliac arteries.
  C. supplies only the vessels of the lower body with blood.
  D. supplies only the vessels of the upper body with blood.

_____ 21. The major artery in the thigh is called the
  A. carotid.   C. radial.
  B. femoral.   D. brachial.

_____ 22. The vessel that carries oxygen-poor blood from the portions of the body
     below the heart and back to the right atrium is called the
  A. posterior tibial.   C. inferior vena cava.
  B. internal jugular.   D. aorta.

_____ 23. The left atrium
  A. receives blood from the veins of the body.
  B. receives blood from the pulmonary veins.
  C. pumps blood to the lungs.
  D. pumps blood to the body.

_____ 24. The fluid that carries the blood cells and nutrients is called
  A. platelets.   C. plasma.
  B. urine.   D. none of the above.

_____ 25. The blood component that is essential to the formation of blood clots
     is called
  A. plasma.   C. white blood cells.
  B. platelets.   D. red blood cells.

_____ 26. The pressure on the walls of an artery when the left ventricle contracts is
     called the _____ pressure.
  A. systolic   C. diastolic
  B. arterial   D. residual

_____ 27. The two main divisions of the nervous system are
  A. central and peripheral.   C. brain and skin.
  B. bones and muscles.   D. spinal cord and brain.

_____ 28. Nerves that carry information from throughout the body to the brain
     are _____ nerves.
  A. motor   C. spinal
  B. cardiac   D. sensory

_____ 29. One of the functions of the skin is to
  A. eliminate excess oxygen into the atmosphere.
  B. regulate the diameter of the blood vessels in the circulation.
  C. protect the body from the environment, bacteria, and other organisms.
  D. allow environmental water to carefully enter the body.

_____ 30. The system that secretes hormones, such as insulin and adrenaline, and
     which is responsible for regulating many body activities, is called
     the _____ system.
  A. integumentary (skin)   C. endocrine
  B. nervous   D. gastrointestinal

COMPLETE THE FOLLOWING

1. List the names of nine arteries in the body.

   A. _____   F. _____

   B. _____   G. _____

   C. _____   H. _____

   D. _____   I. _____

   E. _____

2. List five functions of the skin.

   A. _____   D. _____

   B. _____   E. _____

   C. _____

LABEL THE DIAGRAMS

Fill in the name of each anatomical position on the line provided.

▶ **ANATOMICAL POSTURES**

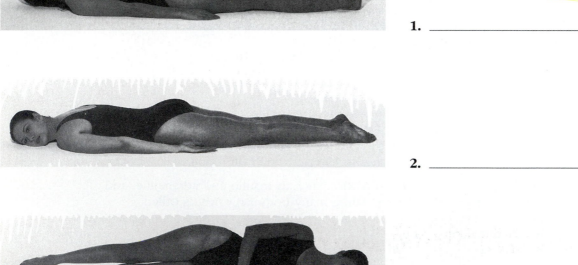

1. _____

2. _____

3. _____

Fill in the appropriate directional term or landmark on the line provided.

▶ **ANATOMICAL POSITION**

Diagram 1

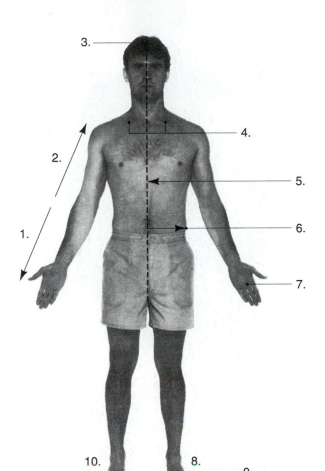

Diagram 2

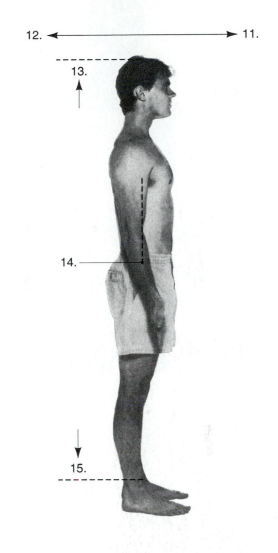

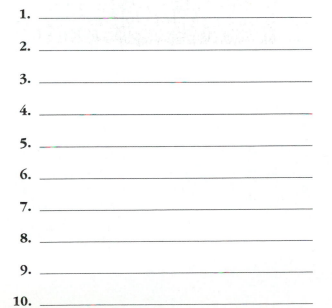

1. _____

2. _____

3. _____

4. _____

5. _____

6. _____

7. _____

8. _____

9. _____

10. _____

11. _____

12. _____

13. _____

14. _____

15. _____

Fill in the name of each body region or structure on the line provided.

▶ **TOPOGRAPHY OF THE TORSO**

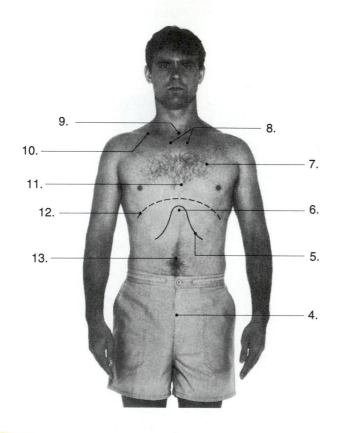
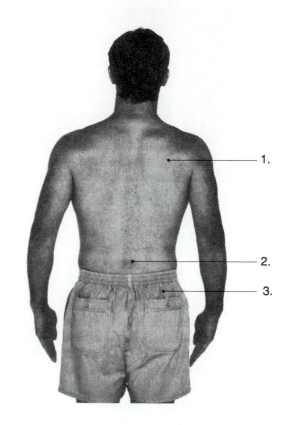

1. _____

2. _____

3. _____

4. _____

5. _____

6. _____

7. _____

8. _____

9. _____

10. _____

11. _____

12. _____

13. _____

VIRTUAL STREET SCENES

(First review the Street Scenes on p. 75 of the textbook. Then answer the questions below.)

1. Why was it necessary to stabilize the patient's head and neck when you got into the car?

2. Since the driver of the truck was walking around, was he still a patient in need of evaluation? Explain your answer.

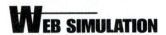

WEB SIMULATION

For interactive case studies that will help you review and practice basic skills, visit the **Emergency Care 9e Companion Website** at www.bradybooks.com/emergencycare.

Chapter Five

LIFTING AND MOVING PATIENTS

MATCH TERMINOLOGY/DEFINITIONS

A. Stretcher, made of a steel wire mesh and tubular steel rim or plastic and steel rim, used to transport patients from one level to another or over rough terrain

B. Portable folding chair with wheels used to transport the patient in a sitting position up or down stairs

C. Aluminum stretcher that splits in halves, which can be pushed together under the patient

D. Method of transferring a patient from bed to stretcher in which two or more rescuers curl the patient to their chests, then reverse the process to lower the patient to the stretcher

E. Patient move that may be made if speed is not priority

F. Method of lifting and carrying a patient in which one rescuer slips hands under the patient's armpits and grasps the wrists, while another rescuer grasps the patient's knees

G. Made from a squatting position with weight to be lifted close to the body, feet apart and flat on ground, body weight on or just behind balls of feet, back locked in

H. Proper use of the body to facilitate lifting and moving and to prevent injury

I. Gripping with as much hand surface as possible the object being lifted, with all fingers bent at the same angle

J. Patient move that should be done quickly yet without any compromise of spinal integrity

K. Method of transferring a patient from bed to stretcher by grasping and pulling the loosened bottom sheet of the bed

L. Line that runs down the center of the body from the top of the head and along the spine

M. Method of lifting and carrying a patient from ground level to a stretcher in which two or more rescuers kneel, curl the patient to their chests, stand, then reverse the process to lower the patient to the stretcher

N. Removal of a patient from a hazardous environment in which safety is the first priority and spinal integrity is second priority

O. Procedure done by three or four rescuers that is designed to move a supine patient onto a long backboard without compromising spinal integrity

_____ 1. Basket stretcher

_____ 2. Body mechanics

_____ 3. Direct carry

_____ 4. Direct ground lift

_____ 5. Draw-sheet method

_____ 6. Emergency move

_____ 7. Extremity lift

_____ 8. Log roll

_____ 9. Long axis

_____ 10. Non-urgent move

_____ 11. Power grip

_____ 12. Power lift

_____ 13. Scoop (orthopedic) stretcher

_____ 14. Stair chair

_____ 15. Urgent move

_____ 1. To assure your own safety when lifting a patient, it is important to
   A. always wear a back brace.
   B. keep the weight as far away from your body as possible.
   C. use your legs, not your back, to lift.
   D. avoid lifting a patient that weighs more than you do.

_____ 2. When lifting a patient, you should do all of the following except
   A. communicate clearly with your partner.
   B. twist while you lift the patient.
   C. know your physical ability and limitations.
   D. communicate frequently with your partner.

_____ 3. When lifting a cot or stretcher,
   A. use an even number of people so that balance is maintained.
   B. keep both of your feet together and flat on the ground.
   C. use a third person positioned on the heaviest side.
   D. if you must use one hand only, compensate by using your back.

_____ 4. When placing all fingers and the palm in contact with the object
being lifted, you are using a
   A. power grip.   C. lock grip.
   B. power lift.   D. grip lift.

_____ 5. When you must push an object,
   A. keep the line of pull through the center of your body by bending
      your knees.
   B. push from an overhead position, keeping your knees locked.
   C. keep the weight you are pushing at least 20 inches away from
      your body.
   D. keep the elbows straight with arms close to your sides.

_____ 6. The situations in which an emergency move would be used include
all of the following except
   A. fire or danger of fire.
   B. explosives or other hazardous chemicals.
   C. inability to protect the patient from other hazards at the scene.
   D. dispatcher is holding another more serious call.

_____ 7. If the patient is on the floor or ground and the EMT-B has decided
that an emergency move is appropriate, the patient can be moved by
   A. rolling her like a log.
   B. using a spine board and strapping her down.
   C. pulling on her clothing in the neck and shoulder area.
   D. using one rescuer on each extremity.

_____ 8. If the patient has an altered mental status, the EMT-B should consider
a(n) _____ move.
   A. emergency   C. non-urgent
   B. urgent   D. immediate

_____ 9. When doing a log roll, lean from your hips and
   A. keep your back curved only while leaning over the patient.
   B. position yourself at least ten inches from the patient.
   C. use your shoulder muscles to help with the roll.
   D. roll the patient as fast as possible.

10. The final step in packaging a patient on a wheeled stretcher is
   A. securing the patient to the stretcher.
   B. placing a towel under the patient's head.
   C. covering the patient with a top sheet.
   D. adjusting the position of the back rest.

11. If you are carrying a patient down stairs, when possible
   A. flex at the waist with bent knees.
   B. keep your lower back muscles loose.
   C. place one hand on the railing for balance.
   D. use a stair chair instead of a stretcher.

12. Which of the following is <u>not</u> recommended for moving a patient with a suspected spinal injury?
   A. wheeled stretcher
   B. scoop stretcher
   C. short spine board
   D. long spine board

13. You have a patient positioned on a scoop-style stretcher and wish to lower the patient from a rooftop. You should
   A. place the stretcher and patient in a plastic basket stretcher.
   B. transfer the patient to a wire basket stretcher.
   C. place the patient in a short spine board.
   D. lower the patient in the scoop stretcher.

14. To avoid trauma to a patient with an injured spine, the best patient-carrying device would be the
   A. long spine board.
   B. wheeled stretcher.
   C. Stokes basket.
   D. portable ambulance stretcher.

15. The direct ground lift is an example of a(n) _____ move for a patient who has no spine injury.
   A. emergency
   B. urgent
   C. immediate
   D. non-urgent

COMPLETE THE FOLLOWING

1. List seven patient carrying devices.

   A. _____

   B. _____

   C. _____

   D. _____

   E. _____

   F. _____

   G. _____

2. List four principles that will help you lift efficiently and prevent injury.

   A. _____

   B. _____

   C. _____

   D. _____

LABEL THE PHOTOGRAPHS

Fill in the name of each lift, move, or drag on the line provided.

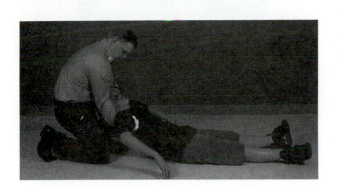

1. _____

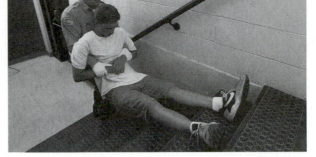

2. _____

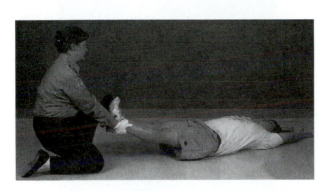

3. _____

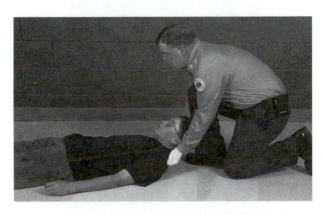

4. _____

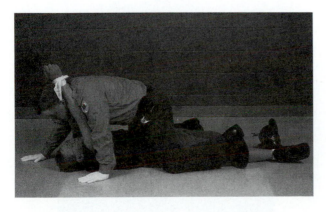

5. _____

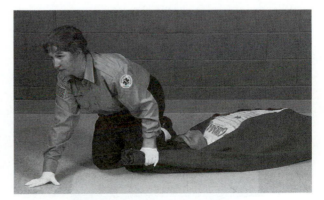

6. _____

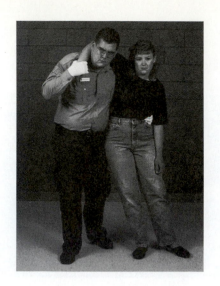

7. _____

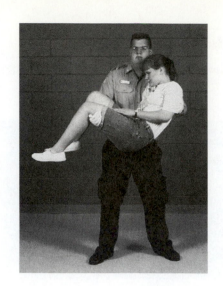

8. _____

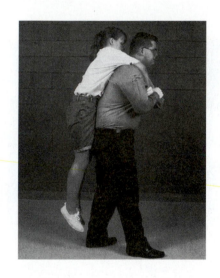
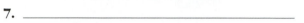

9. _____

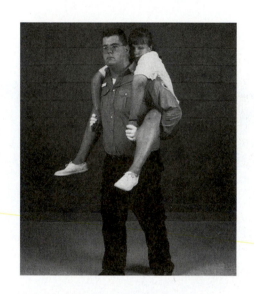

10. _____

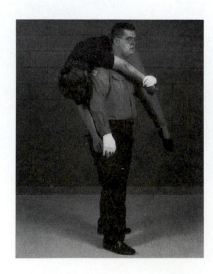

11. _____

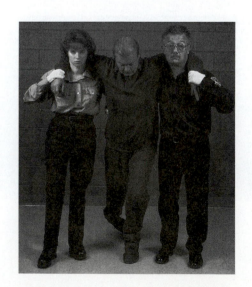

12. _____

VIRTUAL STREET SCENES

(First review the Street Scenes on p.101 of the textbook. Then answer the questions below.)

1. In the call, the patient's weight was not discussed. Suppose the patient weighed 300 lb. Should you consider using a different device to immobilize her?

2. Suppose when it is time to remove the patient from the automobile, the vest-type immobilization device does not go entirely around her and the leg straps are too short. What should you do?

3. After getting the patient out of the car with some extra help, she lies supine in the vest-type immobilization device on a long backboard. She complains that the vest is making it difficult for her to breathe. What can you do?

WEB SIMULATION

For interactive case studies that will help you review and practice basic skills, visit the *Emergency Care 9e Companion Website* at www.bradybooks.com/emergencycare.

EMT-BASIC SKILL PERFORMANCE CHECKLISTS

▶ FIREFIGHTER'S DRAG

❑ Place the patient in the supine position.

❑ Tie patient's hands together with something that will not cut into the skin.

❑ Straddle the patient, facing his head.

❑ Crouch and pass your head through the patient's trussed arms and then raise your body to raise the patient's head, neck, and upper trunk.

❑ Crawl on your hands and knees, dragging the patient and keeping the patient's head low to the ground.

▶ BLANKET DRAG

❑ Gather half of the blanket up against the patient's side.

❑ Roll the patient toward your knees.

❑ Gently roll the patient back onto the blanket.

❑ Roll up the blanket by the patient's head, neck, and shoulders and drag this rolled material, keeping the patient's head low to the ground.

▶ ONE-RESCUER ASSIST

❑ Place the patient's arm around your neck.

❑ Grasp the patient's hand in your hand.

❑ Place your other arm around the patient's waist.

❑ Help the patient walk to safety, communicating with him about obstacles or uneven terrain.

▶ CRADLE CARRY

❑ Place one arm across the patient's back with your hand under his arm.

❑ Place your other arm under his knees and lift.

❑ If the patient is conscious, have him place the near arm over your shoulder.

▶ PACK STRAP CARRY

❑ Have the patient stand.

❑ Turn your back to the patient, bringing his arms over your shoulders to cross your chest.

❑ Keep his arms as straight as possible, his armpits over your shoulders.

❑ Hold the patient's wrists, bend, and pull the patient onto your back.

▶ PIGGY BACK CARRY

❑ Assist the patient to a standing position.

❑ Turn your back to the patient, placing the patient's arms over your shoulders so they cross your chest.

❑ While the patient holds on with his arms, crouch and grasp the patient's thighs.

❑ Use a lifting motion to move the patient onto your back.

❑ Pass your forearms under the patient's knees and grasp his wrists.

▶ FIREFIGHTER'S CARRY

❑ Place your toes against the patient's toes and pull the patient toward you.

❑ Bend at the waist and flex your knees.

❑ Duck and pull the patient across your shoulder, keeping hold of one of his wrists.

❑ Use your free arm to reach between his legs and grasp his thigh.

❑ Let the weight of the patient fall onto your shoulders.

❑ Stand up, transferring your grip on the patient's thigh to his wrist.

▶ TWO-RESCUER ASSIST

❑ Each EMT-B stands at side of the patient.

❑ Each places a patient's arm around his shoulder and grips the patient's hand.

❑ Each EMT-B then places his own free arm around the patient's waist.

❑ They both then help the patient walk to safety.

▶ LOADING THE WHEELED STRETCHER INTO THE AMBULANCE

❑ Lift the rear step of the ambulance if necessary.

❑ Move the stretcher as close to the ambulance as possible.

❑ Make sure the stretcher is locked in its lowest level before lifting (depends on local procedure and type of stretcher).

❑ Position EMT-Bs on opposite sides of the stretcher, bend at the knees, and grasp the lower bar of the stretcher frame.

❑ Both EMT-Bs should come to a full standing position with their backs straight.

❑ Use oblique stepping movements to move the stretcher to the ambulance.

❑ Secure the stretcher into the ambulance, using the appropriate securing device.

❑ Engage both forward and rear catches to hold the stretcher in place.

▶ EXTREMITY CARRY

❑ EMT-B #1 places the patient on his back with his knees flexed.

❑ EMT-B #1 kneels at the patient's head and places his hands under the patient's shoulders.

❑ EMT-B #2 kneels at the patient's feet and grasps the patient's wrists.

❑ EMT-B #2 lifts patient forward while EMT-B #1 slips his arms under the patient's armpits and grasps the patient's wrists.

❑ EMT-B #2 grasps the patient's knees while facing him or turns and grasps the patient's knees while facing away from him.

❑ EMT-B #1 and EMT-B #2 both crouch, then stand at the same time and move as a unit when carrying the patient.

▶ DIRECT GROUND LIFT

❑ Set the stretcher in its lowest position and place opposite the patient.

❑ Two EMT-Bs get inposition along one side of the patient. EMT-B #1 is at the head, and EMT-B #2 is at the foot.

❑ The EMT-Bs drop to one knee facing the patient.

❑ Place patient's arms on his chest.

❑ EMT-B #1 at the head-end cradles the patient's head and neck by sliding one arm under the patient's neck to grasp shoulder; the other arm is placed under the patient's lower back.

❑ EMT-B #2 at the foot-end slides one arm under the patient's knees and the other under the patient above the buttocks.

❑ If a third rescuer is available, he should place both arms under the patient's waist while the two EMT-Bs slide their arms up to the mid-back or down to the buttocks.

❑ On a signal, the crew lifts the patient to his knees.

❑ On a signal, the crew stands and carries the patient to the stretcher. They drop to one knee and roll forward to place the patient onto the mattress.

▶ DRAW-SHEET METHOD

❑ Loosen the bottom sheet of the bed and roll it from both sides toward the patient.

❑ Assure the stretcher is at the same height as the bed and the side rail is down.

❑ Push the stretcher and the bed tightly together.

❑ Firmly grasp the rolled sheet, holding it taut, with an underhand grasp in the area of the head/chest and hip/knee.

❑ On three, EMT-Bs carefully slide the patient onto the stretcher.

▶ DIRECT CARRY

❑ EMT-B #1 and #2: Get in position along one side of patient. EMT-B #1 is at the head-end; EMT-B #2 is at the foot-end.

❑ EMT-B #1 cradles the patient's head and neck by sliding one arm under the patient's neck to grasp the shoulder.

❑ EMT-B #2 slides a hand under the patient's hip and lifts slightly.

❑ EMT-B #1 slides his other arm under the patient's back.

❑ EMT-B #2 places his arms under the patient's hips and calves.

❑ Both EMT-Bs slide the patient to the edge of the bed and bend toward him with their knees slightly bent.

❑ They lift and curl the patient to their chests and return to a standing position.

❑ They rotate and then slide the patient gently onto the stretcher.

Chapter Six
AIRWAY MANAGEMENT

MATCH TERMINOLOGY/DEFINITIONS

▶ PART A

A. The flap of tissue that caps the trachea as you swallow

B. A means of correcting blockage of the airway by the tongue by tilting the head back and lifting the chin

C. The area inside the mouth joining the nasal passageways and the throat

D. The two large tubes that bring air to and from the lungs

E. The voicebox, which contains the epiglottis and vocal cords

F. The ring-shaped structure that forms the lower portion of the trachea

G. The process of breathing in

H. The muscle of breathing that separates the abdomen from the thorax

I. The process of breathing out

J. A means of correcting blockage of the airway by moving the jaw forward without tilting the head or neck

_____ 1. Bronchi

_____ 2. Cricoid cartilage

_____ 3. Diaphragm

_____ 4. Epiglottis

_____ 5. Exhalation

_____ 6. Head-tilt, chin-lift maneuver

_____ 7. Inhalation

_____ 8. Jaw-thrust maneuver

_____ 9. Larynx

_____ 10. Pharynx

▶ PART B

A. A device that uses oxygen under pressure to deliver artificial ventilations

B. A hand-held device with a face mask and self-refilling bag that can be squeezed to provide artificial ventilations to a patient

C. Expansion of the stomach caused by too forceful ventilation pressures, which cause excess air to enter the stomach instead of the lungs

D. Another word for breathing

E. A permanent surgical opening in the neck through which the patient breathes

F. A device connected to the flowmeter to add moisture to the dry oxygen coming from an oxygen cylinder

G. The passageway by which air enters or leaves the body

H. Forcing air or oxygen into the lungs when a patient has stopped breathing or has inadequate breathing

I. A blue or gray skin color resulting from lack of oxygen in the body

J. The breathing in of air or oxygen

_____ 1. Airway

_____ 2. Artificial ventilation

_____ 3. Bag-valve mask

_____ 4. Cyanosis

_____ 5. Flow-restricted, oxygen-powered ventilation device

_____ 6. Gastric distention

_____ 7. Humidifier

_____ 8. Respiration

_____ 9. Stoma

_____ 10. Ventilation

A. A flexible breathing tube inserted through the patient's nose into the pharynx to help maintain an open airway

B. A face mask and reservoir bag device that delivers high concentrations of oxygen. The patient's exhaled air escapes through a valve.

C. A device that delivers low concentrations of oxygen through two prongs that rest in the patient's nostrils

D. A device connected to an oxygen cylinder to reduce cylinder pressure to a safe pressure for delivery of oxygen to a patient

E. A device, usually with a one-way valve, to aid in artificial ventilation. A rescuer breathes through the valve when the device is placed over the patient's face. It also acts as a barrier to prevent contact with a patient's breath or body fluids and can be used with supplemental oxygen when fitted with an oxygen inlet.

F. When breathing completely stops

G. To provide ventilations at a higher rate to compensate for oxygen not delivered during suctioning

H. Container filled with oxygen under pressure

I. Use of a vacuum device to remove blood, vomitus, and other secretions or foreign materials from the airway

J. A rigid curved device inserted through the patient's mouth into the pharynx to help maintain an open airway

K. Vomiting or retching that results when something is placed in the pharynx

L. The reduction of breathing to the point where not enough oxygen is being taken in to sustain life

M. An insufficiency of oxygen in the body's tissues

N. A valve that indicates the flow of oxygen in liters per minute

O. A valve on a BVM designed to blow off excessive pressure; this valve is no longer allowed per AHA standards on any BVM due to the danger of underinflation of the lungs.

_____ **1.** Flowmeter

_____ **2.** Gag reflex

_____ **3.** Hyperventilate

_____ **4.** Hypoxia

_____ **5.** Nasal cannula

_____ **6.** Nasopharyngeal airway

_____ **7.** Nonrebreather mask

_____ **8.** Oropharyngeal airway

_____ **9.** Oxygen cylinder

_____ **10.** Pocket face mask

_____ **11.** Pop-off valve

_____ **12.** Pressure regulator

_____ **13.** Respiratory arrest

_____ **14.** Respiratory failure

_____ **15.** Suctioning

MULTIPLE-CHOICE REVIEW

_____ **1.** During respiration,
   A. oxygen enters the body during each inspiration.
   B. carbon dioxide enters the body during each expiration.
   C. oxygen exits the body on each expiration.
   D. carbon dioxide does not enter the body.

_____ **2.** Respiratory failure is
   A. the cessation of breathing.
   B. the reduction of breathing to a point where oxygen intake is not sufficient to support life.
   C. the same as respiratory arrest.
   D. caused by electrocution.

_____ **3.** Which of the following is <u>not</u> a sign of adequate breathing?
  A. air moving out of the nose and mouth
  B. equal expansion of both sides of the chest
  C. breathing limited to abdominal movement
  D. absence of blue or gray skin coloration

_____ **4.** Signs of inadequate breathing in children may include
  A. cyanotic skin, lips, tongue, or earlobes.
  B. retractions between the ribs.
  C. nasal flaring.
  D. all of the above.

_____ **5.** Each of the following are signs of inadequate breathing <u>except</u>
  A. inspirations or expirations that are prolonged.
  B. breathing rate in an adult of 14–18 breaths per minute.
  C. breathing is very shallow, very deep, or appears labored.
  D. the patient is unable to speak in full sentences.

_____ **6.** Additional signs of inadequate breathing include all of the following <u>except</u>
  A. absent chest movement.
  B. air that can be felt at the nose or mouth.
  C. diminished breath sounds.
  D. noises such as wheezing or crowing.

_____ **7.** Inadequate breathing in a child is defined as
  A. less than 15 breaths per minute.
  B. more than 30 breaths per minute.
  C. both of the above.
  D. neither of the above.

_____ **8.** When at rest, the normal adequate breathing rate for an adult is _____ times per minute.
  A. 12 to 20   **C.** 60 to 80
  B. 30 to 40   **D.** 75 to 100

_____ **9.** Cyanosis can be checked by observing the patient's
  A. tongue.   **C.** nail beds.
  B. earlobes.   **D.** tongue, nail beds, and earlobes.

_____ **10.** One indication that a patient is experiencing inadequate breathing is that she
  A. has a headache.   **C.** talks in short, choppy sentences.
  B. complains of nausea.   **D.** is dizzy when standing.

_____ **11.** The very first step to aid a patient who is not breathing is to
  A. clear the mouth.   **C.** apply positive ventilation.
  B. administer oxygen.   **D.** open the airway.

_____ **12.** What is the importance of mechanism of injury to airway care?
  A. An injured patient will need more oxygen.
  B. The procedure for opening the patient's airway is different in trauma.
  C. Patients without a mechanism of injury will have an open airway.
  D. An injury can make airway care easier to manage than a medical emergency.

_____ **13.** To open the airway of a patient with no suspected head, neck, or spine injury, the EMT-B should use a _____ maneuver.
  A. jaw-thrust   **C.** head-tilt, neck-lift
  B. head-tilt, chin-lift   **D.** modified chin-thrust

_____ **14.** When performing the head-tilt, chin-lift maneuver, the EMT-B should
  A. not allow the patient's mouth to close.
  B. position himself at the top of the patient's head.
  C. tilt the head by applying pressure to the patient's chin.
  D. use fingertips to lift the neck.

_____ **15.** When performing the jaw-thrust maneuver, the EMT-B should do each one of the following except
  A. kneel at the top of the patient's head.
  B. stabilize the patient's head with forearms.
  C. use the index fingers to push the angles of the patient's lower jaw forward.
  D. tilt the head by applying gentle pressure to the patient's forehead.

_____ **16.** The main purpose of the jaw-thrust maneuver is to
  A. open the mouth with only one hand.
  B. open the airway without moving the head or neck.
  C. create an airway for the medical patient.
  D. create an airway when it is not possible to jut the jaw.

_____ **17.** Various techniques the EMT-B can use to provide artificial ventilation are listed below.
  1) one-rescuer bag-valve mask
  2) flow-restricted, oxygen-powered ventilation device
  3) two-rescuer bag-valve mask with high flow supplemental oxygen at 15 LPM
  4) mouth-to-mask without supplemental oxygen

  What is the most effective of these techniques?
  A. 1   **C.** 3
  B. 2   **D.** 4

_____ **18.** All of the following are signs of inadequate artificial ventilations except
  A. chest does not rise and fall with ventilation.
  B. rate of ventilation is too slow or too fast.
  C. patient's color changes from cyanotic to pink.
  D. patient's heart rate does not return to normal with ventilations.

_____ **19.** When performing mouth-to-mask ventilation on an adult patient, ventilations should be delivered over _____ seconds.
  A. 1 to 1½   **C.** 4
  B. 2½ to 3   **D.** 5

_____ **20.** The bag-valve mask on your ambulance should have
  A. a non-refilling shell that is easily cleaned.
  B. a non-jam valve with an oxygen inlet.
  C. a standard 9/12 mm fitting.
  D. manual disabling pop-off valve.

_____ **21.** The bag-valve mask should be capable of
  A. withstanding cold temperatures.
  B. providing a high pressure in the chest and airway.
  C. blowing off at pressures above 40 mm of water pressure.
  D. receiving an oxygen inlet flow of 25 liters per minute.

_____ **22.** When ventilating a suspected trauma patient with a bag-valve mask, it is most effective to do all of the following except
  A. use a device with a volume of 1,000–1,600 mL.
  B. use two EMT-Bs to perform the procedure.
  C. position the EMT-B who is maintaining the mask seal at the patient's head.
  D. maintain the head-tilt, chin-lift maneuver.

_____ 23. When ventilating an unconscious patient, a bag-valve mask is complete if it is used with
A. a reservoir bag.
B. an oral airway.
C. an oxygen tank and liter flow regulator.
D. all of the above.

_____ 24. If the patient's chest does not rise and fall when using a bag-valve mask, the EMT-B should do all of the following except
A. reposition the head and re-attempt ventilations.
B. check for escape of air around the mask.
C. use an alternative method of artificial ventilation.
D. increase the rate at which the bag is squeezed.

_____ 25. If the patient has a _____ and needs ventilatory assistance, the best device to use is a _____ .
A. stoma : pocket mask
B. tracheotomy : positive-pressure ventilator
C. stoma : bag-valve mask
D. tracheotomy : nasal airway

_____ 26. The flow-restricted, oxygen-powered ventilation device should
A. operate in both ordinary and extreme environmental conditions.
B. have an audible alarm when the relief valve is activated.
C. have a trigger so two hands can be used to seal the mask.
D. do all of the above.

_____ 27. An oral or nasal airway should be
A. cleaned for re-use after the call.
B. inserted in all critically injured patients.
C. used to keep the tongue from blocking the airway.
D. used in order to prevent the need for suctioning.

_____ 28. If something is placed in the patient's throat, the gag reflex causes the patient to
A. take deep breaths.
B. pass out.
C. vomit or retch.
D. all of the above.

_____ 29. An oropharyngeal airway of proper size will extend from the
A. corner of the patient's mouth to the tip of the earlobe.
B. lips to the larynx.
C. nose to the angle of the jaw.
D. none of the above.

_____ 30. An oral airway should be inserted
A. upside down, with the tip toward the roof of the mouth, then flipped 180 degrees over the tongue.
B. right side up, using a tongue depressor to press the tongue down and forward to keep it from obstructing the airway.
C. both of the above.
D. neither of the above.

_____ 31. A nasopharyngeal airway should be
A. inserted with the bevel on the lateral side of the nostril.
B. measured from the patient's nostril to the earlobe.
C. inserted in the left nostril when possible.
D. turned 180 degrees with the tip facing the roof of the mouth.

_____ 32. When inserting a nasopharyngeal airway, lubricate the outside of the tube with a(n)
A. petroleum jelly.
B. oil-based lubricant.
C. silicone-based gel.
D. water-based lubricant.

_____ **33.** The purpose(s) of suctioning include removal of
  A. teeth and large pieces of solid material.
  B. excess oxygen from the patient.
  C. blood, vomitus, and other secretions.
  D. all of the above.

_____ **34.** When a patient begins to vomit, it is essential that you have a(n) _____ ready to go at the patient's side.
  A. suction unit   **C.** blood pressure cuff
  B. oxygen tank   **D.** pocket mask

_____ **35.** Which of the following is <u>not</u> true of the Yankauer suction tip?
  A. It has a rigid tip.
  B. It allows for excellent control over the distal end of the device.
  C. It is most successfully used with responsive patients.
  D. It has a larger bore than flexible catheters.

_____ **36.** When using a soft, flexible-tip catheter,
  A. measure so that it is inserted only as far as the base of the tongue.
  B. never pass the catheter through a nasal tube.
  C. insert the device with the suction turned on.
  D. do none of the above.

_____ **37.** When suctioning an adult patient who is unconscious, never suction for longer than _____ seconds at a time.
  A. 5   **C.** 15
  B. 10   **D.** 20

_____ **38.** When inserting a rigid-tip suction catheter,
  A. insert the device only as far as you can see.
  B. measure from the nose to the earlobe.
  C. slide the device along the palate in children.
  D. insert the device with the suction on.

_____ **39.** Atmospheric air contains _____ oxygen.
  A. 10%   **C.** 21%
  B. 16%   **D.** 25%

_____ **40.** A fully pressurized oxygen tank should have approximately _____ psi.
  A. 1,000   **C.** 2,000
  B. 1,500   **D.** 2,500

_____ **41.** Which <u>portable</u> oxygen cylinder, when full, will last the longest?
  A. D   **C.** A
  B. E   **D.** M

_____ **42.** Before connecting a regulator to an oxygen supply cylinder, the EMT-B should
  A. remove the protective seal and then open the valve.
  B. stand to the side of the main valve opening and crack the cylinder valve slightly.
  C. attach the nonrebreather mask to the flow meter; then attach to the tank.
  D. do all of the above.

_____ **43.** Humidified oxygen is
  A. not possible in an ambulance.
  B. not used for patients on chronic oxygen therapy.
  C. not needed in adult patients being transported for short distances.
  D. habit forming.

_____ **44.** Concerns about the dangers of giving too much oxygen to patients with COPD
  A. are invalid in the prehospital setting.
  B. have been understated and proven with research.
  C. are invalid when the patient is over the age of 60.
  D. are dealt with by using a nonrebreather mask at low flow rates.

_____ **45.** The best method for EMT-Bs to use when giving a high concentration of oxygen to breathing patients is a
  A. nasal cannula.
  B. venturi mask.
  C. simple face mask
  D. nonrebreather mask.

_____ **46.** The oxygen concentration of a nonrebreather mask is between
  A. 20% and 40%.
  B. 40% and 60%.
  C. 60% and 80%.
  D. 80% and 100%.

_____ **47.** The flow rate of a nonrebreather mask should be
  A. adjusted so that when the patient inhales, the bag deflates by two-thirds.
  B. 12 to 15 liters per minute.
  C. adjusted to 6 liters per minute.
  D. all of the above.

_____ **48.** The oxygen concentration of a nasal cannula is between
  A. 4% and 6%.
  B. 8% and 20%.
  C. 24% and 44%.
  D. 50% and 65%.

COMPLETE THE FOLLOWING

1. List at least six of the signs of inadequate breathing.

  A. _____

  B. _____

  C. _____

  D. _____

  E. _____

  F. _____

2. List in order of preference the four techniques available to the EMT-B to provide artificial ventilations.

  A. _____

  B. _____

  C. _____

  D. _____

LABEL THE DIAGRAM

Write the name of each part of the respiratory system on the line provided.

1. _____

2. _____

3. _____

4. _____

5. _____

6. _____

7. _____

8. _____

9. _____

10. _____

11. _____

12. _____

13. _____

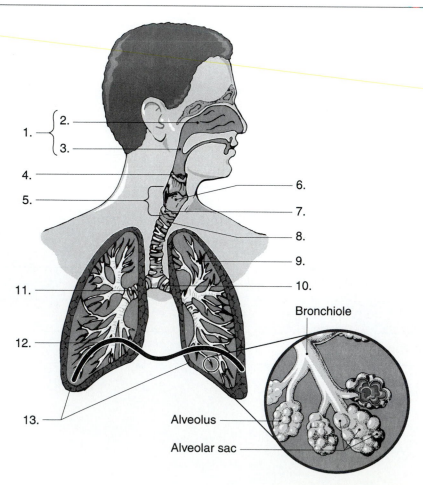

VIRTUAL STREET SCENES

(First review the Street Scenes on p. 140 of your textbook. Then answer the questions below.)

1. If the patient had no gag reflex, what airway adjunct would you consider using? How would you insert it?

2. If the patient vomits during BVM ventilation, what should you do?

3. If the patient's pulse had not increased so quickly, should you have called for an ALS intercept? Why or why not?

WEB SIMULATION

For interactive case studies that will help you review and practice basic skills, visit the *Emergency Care 9e Companion Website* at www.bradybooks.com/emergencycare.

EMT-BASIC SKILL PERFORMANCE CHECKLISTS

▶ HEAD-TILT, CHIN-LIFT MANEUVER

❑ Take BSI precautions.

❑ Once patient is supine, place one hand on the forehead. Place the fingertips of your other hand under the bony area at the center of the patient's lower jaw.

❑ Tilt the head by applying gentle pressure to the patient's forehead.

❑ Use your fingertips to lift the chin and to support the lower jaw. Move the jaw forward to a point where the lower teeth are almost touching the upper teeth. Do not compress the soft tissues under the lower jaw.

❑ Do not close the patient's mouth. It is best to insert an oral airway if the patient has no gag reflex.

▶ Jaw-Thrust Maneuver

❑ Take BSI precautions.

❑ Carefully keep the patient's head, neck, and spine aligned, moving him as a unit as you place him in the supine position.

❑ Kneel approximately 18 inches above the head of the supine patient.

❑ Reach forward and gently place one hand on each side of the patient's lower jaw. Run your fingers along the jaw until you just pass the angle of the jaw.

❑ Stabilize the patient's head with your palms and forearms.

❑ Using your index fingers, push the angles of the patient's lower jaw forward.

❑ To keep the mouth open, use an oropharyngeal airway on a patient with no gag reflex.

❑ Do not tilt or rotate the patient's head.

NOTE: Remember the purpose of the jaw-thrust manuever is to open the airway without moving the head or neck from the nuetral position.

▶ Oropharyngeal (Oral) Airway Insertion

❑ Take BSI precautions.

❑ Select appropriate size airway.

❑ Measure airway (center of mouth to angle of jaw, or corner of mouth to tip of earlobe).

❑ Insert airway without pushing the tongue posteriorly. Insert upside down and flip 180 degrees over the tongue, or straight in with a tongue blade holding tongue forward.

❑ Remove oropharyngeal airway quickly if patient gags.

▶ Nasopharyngeal (Nasal) Airway Insertion

❑ Take BSI precautions.

❑ Select appropriate size airway (diameter of patient's little finger). An alternative method is to measure from patient's nostril to earlobe or to angle of jaw.

❑ Measure airway (nostril to earlobe).

❑ Lubricate nasopharyngeal airway with water-soluble gel.

❑ Fully insert the airway with the bevel facing the nasal septum.

▶ Mouth-to-Mask with Supplemental Oxygen

❑ Take BSI precautions.

❑ Connect one-way valve to mask.

❑ Connect oxygen to the inlet on the face mask. Oxygen should be run at 15 liters per minute.

❑ Kneel about 18 inches above head of the supine patient.

❑ Open airway (manually or with adjunct).

❑ Position the mask on the patient's face so that the apex is over the bridge of the nose and the base is between the lower lip and the prominence of the chin.

(continued next page)

❑ Establish and maintain a proper mask-to-face seal (jaw-thrust maneuver) by placing both thumbs on the sides of the mask and with the index, third, and fourth fingers of each hand grasping the lower jaw on each side, between the angle of the jaw and the earlobe, to jut the jaw forward.

❑ Ventilate the patient at the proper volume and rate (600–800 mL per breath, or greater amounts if necessary to cause obvious chest rise, 12 breaths per minute, 1 to 1½ seconds for each adult breath).

❑ Remove your mouth from the port to allow for passive exhalation.

NOTE: If oxygen is not immediately available, do not delay mouth-to-mask ventilations.

▶ OROPHARYNGEAL SUCTIONING

❑ Take BSI precautions.

❑ Position yourself at the patient's head and turn the patient onto his side.

❑ Measure flexible suction catheter: the distance between the patient's earlobe and the corner of the mouth, or center of the mouth to the angle of the jaw. A rigid tip (Yankauer) does not need to be measured. This is the preferred device. But do not lose sight of the tip.

❑ Turn the suction unit on. Attach the catheter and test for suction.

❑ Open and clear the patient's mouth.

❑ Place the rigid pharyngeal tip so that the convex (bulging-out) side is against the roof of the patient's mouth. Insert the tip just to the base of the tongue. Do not push the tip down into the throat or into the larynx.

❑ Apply suction only after the tip of the catheter or the rigid tip is in place, suctioning on the way out, moving the tip from side to side.

❑ Hyperventilate the patient with 100% oxygen.

▶ TWO-RESCUER BVM VENTILATION

❑ Take BSI precautions.

❑ Open the medical patient's airway, using the head-tilt, chin-lift maneuver.

❑ Suction and insert an oral airway.

❑ Select the correct bag-valve mask size (adult, child, or infant). A pop-off valve is not acceptable!

❑ Kneel approximately 18 inches above the head of the supine patient.

❑ Position the mask on the patient's face so that the apex is over the bridge of the nose and the base is between the lower lip and the prominence of the chin.

❑ Position your thumbs over the top half of the mask, index and middle fingers over the bottom half.

❑ Use the ring and middle fingers to bring the patient's jaw up to the mask and maintain the head-tilt, chin-lift. Tilt the head back as if you were trying to stand the patient on his head!

(continued next page)

❑ The second EMT-B should connect the bag to mask if not already done. While you maintain the mask seal, the second EMT-B should squeeze the bag with two hands until the patient's chest rises. Ventilate the patient at the proper volume and rate (400–600 mL per breath, or greater amounts if necessary to cause obvious chest rise, 10 to 12 breaths per minute, 1 to 1½ seconds for each adult breath).

❑ The second EMT-B should release pressure on the bag and let the patient exhale passively. While this occurs, the bag from the oxygen reservoir is refilling.

❑ Patient can be hyperventilated if his condition warrants it.

NOTE: This technique may be used for a trauma patient by combining a jaw-thrust maneuver with manual stabilization of the head and neck.

▶ PREPARING THE OXYGEN DELIVERY SYSTEM

❑ Select desired cylinder. Check label and hydrostat date.

❑ Place the cylinder in an upright position and stand to one side.

❑ Remove the plastic wrapper or cap protecting the cylinder outlet.

❑ Keep the plastic washer (some setups).

❑ Crack the main valve for one second to clean it out.

❑ Select the correct pressure regulator and flowmeter.

❑ Place cylinder valve gasket on regulator oxygen port.

❑ Make certain that the pressure regulator is closed.

❑ Align pins or thread by hand.

❑ Tighten T-screw for pin yoke.

❑ Tighten with a wrench for a threaded outlet.

❑ Attach tubing and delivery device.

▶ OXYGEN ADMINISTRATION—NONREBREATHER MASK

❑ Take BSI precautions.

❑ Assemble regulator onto tank.

❑ Open main valve on tank.

❑ Check for leaks.

❑ Check tank pressure.

❑ Attach nonrebreather mask.

❑ Adjust liter flow to 12 to 15 liters per minute.

❑ Prefill reservoir.

❑ Apply and adjust mask to the patient's face, expaining the need for oxygen.

❑ Secure tank during transport.

▶ OXYGEN ADMINISTRATION—NASAL CANNULA

- ❑ Take BSI precautions.
- ❑ Assemble regulator onto tank.
- ❑ Open main valve on tank.
- ❑ Check for leaks.
- ❑ Check tank pressure.
- ❑ Attach nasal cannula to regulator.
- ❑ Place nasal prongs into the patient's nose, and adjust tubing for comfort.
- ❑ Adjust liter flow to 1 to 6 liters per minute.
- ❑ Secure tank during transport.

▶ DISCONTINUING OXYGEN ADMINISTRATION

- ❑ Remove delivery device from patient.
- ❑ Turn off the liter flow rate.
- ❑ Close the main valve.
- ❑ Remove the delivery tubing.
- ❑ Bleed the flowmeter.
- ❑ Change the tank before the volume reaches 200 psi or less.

▶ REPOSITIONING THE ADULT PATIENT FOR BASIC LIFE SUPPORT

- ❑ Take BSI precautions.
- ❑ Straighten the patient's legs and position arm closest to you above his head.
- ❑ Cradle the patient's head and neck. Grasp under the distant armpit.
- ❑ Move the patient as a unit onto his side.
- ❑ Move the patient onto back and reposition the extended arm.

NOTE: This maneuver is used to initiate airway evaluation, artificial ventilation, or CPR when the EMT-B must act alone. When trauma is suspected, the four-rescuer log roll is the preferred technique.

CASE STUDY

▶ **THE COMPLICATED AIRWAY: THE SELF-INFLICTED SHOOTING**

Your unit and the police are dispatched to the scene of an attempted suicide with shots fired. Apparently the call was received by a family member who was called by the patient threatening to do harm to himself with a handgun. The police arrive before you and advise that the scene is secure (safe) and that you should respond directly to the scene, which is a private home in a suburban community. Upon arrival, you find a 45-year-old male lying with his face covered with blood. He is moaning, and his chest and abdomen appear to be moving as he breathes. After donning protective gloves, mask, and goggles, both you and your partners carefully provide manual stabilization of the neck and log roll the patient onto a long backboard.

What you reveal is a mandible and tongue that are severely lacerated, and the mouth and nose are bubbling with blood as the patient attempts to breathe.

1. How should you open the airway of this patient?

2. **A)** Does this patient need to be suctioned? **B)** If so, what is the maximum amount of time to accomplish this procedure?

   A. _____

   B. _____

3. Should an airway adjunct be used on this patient?

Once the patient's airway is opened and cleared, you need to oxygenate this patient. He has no other obvious injuries, yet you are treating him for a possible spinal injury due to the impact of the bullet and his backward fall from his desk chair during the incident. The police think that this is why he shot his chin instead of his brain during the suicide attempt. You evaluate the patient's breathing rate as 28, shallow and labored, and his pulse as 120, weak and regular.

4. What device should be used to administer oxygen to this patient?

5. What is the proper liter flow to set the regulator for the device you chose in Number 4?

6. Your portable D cylinder was full at the beginning of the shift and this is your first call. **A)** How many liters are in the tank? **B)** How much pressure is in it? **C)** How much time can you expect to get out of the tank, considering your service's policy is to refill tanks at 200 psi?

   A. _____

   B. _____

   C. _____

7. As you prepare to transport the patient, you continue to suction him, making sure not to exceed **A)** _____ seconds per attempt because as you suction you are also removing **B)** _____ . **C)** Which would be better to use, a rigid tip or a flexible catheter?

   A. _____

   B. _____

   C. _____

8. The patient has a blood pressure of 100/70, so you decide his priority is **A)** [high, low]. The major problem with this patient is his **B)** _____ . He should be transported **C)** [right away, in a few minutes] to the **D)** [local hospital, trauma center].

   A. _____

   B. _____

   C. _____

   D. _____

9. From your knowledge of your EMS system, what ALS (advanced life support) treatment might be helpful to this patient if you can arrange for an ALS intercept?

10. What should you do if you hear hissing or bubbling around the mask as you ventilate?

Interim Exam One

Use the answer sheet on pages 60–61 to complete this exam. It is perforated so it can be easily removed from this book.

1. Most EMT-B training programs are based on standards developed by the
   A. American Red Cross (ARC).
   B. American Heart Association (AHA).
   C. United States Department of Transportation (DOT).
   D. National Institute of Health (NIH).

2. An EMT-B can inspire patient confidence and cooperation by
   A. transporting the patient from the scene to a hospital.
   B. providing patient care without regard for her own personal safety.
   C. telling the patient that everything will be all right.
   D. being pleasant, cooperative, sincere, and a good listener.

3. If an on-duty EMT-B fails to provide the standard of care and if this failure causes harm or injury to the patient, the EMT-B may be accused of
   A. assault.
   B. abandonment.
   C. negligence.
   D. breach of promise.

4. A conscious and mentally competent adult patient has the right to refuse care. This refusal must be _____ and documented.
   A. implied   C. involuntary
   B. actual   D. informed

5. The EMT-B can treat and transport an unconscious patient because of the legal consideration known as _____ consent.
   A. applied   C. triage
   B. implied   D. immunity

6. A child falls off a trampoline at an elementary school and twists her ankle. Since the parents are not present, the child's consent is
   A. not needed.   C. implied.
   B. actual.   D. meaningless.

7. _____ help protect the off-duty EMT-B from lawsuits when stopping at the scene of a collision to offer assistance.
   A. Professional associations
   B. Blanket insurance policies
   C. Good Samaritan laws
   D. Abandonment laws

8. Each of the following is the responsibility of an EMT-B at a hazardous-materials incident except
   A. entering hazmat scenes with SCBA.
   B. protecting yourself and others.
   C. recognizing potential problems.
   D. notifying hazardous-materials response team.

9. The form of infection control that assumes that all body fluids should be considered potentially infectious is
   A. infectious disease.
   B. body substance isolation.
   C. immunity.
   D. universal precautions.

10. When planning to lift, all of the following are important considerations except
    A. the weight of the object.
    B. one's physical characteristics.
    C. communicating with one's partner.
    D. the distance the object is to be carried.

11. When lifting, the EMT-B should
    A. keep the back loose and knees locked.
    B. twist or attempt to make moves other than the lift.
    C. use the leg muscles to do the lift.
    D. try not to talk to his partner.

12. When carrying a conscious patient on the stairs, the EMT-B should
    A. keep the stretcher as level as possible.
    B. use a long backboard at all times.
    C. use a stair chair whenever possible.
    D. do all of the above.

13. Ways an EMT-B can avoid a potential back injury include all the following except
    A. push, rather than pull, a load.
    B. keep back locked-in while lifting.
    C. keep arms straight when pulling.
    D. push or pull from a kneeling position if the weight is below waist level.

14. An emergency move is required in each of the following situations except when
    A. the scene is hazardous.
    B. care of life-threatening conditions requires repositioning.
    C. other patients must be reached who have life threats.
    D. the patient is unconscious.

15. Which of the following is the greatest danger to the patient in an emergency move?
    A. A spinal injury may be aggravated.
    B. Bleeding may increase after movement.
    C. The airway may become obstructed.
    D. There is no danger associated with an emergency move.

16. A method of lifting and carrying a patient in which one EMT-B slips hands under the patient's armpits and grasps the wrists while another EMT-B grasps the patient's knees is called the
    A. direct ground lift.
    B. extremity lift.
    C. draw sheet method.
    D. direct carry method.

17. When moving a patient from the ambulance stretcher to the hospital stretcher, you probably will use the
    A. cradle carry.
    B. modified draw sheet method.
    C. direct ground lift.
    D. extremity lift.

18. To load the wheeled ambulance stretcher into the ambulance, the two EMT-Bs should position themselves on _____ of the stretcher.
    A. opposite sides
    B. opposite ends
    C. the same side
    D. one end and one side

19. Move a patient who has no broken bones or spinal injury from the floor to a stair chair using the
    A. indirect carry.   C. slide transfer.
    B. extremity lift.   D. chair lift.

20. Drags are used only in emergencies because they
    A. do not protect the patient's neck and spine.
    B. require excessive energy from the EMT-B.
    C. may injure the EMT-B's back.
    D. provide full immobilization.

21. In order to maintain balance when lifting a patient carrying device, it is best to use _____ rescuers to carry the device.
    A. three
    B. an even number of
    C. an odd number of
    D. bystanders and

22. The driver of a vehicle involved in a collision requires immediate airway and bleeding control. You are unable to provide this treatment in the vehicle. You should
    A. check the patient's vital signs.
    B. make an urgent move.
    C. remove the patient on a short backboard.
    D. do all of the above.

23. Which carry is considered very difficult to use with an unconscious person?
    A. cradle   C. shoulder
    B. three-rescuer   D. piggyback

24. The _____ carry must be performed in one unbroken sweep.
    A. pack strap
    B. front piggyback
    C. firefighter's
    D. four-rescuer

25. A canvas or rubberized stretcher that can be used to move a patient through a narrow hallway or restricted area is called a _____ stretcher.
    A. basket
    B. portable
    C. flexible
    D. wheeled-ambulance

26. A victim with obvious spinal injuries is found on the floor of a burning building. The EMT-B rates the situation hazardous, but not yet dire. Alone and without special equipment, the EMT-B should use the
    A. cradle carry.
    B. clothes drag.
    C. firefighter's carry.
    D. pack-strap method.

27. The patient carrying device of choice for the uninjured patient is the _____ stretcher.
    A. portable ambulance
    B. wire basket
    C. wheeled ambulance
    D. slat

28. If you are an EMT-B with a service that does not provide the appropriate personal protective equipment, why should you serve as an advocate for this equipment?
    A. Your crew members could be injured unnecessarily.
    B. You could be seriously injured.
    C. An injured EMT-B is of little help to the patient.
    D. All of the above.

29. During an EMS call, a lethal threat is recognized. The EMT-B should first
    A. retreat to a safe area.
    B. radio for assistance.
    C. re-evaluate the situation.
    D. remedy the situation.

30. Of the different types of stress, which is a positive form that helps the EMT-B work under pressure and respond effectively?
    A. cumulative stress
    B. eustress
    C. distress
    D. critical incident stress

31. When responding to a violent situation, observation begins when you
    A. enter the scene.
    B. exit the ambulance.
    C. enter the neighborhood.
    D. arrive at the patient's side.

32. To ensure crew safety, one member of the crew should always
    A. remain in the ambulance.
    B. carry a portable radio.
    C. wear a bulletproof vest.
    D. carry a canister of "pepper gas."

33. While treating a patient with a severely bleeding forearm, the patient's pet dog appears. The patient states, "He won't hurt you. He's very friendly." Your best course of action would be to
    A. have your partner observe the dog closely while you treat the patient.
    B. quickly control the bleeding; then have the dog locked in another room.
    C. ignore the dog since the patient assures it is friendly and will not harm you.
    D. do all of the above.

34. If a patient refuses care and then becomes unconscious, it is best for the EMT-B to
    A. refuse to treat or transport the patient.
    B. ask a family member for permission to treat.
    C. treat life-threatening problems and transport.
    D. contact medical direction for advice.

35. An advantage of the "advance directive" is that
    A. the patient is not involved in making a decision about her treatment.
    B. the patient's expressed wishes may be followed.
    C. no matter what the family says, CPR is not given.
    D. it protects the EMT-B from charges of negligence.

36. In most cases, the oral wishes of the patient's family to withhold care are
    A. all that is needed to stop CPR from being initiated.
    B. all that is needed to stop CPR once it is initiated.
    C. not a reason to withhold medical care.
    D. not sufficient unless they are given in writing.

37. You can prevent most lawsuits if you
    A. provide care within the scope of your practice.
    B. properly document your care.
    C. are courteous and respectful to all your patients.
    D. do all of the above.

38. The negligent EMT-B may be required to pay for all of the following except the patient's
    A. lost wages.
    B. medical expenses.
    C. pain and suffering.
    D. health insurance costs.

39. Which of the following is not a function of the musculoskeletal system?
    A. It gives the body shape.
    B. It protects the internal organs.
    C. It provides for body movement.
    D. It regulates body temperature.

40. The superior portion of the sternum is called the
    A. xiphoid process.   C. manubrium.
    B. sternal body.   D. clavicle.

41. A young girl fell while ice skating, injuring the protrusion on the inside of the ankle. The medical term for this location is the
    A. acromion.   C. lateral malleolus.
    B. medial malleolus.   D. calcaneus.

42. The heart muscle has a property called _____ . This means that the heart has the ability to generate and conduct electrical impulses on its own.
    A. contractility
    B. automaticity
    C. involuntary contraction
    D. conductibility

43. A division of the peripheral nervous system that controls involuntary motor functions is called the _____ nervous system.
    A. autonomic   C. sensory
    B. central   D. motor

44. When in the anatomical position, the person will be facing
    A. away from you.   C. face down.
    B. forward.   D. face up.

45. In the anatomical position, the person's palms will be facing
  A. forward.
  B. backward.
  C. upward.
  D. downward.

46. An anatomical term that is occasionally used to refer to the sole of the foot is
  A. calcaneus.
  B. ventral.
  C. dorsal.
  D. plantar.

47. The bones of the cheek are called the _____ bones.
  A. orbit
  B. maxillae
  C. zygomatic
  D. mandible

48. The heart is _____ to the stomach.
  A. distal
  B. medial
  C. proximal
  D. superior

49. When comparing body structure positions, the knees are said to be _____ to the toes, and the toes are _____ to the knees.
  A. inferior : superior
  B. proximal : distal
  C. distal : dorsal
  D. anterior : posterior

50. A patient found lying on her back is in the _____ position.
  A. anatomical
  B. prone
  C. supine
  D. lateral recumbent

51. To assist in describing the location of abdominal pain, we divide the abdomen into _____ parts.
  A. two
  B. three
  C. four
  D. five

52. The torso of the body is composed of the abdomen, pelvis, and
  A. thorax.
  B. upper arms and legs.
  C. extremities.
  D. head.

53. The heart is located in the center of the _____ cavity.
  A. thoracic
  B. cranial
  C. pelvic
  D. cardiac

54. The structure that divides the chest cavity from the abdominal cavity is the
  A. meninges.
  B. duodenum.
  C. diaphragm.
  D. spinal column.

55. The anatomical name for the kneecap is the
  A. ilium.
  B. malleolus.
  C. patella.
  D. phalange.

56. The cranium consists of the
  A. facial bones.
  B. mandible and maxillae.
  C. top, back, and sides of the skull.
  D. zygomatic bones.

57. The highest point in the shoulder is the
  A. acromion process.
  B. humerus.
  C. metatarsal.
  D. clavicle.

58. At the scene of an accident, an off-duty EMT-B provides care to the patient, acting in good faith and to the best of her abilities. In many states, this EMT-B is protected from care-related lawsuits by _____ laws.
  A. applied consent
  B. total immunity
  C. Good Samaritan
  D. jeopardy

59. When confronted with an unconscious minor without parents or a legal guardian present, the EMT-B should
  A. seek a physician's approval before beginning care.
  B. consider consent for care to be implied and begin care.
  C. ask the child for consent and begin care.
  D. consider consent to be applied and begin care.

60. The legal concept of negligence requires that three circumstances must be demonstrated. Which of the following is <u>not</u> one of the three circumstances?
  A. The EMT had a duty to act.
  B. The EMT committed a breach of duty.
  C. The EMT had a local duty.
  D. The breach of duty caused harm.

61. A person lying on his stomach with his face down is in the _____ position.
  A. supine
  B. prone
  C. coma
  D. recovery

62. In a trauma center, surgery teams are
  A. on call 12 hours a day.
  B. available most of the time.
  C. available 24 hours a day.
  D. supervised by the Medical Director.

63. In 1970, the _____ was founded to establish professional standards for EMS personnel.
  A. American Medical Association
  B. National Registry of Emergency Medical Technicians
  C. National Highway Traffic Safety Administration
  D. U.S. Department of Transportation

64. Safe, reliable transportation is a critical component of an EMS system. Most patients can be effectively transported by
  A. airplane.
  B. helicopter.
  C. rescue vehicle.
  D. ambulance.

65. An _____ is a national level EMT who has been trained to start IVs, perform advanced airway techniques, and administer some medicines beyond the EMT-B.
    A. EMT-First Responder
    B. EMT-Intermediate
    C. EMT-Critical Care
    D. EMT-Paramedic

66. A continuous self-review with the purpose of identifying and correcting aspects of the EMS system that require improvement is called
    A. standing orders.
    B. quality improvement.
    C. protocols.
    D. medical direction.

67. A physician who assumes the ultimate responsibility for the patient care aspects of the EMS system is called the
    A. Designated Agent.
    B. Medical Director.
    C. Off-line Director.
    D. Primary Care Physician.

68. A common cause of lawsuits against EMS agencies is
    A. patients who refuse care.
    B. on-scene deaths.
    C. cardiac arrest cases.
    D. pedestrians struck by cars.

69. The legal extent or limits of the EMT-B's job are formally defined by the
    A. patient.
    B. DOT curriculum.
    C. state.
    D. scope of practice.

70. Which is not generally considered a sign or symptom of stress?
    A. decisiveness
    B. guilt
    C. loss of interest in work
    D. difficulty sleeping

71. All of the following are types of calls that have a high potential for causing excessive stress except
    A. calls involving infants and children.
    B. patients with severe injuries.
    C. cases of abuse and neglect.
    D. motor-vehicle collisions.

72. Life-style changes that can help the EMT-B deal with stress include all of the following except
    A. exercise to burn off tension.
    B. increased consumption of fatty foods.
    C. decreased caffeine consumption.
    D. decreased consumption of alcohol.

73. Changes in your professional life to reduce and prevent stress could include
    A. requesting a change of shift or location.
    B. taking on another part-time position.
    C. working additional overtime shifts.
    D. requesting a busier location.

74. After a CISD,
    A. management investigates the call.
    B. performance appraisals are initiated.
    C. the peer team writes a detailed critique.
    D. the peer team offers support.

75. Stress after a major EMS incident is
    A. unusual and unexpected.
    B. a sign of weakness.
    C. normal and to be expected.
    D. part of the grieving process.

76. Retreating to a world of one's own after hearing one is going to die is a result of the stage of grief called
    A. bargaining.   C. denial.
    B. depression.   D. anxiety.

77. All of the following communicable diseases should be of particular concern to the EMT-B except
    A. hepatitis B.   C. HIV/AIDS.
    B. tuberculosis.   D. PPD.

78. A disease that is spread by exposure to an open wound or sore of an infected individual is caused by a(n) _____ pathogen.
    A. universal   C. bloodborne
    B. airborne   D. infectious

79. An infection that causes inflammation of the liver is called
    A. meningitis.   C. typhoid.
    B. tuberculosis.   D. hepatitis.

80. A disease spread by inhaling or absorbing droplets from the air through the eyes, nose, or mouth is considered
    A. bloodborne.
    B. noncommunicable.
    C. airborne.
    D. viral.

81. The communicable disease that kills the most health workers every year in the United States is
    A. tuberculosis.   C. meningitis.
    B. HIV/AIDS.   D. hepatitis B virus.

82. Always assume that any patient with a
    A. cold has a bloodborne disease.
    B. productive cough has TB.
    C. fever has typhoid.
    D. rash has measles.

83. Which of the following is <u>not</u> true about the human immunodeficiency virus (HIV)?
   A. It attacks the immune system.
   B. It doesn't survive well outside the human body.
   C. It can be introduced through puncture wounds.
   D. It is an airborne pathogen.

84. Your patient has hepatitis B. You are accidentally stuck with a needle that has some of this patient's infected blood on it. Your chance of contracting the disease is about
   A. 10%.   C. 30%.
   B. 20%.   D. 40%.

85. Your patient has HIV. You are accidentally stuck with a needle that has some infected blood on it. Your chance of contracting the disease is about
   A. 0.5%.   C. 10%.
   B. 5%.   D. 15%.

86. If you think your patient has TB, you should wear the usual personal protective equipment plus a
   A. surgeon's mask.   C. HEPA respirator.
   B. gown.   D. Tyvek suit.

87. When alone, instead of providing mouth-to-mouth ventilations on the nonbreathing patient, the EMT-B should use a
   A. pocket mask with a one-way valve.
   B. one-way valve.
   C. bag-valve mask.
   D. endotracheal tube.

88. Which method of infection control will reduce exposure to yourself, your crew, and your next patient?
   A. wearing a HEPA respirator
   B. taking universal precautions
   C. handwashing after each patient contact
   D. none of the above

89. An act that establishes procedures through which emergency response workers can find out if they have been exposed to life-threatening infectious diseases is called
   A. OSHA 1910.1030.
   B. Ryan White CARE Act.
   C. AIDS Protection Act.
   D. OSHA 1910.120.

90. Each emergency response employer must develop a plan that identifies and documents job classifications and tasks in which there is the possibility of exposure to potentially infectious body fluids. This is required by
   A. OSHA 1910.1030.
   B. Ryan White CARE Act.
   C. AIDS Protection Act.
   D. OSHA 1910.120.

91. Every employer of EMT-Bs must provide free of charge
   A. a yearly physical examination.
   B. a life insurance policy.
   C. universal health insurance.
   D. a hepatitis B vaccination.

92. Engineering controls that prevent the spread of bloodborne diseases include
   A. pocket masks.
   B. needle containers.
   C. disposable airway equipment.
   D. all of the above.

93. Which of the following is <u>not</u> required by the OSHA bloodborne pathogen standard?
   A. post-exposure evaluation and follow-up
   B. personal protective equipment
   C. HEPA respirator
   D. housekeeping controls and labeling

94. Which of the following is <u>not</u> considered a high risk area for TB?
   A. correctional facilities
   B. day care centers
   C. homeless shelters
   D. nursing homes

95. As you near an emergency scene, you should
   A. sound your siren to broadcast your arrival.
   B. go straight to the front door.
   C. secure the scene as quickly as possible.
   D. turn off your lights and siren.

96. If anyone at the scene is in possession of a weapon, the EMT-B should
   A. notify the police immediately.
   B. ask the person to give it to you.
   C. ignore the person with the weapon.
   D. advise the person to leave the scene.

97. The reduction of breathing to the point where oxygen intake is not sufficient to support life is called
   A. respiratory failure.
   B. anoxic metabolism.
   C. respiratory arrest.
   D. respiratory support.

98. Adequate signs of breathing include all of the following <u>except</u>
   A. equal expansion of both sides of the chest.
   B. air moving in and out of the nose.
   C. blue or gray skin coloration.
   D. present and equal breath sounds.

99. The widening of the nostrils of the nose with respirations is called
   A. hyperventilating.   C. nasal gurgling.
   B. nasal flaring.   D. wheezing.

100. The condition in which a patient's skin or lips are blue or gray is called.
   A. stridor.   C. pallor.
   B. cyanosis.   D. anemia.

101. If a patient is unable to speak in full sentences, this could be a sign of
   A. complete airway blockage.
   B. snoring.
   C. shortness of breath.
   D. respiratory arrest.

102. The procedures by which life-threatening respiratory problems are initially treated by the EMT-B include all of the following except
   A. opening and maintaining the airway.
   B. inserting an endotracheal tube immediately.
   C. providing supplemental oxygen to the breathing patient.
   D. assuring a clear airway with frequent suctioning.

103. Most airway problems are caused by
   A. the tongue.   C. shock.
   B. asthma.   D. the epiglottis.

104. Which maneuver is most appropriate for an unconscious patient found lying at the bottom of a stairwell?
   A. head-tilt, chin-lift
   B. head-tilt, neck-lift
   C. jaw-pull lift
   D. jaw-thrust

105. When choosing a means of ventilating a patient, your last choice would be
   A. flow-restricted, oxygen-powered ventilation device.
   B. one-rescuer bag-valve mask.
   C. two-rescuer bag-valve mask.
   D. mouth-to-mask with high-flow supplemental oxygen.

106. Artificial ventilation may be inadequate if the
   A. chest rises with each ventilation.
   B. heart rate returns to normal.
   C. rate of ventilation is too fast or too slow.
   D. skin becomes warm and dry.

107. The standard respiratory fitting on a bag-valve mask that ensures a proper fit with other respiratory equipment is
   A. 15/22 mm.   C. 5/20 mm.
   B. 10/14 mm.   D. 20/26 mm.

108. A bag-valve mask should have all of the following except
   A. self-refilling shell.
   B. a clear face mask.
   C. be easily cleared and sterilized.
   D. a pop-off valve.

109. The proper oxygen flow rate when ventilating a patient with a BVM is _____ liters per minute.
   A. 5   C. 15
   B. 10   D. 20

110. According to the American Heart Association guidelines, at least _____ milliliters of air must be delivered to the patient when ventilating with a BVM attached to supplemental oxygen.
   A. 400   C. 800
   B. 600   D. 1,000

111. The first step in providing artificial ventilation of a stoma breather is to
   A. leave the head and neck in a neutral position.
   B. ventilate at the appropriate rate for the patient's age.
   C. clear any mucus or secretions obstructing the stoma.
   D. establish a seal using a pediatric-sized mask.

112. A flow-restricted, oxygen-powered ventilation device should have all of the following features except
   A. an audible alarm when ventilation is activated.
   B. a trigger that enables the rescuer to use both hands.
   C. a peak flow rate of up to 40 liters per minute.
   D. a rugged design and construction.

113. The two most common airway adjuncts for the EMT-B to use are the oropharyngeal airway and the
   A. nasal cannula.
   B. nasopharyngeal airway.
   C. endotracheal tube.
   D. Yankauer.

114. An oropharyngeal airway should be inserted in
   A. all patients with inadequate breathing.
   B. trauma patients with a gag reflex.
   C. medical patients with a gag reflex.
   D. all unconscious patients with no gag reflex.

115. When suctioning a patient, the EMT-B should
   A. suction on the way in and way out.
   B. avoid using eye wear or a mask.
   C. never suction for longer than 15 seconds.
   D. hypoventilate prior to suctioning.

116. The emergency situation in which there is a failure of the cardiovascular system to provide sufficient blood to all the vital tissues is called
   A. respiratory arrest.
   B. respiratory failure.
   C. shock.
   D. cardiac arrest.

117. An insufficiency in the supply of oxygen to the body's tissues is called
   A. anoxia.   C. hypoxia.
   B. no-oxia.   D. cyanosis.

118. Before the oxygen cylinder's pressure gauge reads _____ psi, you must switch to a fresh cylinder.
   A. 200   C. 800
   B. 400   D. 1,000

119. When handling oxygen cylinders, the EMT-B should do all of the following except
   A. have the cylinders hydrostatically tested every 5 years.
   B. ensure that valve seat inserts and gaskets are in good condition.
   C. store reserve cylinders in a warm, humid room.
   D. use medical grade oxygen in all cylinders.

120. The best way to deliver high-concentration oxygen to a breathing patient is to use a
   A. nonrebreather mask.
   B. partial rebreather mask.
   C. bag-valve mask.
   D. nasal cannula.

121. A nasal cannula provides between _____ % and _____ % oxygen concentrations.
   A. 10 : 21   C. 36 : 58
   B. 24 : 44   D. 72 : 96

122. If the patient has dentures, during airway procedures the EMT-B should
   A. remove them right away.
   B. leave them in unless they are loose.
   C. remove the teeth one at a time.
   D. hold them in place with a free hand.

123. When managing an airway of a child, an airway consideration you should remember is the
   A. mouth and nose are smaller and more easily obstructed.
   B. chest wall is firmer in a child.
   C. trachea is wider and less easily obstructed.
   D. all of the above.

124. When breathing stops completely, the patient is in
   A. respiratory arrest.
   B. ventilatory reduction.
   C. artificial ventilation.
   D. respiratory failure.

125. Which ventilation device is contraindicated in infants and children?
   A. bag-valve mask
   B. pediatric pocket mask
   C. flow-restricted, oxygen-powered ventilation device
   D. nonrebreather mask

126. A device that allows the control of oxygen in liters per minute is called a
   A. flowmeter.   C. humidifier.
   B. G tank.   D. reservoir.

127. A type of flowmeter that has no gauge and allows for the adjustment of flow in liters per minute in stepped increments is called a
   A. Bourdon gauge flowmeter.
   B. constant flow selector valve.
   C. humidifier.
   D. pressure compensated flowmeter.

128. Why do some systems use humidified oxygen?
   A. Lack of humidity can dry out the patient's mucous membranes.
   B. It provides a reservoir for the oxygen.
   C. It limits the risk of infection.
   D. It is helpful when transporting patients short distances.

129. A patient in the end stage of a respiratory disease may have switched over to
   A. hyperventilation syndrome.
   B. hyperbaric therapy.
   C. hypoxic drive.
   D. carbon dioxide drive.

130. What is COPD?
   A. type of shock
   B. type of ventilation
   C. mechanism of breathing
   D. chronic pulmonary disease

Chapter Exam One Answer Sheet

Fill in the correct answer for each item. When scoring, note there are 130
questions valued at 0.769 points each.

1.	[ ] A	[ ] B	[ ] C	[ ] D	36.	[ ] A	[ ] B	[ ] C	[ ] D
2.	[ ] A	[ ] B	[ ] C	[ ] D	37.	[ ] A	[ ] B	[ ] C	[ ] D
3.	[ ] A	[ ] B	[ ] C	[ ] D	38.	[ ] A	[ ] B	[ ] C	[ ] D
4.	[ ] A	[ ] B	[ ] C	[ ] D	39.	[ ] A	[ ] B	[ ] C	[ ] D
5.	[ ] A	[ ] B	[ ] C	[ ] D	40.	[ ] A	[ ] B	[ ] C	[ ] D
6.	[ ] A	[ ] B	[ ] C	[ ] D	41.	[ ] A	[ ] B	[ ] C	[ ] D
7.	[ ] A	[ ] B	[ ] C	[ ] D	42.	[ ] A	[ ] B	[ ] C	[ ] D
8.	[ ] A	[ ] B	[ ] C	[ ] D	43.	[ ] A	[ ] B	[ ] C	[ ] D
9.	[ ] A	[ ] B	[ ] C	[ ] D	44.	[ ] A	[ ] B	[ ] C	[ ] D
10.	[ ] A	[ ] B	[ ] C	[ ] D	45.	[ ] A	[ ] B	[ ] C	[ ] D
11.	[ ] A	[ ] B	[ ] C	[ ] D	46.	[ ] A	[ ] B	[ ] C	[ ] D
12.	[ ] A	[ ] B	[ ] C	[ ] D	47.	[ ] A	[ ] B	[ ] C	[ ] D
13.	[ ] A	[ ] B	[ ] C	[ ] D	48.	[ ] A	[ ] B	[ ] C	[ ] D
14.	[ ] A	[ ] B	[ ] C	[ ] D	49.	[ ] A	[ ] B	[ ] C	[ ] D
15.	[ ] A	[ ] B	[ ] C	[ ] D	50.	[ ] A	[ ] B	[ ] C	[ ] D
16.	[ ] A	[ ] B	[ ] C	[ ] D	51.	[ ] A	[ ] B	[ ] C	[ ] D
17.	[ ] A	[ ] B	[ ] C	[ ] D	52.	[ ] A	[ ] B	[ ] C	[ ] D
18.	[ ] A	[ ] B	[ ] C	[ ] D	53.	[ ] A	[ ] B	[ ] C	[ ] D
19.	[ ] A	[ ] B	[ ] C	[ ] D	54.	[ ] A	[ ] B	[ ] C	[ ] D
20.	[ ] A	[ ] B	[ ] C	[ ] D	55.	[ ] A	[ ] B	[ ] C	[ ] D
21.	[ ] A	[ ] B	[ ] C	[ ] D	56.	[ ] A	[ ] B	[ ] C	[ ] D
22.	[ ] A	[ ] B	[ ] C	[ ] D	57.	[ ] A	[ ] B	[ ] C	[ ] D
23.	[ ] A	[ ] B	[ ] C	[ ] D	58.	[ ] A	[ ] B	[ ] C	[ ] D
24.	[ ] A	[ ] B	[ ] C	[ ] D	59.	[ ] A	[ ] B	[ ] C	[ ] D
25.	[ ] A	[ ] B	[ ] C	[ ] D	60.	[ ] A	[ ] B	[ ] C	[ ] D
26.	[ ] A	[ ] B	[ ] C	[ ] D	61.	[ ] A	[ ] B	[ ] C	[ ] D
27.	[ ] A	[ ] B	[ ] C	[ ] D	62.	[ ] A	[ ] B	[ ] C	[ ] D
28.	[ ] A	[ ] B	[ ] C	[ ] D	63.	[ ] A	[ ] B	[ ] C	[ ] D
29.	[ ] A	[ ] B	[ ] C	[ ] D	64.	[ ] A	[ ] B	[ ] C	[ ] D
30.	[ ] A	[ ] B	[ ] C	[ ] D	65.	[ ] A	[ ] B	[ ] C	[ ] D
31.	[ ] A	[ ] B	[ ] C	[ ] D	66.	[ ] A	[ ] B	[ ] C	[ ] D
32.	[ ] A	[ ] B	[ ] C	[ ] D	67.	[ ] A	[ ] B	[ ] C	[ ] D
33.	[ ] A	[ ] B	[ ] C	[ ] D	68.	[ ] A	[ ] B	[ ] C	[ ] D
34.	[ ] A	[ ] B	[ ] C	[ ] D	69.	[ ] A	[ ] B	[ ] C	[ ] D
35.	[ ] A	[ ] B	[ ] C	[ ] D	70.	[ ] A	[ ] B	[ ] C	[ ] D

71.	[ ] A	[ ] B	[ ] C	[ ] D		
72.	[ ] A	[ ] B	[ ] C	[ ] D		
73.	[ ] A	[ ] B	[ ] C	[ ] D		

71. [ ] A [ ] B [ ] C [ ] D
72. [ ] A [ ] B [ ] C [ ] D
73. [ ] A [ ] B [ ] C [ ] D
74. [ ] A [ ] B [ ] C [ ] D
75. [ ] A [ ] B [ ] C [ ] D
76. [ ] A [ ] B [ ] C [ ] D
77. [ ] A [ ] B [ ] C [ ] D
78. [ ] A [ ] B [ ] C [ ] D
79. [ ] A [ ] B [ ] C [ ] D
80. [ ] A [ ] B [ ] C [ ] D
81. [ ] A [ ] B [ ] C [ ] D
82. [ ] A [ ] B [ ] C [ ] D
83. [ ] A [ ] B [ ] C [ ] D
84. [ ] A [ ] B [ ] C [ ] D
85. [ ] A [ ] B [ ] C [ ] D
86. [ ] A [ ] B [ ] C [ ] D
87. [ ] A [ ] B [ ] C [ ] D
88. [ ] A [ ] B [ ] C [ ] D
89. [ ] A [ ] B [ ] C [ ] D
90. [ ] A [ ] B [ ] C [ ] D
91. [ ] A [ ] B [ ] C [ ] D
92. [ ] A [ ] B [ ] C [ ] D
93. [ ] A [ ] B [ ] C [ ] D
94. [ ] A [ ] B [ ] C [ ] D
95. [ ] A [ ] B [ ] C [ ] D
96. [ ] A [ ] B [ ] C [ ] D
97. [ ] A [ ] B [ ] C [ ] D
98. [ ] A [ ] B [ ] C [ ] D
99. [ ] A [ ] B [ ] C [ ] D
100. [ ] A [ ] B [ ] C [ ] D

101. [ ] A [ ] B [ ] C [ ] D
102. [ ] A [ ] B [ ] C [ ] D
103. [ ] A [ ] B [ ] C [ ] D
104. [ ] A [ ] B [ ] C [ ] D
105. [ ] A [ ] B [ ] C [ ] D
106. [ ] A [ ] B [ ] C [ ] D
107. [ ] A [ ] B [ ] C [ ] D
108. [ ] A [ ] B [ ] C [ ] D
109. [ ] A [ ] B [ ] C [ ] D
110. [ ] A [ ] B [ ] C [ ] D
111. [ ] A [ ] B [ ] C [ ] D
112. [ ] A [ ] B [ ] C [ ] D
113. [ ] A [ ] B [ ] C [ ] D
114. [ ] A [ ] B [ ] C [ ] D
115. [ ] A [ ] B [ ] C [ ] D
116. [ ] A [ ] B [ ] C [ ] D
117. [ ] A [ ] B [ ] C [ ] D
118. [ ] A [ ] B [ ] C [ ] D
119. [ ] A [ ] B [ ] C [ ] D
120. [ ] A [ ] B [ ] C [ ] D
121. [ ] A [ ] B [ ] C [ ] D
122. [ ] A [ ] B [ ] C [ ] D
123. [ ] A [ ] B [ ] C [ ] D
124. [ ] A [ ] B [ ] C [ ] D
125. [ ] A [ ] B [ ] C [ ] D
126. [ ] A [ ] B [ ] C [ ] D
127. [ ] A [ ] B [ ] C [ ] D
128. [ ] A [ ] B [ ] C [ ] D
129. [ ] A [ ] B [ ] C [ ] D
130. [ ] A [ ] B [ ] C [ ] D

Chapter Seven

SCENE SIZE-UP

MATCH TERMINOLOGY/DEFINITIONS

A. Force or forces that may have caused injury

B. Injury caused by an object that passes through the skin and other body tissues

C. Steps taken by EMS crew when approaching, arriving, and attending at the scene of an emergency call to ensure the safety of the crew, the patient, and bystanders

D. Area around the wreckage of a vehicle collision or other incident within which special safety precautions should be taken

E. Principle that a body in motion will remain in motion unless acted on by an outside force

F. Keen awareness that a person may have injuries

G. Agency that provides advice on hazardous materials via a hotline

H. Injury caused by a blow that does not penetrate through the skin or body tissues

I. Material available for rescuers to obtain quick information about hazardous materials

J. Violence in the home

_____ 1. Blunt-force trauma

_____ 2. CHEMTREC

_____ 3. Danger zone

_____ 4. Domestic violence

_____ 5. High index of suspicion

_____ 6. Law of inertia

_____ 7. Mechanism of injury

_____ 8. *North American Emergency Response Guidebook*

_____ 9. Penetrating trauma

_____ 10. Scene size-up

MULTIPLE-CHOICE REVIEW

_____ 1. Your top priority when conducting a scene size-up is determining
   A. patient safety.
   B. personal safety.
   C. number of injured.
   D. mechanism of injury.

_____ 2. Which of the following is the most accurate statement about scene size-up?
   A. It takes place as you are approaching the scene.
   B. It is replaced by patient care once you arrive at the scene.
   C. It is confined to the first part of the assessment process.
   D. It is an ongoing process throughout the call.

_____ 3. If you arrive at a collision scene where there are police, fire vehicles, and other ambulances already present, you should
   A. immediately begin patient care.
   B. conduct your own scene size-up.
   C. ensure that no bystanders are injured.
   D. do all of the above.

_____ 4. Which of the following is <u>not</u> an appropriate action when you near the scene of a traffic collision?
   A. Look and listen for other EMS units as you near intersections.
   B. Look for signs of collision-related power outages.
   C. Observe traffic flow to anticipate blockage at the scene.
   D. Attempt to park your vehicle downhill from the scene.

_____ 5. When you are in sight of the collision scene, you should watch for the signals of police officers and other emergency service personnel because
   A. they may have information about hazards or the location of injured persons.
   B. the first ones on the scene are considered to be in charge.
   C. federal law requires you to follow the command of other responders.
   D. they are considered the medical-care experts on the scene.

_____ 6. When there are no apparent hazards, consider the danger zone to extend _____ feet in all directions from the wreckage.
   A. 25   C. 100
   B. 50   D. 200

_____ 7. When a collision vehicle is on fire, consider the danger zone to extend at least _____ feet in all directions, even if the fire appears small and limited to the engine compartment.
   A. 25   C. 100
   B. 50   D. 200

_____ 8. A good scene size-up should identify
   A. the potential for a violent situation.
   B. the name and amount of toxic substances.
   C. the number of patients and their diagnoses.
   D. all of the above.

_____ 9. The EMT-B's BSI equipment during the scene size-up may include all of the following <u>except</u>
   A. eye protection.   C. mask.
   B. disposable gloves.   D. oxygen mask.

_____ 10. The key element of BSI precautions is to
   A. always wear all the protective clothing.
   B. always have personal protective equipment readily available.
   C. place equipment on the patient as well as the rescuer.
   D. determine which body fluids are a danger to the EMT-B.

_____ 11. Injuries to bones and joints are usually associated with
   A. fights and drug usage.   C. fires and explosions.
   B. falls and vehicle collisions.   D. bullet wounds.

_____ 12. Knowing the mechanism of injury assists the EMT-B in
   A. immobilizing the patient's spine.
   B. determining which BSI precautions to use.
   C. predicting various injury patterns.
   D. all of the above.

_____ 13. The law of inertia states that
   A. the faster you enter a turn the more your vehicle will be pulled straight.
   B. the slower the speed the greater is the energy loss.
   C. a body in motion will remain in motion unless acted upon by an outside force.
   D. the mass or weight of an object is the most important contributor to an injury.

_____ **14.** An unrestrained driver involved in a head-on, up-and-over collision is
likely to sustain injuries to the
  A. skull.
  B. fibula.
  C. knees.
  D. femur.

_____ **15.** Which of the following is least likely to be considered a mechanism of
injury in up-and-over and down-and-under head-on collisions?
  A. steering wheel
  B. windshield
  C. brake pedal
  D. dashboard

_____ **16.** Knee, leg, and hip injuries are common in a _____ collision.
  A. head-on, up-and-over
  B. rear-end
  C. head-on, down-and-under
  D. rotational impact

_____ **17.** Which type of collision is most serious because it has the potential for
multiple impacts?
  A. side impact
  B. rear-end impact
  C. head-on, up-and-over
  D. roll-over

_____ **18.** All of the following are examples of mechanisms of injury <u>except</u> a
  A. patient who fell three times her height.
  B. spiderweb crack in the windshield.
  C. broken steering column in a collision.
  D. flat rear tire.

_____ **19.** A severe fall for an adult is
  A. over 15 feet.
  B. often accompanied by an amputation.
  C. less than 10 feet.
  D. always fatal.

_____ **20.** A penetrating injury that is usually limited to the penetrated area is called
a _____ injury.
  A. low-velocity
  B. medium-velocity
  C. high-velocity
  D. super-velocity

_____ **21.** The pressure wave around the bullet's tract through the body is called
  A. exsanguination.
  B. gas penetration.
  C. cavitation.
  D. pressure damage.

_____ **22.** An injury caused by a blow that strikes the body but does not penetrate
the skin is called
  A. inertia trauma.
  B. cavitation.
  C. blunt-force trauma.
  D. rotational impact.

_____ **23.** In which of the following situations would it be necessary for you and
your partner to call for additional assistance?
  A. You are treating a patient who has flu-like symptoms who also has a
toddler with similar symptoms.
  B. Your patient is a 350-pound male who fell down the stairs and has a
broken leg.
  C. You are treating a patient with a deep laceration in his right forearm.
  D. Your patient loses consciousness while you are carrying her to the
ambulance.

_____ **24.** While in the living room of a private house treating a patient for nausea,
headache, and general body weakness, your eyes begin to tear. Three
family members have the same symptoms. You should immediately
  A. evacuate all people from the building.
  B. call for three additional ambulances.
  C. notify the police department.
  D. begin to flush out everyone's eyes.

_____ **25.** If the number of patients is more than the responding units can effectively handle, the EMT-B should
   A. involve bystanders in care of the injured.
   B. call for additional EMS resources immediately.
   C. advise medical direction that assistance is needed.
   D. do all of the above.

COMPLETE THE FOLLOWING

1. List the four parts of the scene size-up.

   A. _____

   B. _____

   C. _____

   D. _____

2. List five signs of danger from violence that you may observe as you approach the scene.

   A. _____

   B. _____

   C. _____

   D. _____

   E. _____

3. List five types of motor-vehicle collisions.

   A. _____

   B. _____

   C. _____

   D. _____

   E. _____

VIRTUAL STREET SCENES

(First review the Street Scenes on pp. 158–159 of the textbook. Then answer the questions below.)

1. Suppose the situation played out in a different way. On arrival at the scene, the driver of the truck comes running up to your ambulance and says, "My truck is overturned and leaking toxic chemicals all over the place." What should you do next?

2. Instead of a hazardous-materials incident, suppose upon arrival you find the driver of the truck is acting as if he is intoxicated. He also is holding a rifle in his lap with his right hand in position for firing. What should you do?

WEB SIMULATION

For interactive case studies that will help you review and practice basic skills, visit the *Emergency Care 9e Companion Website* at www.bradybooks.com/emergencycare.

Chapter Eight
THE INITIAL ASSESSMENT

MATCH TERMINOLOGY/DEFINITIONS

A. Steps taken by the EMT-B for the purpose of discovering and dealing with a patient's life-threatening problems

B. Level of a patient's responsiveness

C. Method of assessing circulation in a pediatric patient

D. Reason EMS was called

E. Part of the EMT-B's evaluation that includes assessment of the environment and the patient's chief complaint and appearance

F. Memory aid to keep the levels of responsiveness in mind

G. Actions taken to correct a patient's problems

H. Awake and oriented

I. Lack of response to any stimuli

J. Ability to respond to stimuli

_____ 1. Alert

_____ 2. AVPU

_____ 3. Capillary refill

_____ 4. Chief complaint

_____ 5. General impression

_____ 6. Initial assessment

_____ 7. Interventions

_____ 8. Mental status

_____ 9. Responsive

_____ 10. Unresponsive

MULTIPLE-CHOICE REVIEW

_____ 1. Which of the following steps is not a part of the initial assessment of a responsive patient with a medical problem?
   A. Assess the patient's mental status.
   B. Assess the adequacy of breathing.
   C. Determine the patient's priority.
   D. Obtain the blood pressure.

_____ 2. The general impression is an evaluation of all of the following except
   A. chief complaint.   C. environment.
   B. appearance.   D. past medical history.

_____ 3. An example of a patient's environment providing information about the patient's condition is
   A. a bruise on the patient's chest.   C. drug-use paraphernalia.
   B. an alleyway that is not well lit.   D. a medical history of asthma.

_____ 4. Clinical judgment is also referred to as a(n)
   A. license to diagnose what is wrong with the patient.
   B. sixth sense that provides clues to the severity of a patient's condition.
   C. reliance on medical direction to recommend treatment.
   D. ability to judge the patient's mental status without using AVPU.

_____ **5.** During the general impression, the EMT-B should
   A. look.   **C.** smell.
   B. listen.   **D.** do all of the above.

_____ **6.** One way to determine the patient's level of responsiveness is to
   A. put ammonia inhalants into each nostril.
   B. rub the patient's sternum briskly.
   C. place the patient's hands in water.
   D. press on the patient's nail beds.

_____ **7.** The "A" in AVPU stands for
   A. action.   **C.** assess.
   B. airway.   **D.** alert.

_____ **8.** The "V" in AVPU stands for
   A. violent.   **C.** verbal.
   B. very painful.   **D.** venous.

_____ **9.** The "P" in AVPU stands for
   A. priority.   **C.** position.
   B. painful.   **D.** patient.

_____ **10.** One major difference between the initial assessment of a responsive trauma patient and the initial assessment of an unresponsive trauma patient is
   A. the initial assessment is done more quickly on the responsive patient.
   B. the unresponsive patient is a higher priority for immediate transport.
   C. there is no difference between the two assessments.
   D. a jaw-thrust maneuver should always be used on the responsive patient.

_____ **11.** If a patient is not alert and his breathing rate is slower than 8, the EMT-B should
   A. give high-concentration oxygen via nonrebreather mask.
   B. quickly evaluate the circulation and treat for shock.
   C. suction the patient and perform rescue breathing.
   D. provide positive pressure ventilations with 100% oxygen.

_____ **12.** During the initial assessment, if the patient is alert and the breathing rate is faster than 24, provide the patient with
   A. positive pressure ventilations with 100% oxygen.
   B. high-concentration oxygen via nonrebreather mask.
   C. low-concentration oxygen via bag-valve mask.
   D. medium-concentration oxygen via nasal cannula.

_____ **13.** In the initial assessment, the circulation assessment includes evaluating all of the following except
   A. pulse.   **C.** severity of bleeding.
   B. skin.   **D.** blood pressure.

_____ **14.** If a patient's skin is warm, dry, and a normal color, it indicates
   A. a serious sunburn.   **C.** alcohol abuse.
   B. heat exposure.   **D.** good circulation.

_____ **15.** If a patient's skin is cool, pale, and moist, it indicates
   A. increased perfusion. **C.** poor circulation.
   B. high blood pressure. **D.** cold exposure.

_____ **16.** In order to evaluate skin color in a dark-skinned patient, the EMT-B should also
   A. evaluate the tissues of the lips or nail beds.
   B. evaluate the tissues of the heels of the feet.
   C. check the pupils of the eyes.
   D. do all of the above.

_____ **17.** When assessing the circulation, you should check for and control severe bleeding because
    A. open wounds can become infected.
    B. it may lead to long-term complications.
    C. a patient can bleed to death in minutes.
    D. the blood pressure may drop over time.

_____ **18.** When a life threat is observed in the initial assessment, the EMT-B should
    A. complete the assessment, then treat.
    B. treat it immediately.
    C. determine the patient's priority, then treat.
    D. package the patient for transport.

_____ **19.** High priority conditions include
    A. poor general impression.   **C.** shock (hypoperfusion).
    B. unresponsiveness.   **D.** all of the above.

_____ **20.** All of the following would be considered high-priority conditions <u>except</u>
    A. difficulty breathing.
    B. responsive but not following commands.
    C. an uncomplicated childbirth.
    D. chest pain with systolic pressure less than 100.

COMPLETE THE FOLLOWING

1. List the six steps of the initial assessment.

    A. _____

    B. _____

    C. _____

    D. _____

    E. _____

    F. _____

2. State what the letters in AVPU stand for.

    A _____

    V _____

    P _____

    U _____

3. List five high-priority conditions.

    A. _____

    B. _____

    C. _____

    D. _____

    E. _____

EMT-BASIC SKILL PERFORMANCE CHECKLIST

▶ INITIAL ASSESSMENT

❑ Take BSI precautions.

❑ Form a general impression based on assessment of the environment and the patient's chief complaint and appearance.

❑ Assess mental status using AVPU (alert, verbal, painful, unresponsive).

❑ Assess the airway. If it is not open or if it is endangered, take measures to open it.

❑ Assess breathing. If needed, initiate any appropriate oxygen therapy and assure adequate ventilation.

❑ Assess circulation (pulse, skin, and bleeding). Control severe bleeding immediately.

❑ Determine a patient's priority for immediate transport vs. further on-scene assessment and care.

NOTE: Apply manual stabilization upon first contact with any patient who you suspect may have an injury to the spine.

VIRTUAL STREET SCENES

(First review the Street Scenes on p. 175 of the textbook. Then answer the questions below.)

1. Imagine that your 78-year-old patient, who fell to the floor, does not wake up and his respirations continue with gurgling sounds due to blood in the back of his throat. What should you do?

2. What priority would this patient be? Would ALS be appropriate to call for?

3. Look again at the third patient encounter. Is it necessary to take this patient to the hospital? Explain.

WEB SIMULATION

For interactive case studies that will help you review and practice basic skills, visit the *Emergency Care 9e Companion Website* at www.bradybooks.com/emergencycare.

Chapter Nine

VITAL SIGNS AND SAMPLE HISTORY

MATCH TERMINOLOGY/DEFINITIONS

▶ **PART A**

A. Pressure remaining in the arteries when the left ventricle of the heart relaxes and refills

B. Slow pulse; any pulse rate below 60 beats per minute

C. Force of blood against the walls of the blood vessels

D. Pulse felt along the large artery on either side of the neck

E. Feeling with the fingertips

F. Number of pulse beats per minute

G. Reacting to light by changing size such as occurs in the pupils of the eyes

H. Rhythmic beats felt as the heart pumps blood through the arteries

I. Rhythm (regular or irregular) and force (strong or weak) of the pulse

J. Major artery of the arm

K. Black center of the eye

L. When a stethoscope is used to listen for characteristic sounds

M. To get larger

N. To get smaller

O. Pulse felt at the wrist on the lateral (thumb) side

_____ 1. Auscultation

_____ 2. Blood pressure

_____ 3. Brachial artery

_____ 4. Bradycardia

_____ 5. Carotid pulse

_____ 6. Constrict

_____ 7. Dilate

_____ 8. Diastolic blood pressure

_____ 9. Palpation

_____ 10. Pulse

_____ 11. Pulse quality

_____ 12. Pulse rate

_____ 13. Pupil

_____ 14. Radial pulse

_____ 15. Reactivity

PART B

A. Normal or abnormal (shallow, labored, noisy) character of breathing

B. Number of breaths a person takes in one minute

C. Rapid pulse; any pulse rate above 100 beats per minute

D. Pressure created when the heart contracts and forces blood into the arteries

E. Regular or irregular spacing of breaths

F. Information about the present problem (signs and symptoms) and past medical history of the patient

G. An indication of a patient's condition that is objective—something you see, hear, feel, or smell

H. An indication of a patient's condition that cannot be observed by another person but rather is subjective—something felt and reported by the patient

I. Cuff and gauge used to measure blood pressure

J. Outward signs of what is going on inside the body, including respiration; pulse; skin color, temperature, and condition; pupils; and blood pressure

_____ **1.** Respiratory quality

_____ **2.** Respiratory rate

_____ **3.** Respiratory rhythm

_____ **4.** SAMPLE history

_____ **5.** Sign

_____ **6.** Sphygmomanometer

_____ **7.** Symptom

_____ **8.** Systolic pressure

_____ **9.** Tachycardia

_____ **10.** Vital signs

MULTIPLE-CHOICE REVIEW

_____ **1.** The assessed components of the vital signs include all of the following except
   A. respiratory rate and quality.
   B. skin color and condition.
   C. pulse rate and quality.
   D. pulse oximetry.

_____ **2.** A sign that gives important information about the patient's condition but is not considered a "vital sign" is
   A. blood pressure.
   B. mental status.
   C. pulse rate.
   D. respiratory rhythm.

_____ **3.** Why is it essential that vital signs be recorded as they are obtained?
   A. to avoid having to take them more than once
   B. to prevent forgetting them and to note the time they were taken
   C. to give the patient a chance to calm down
   D. because they will always change quickly

_____ **4.** When a patient's pulse rate exceeds 100 beats per minute, this is called
   A. normal.
   B. regular.
   C. bradycardia.
   D. tachycardia.

_____ **5.** Based upon the pulse alone, a sign that something may be seriously wrong with a patient could be
   A. a sustained rate below 50 beats per minute.
   B. a sustained rate above 120 beats per minute.
   C. a rate above 150 beats per minute.
   D. all of the above.

_____ **6.** In addition to the answer to Number 5, another serious indicator found in the pulse may be a(n)
   A. regular strong rhythm.
   B. irregular rhythm.
   C. athlete with a pulse of 50.
   D. increase in rate after exercise.

_____ 7. The quality of the pulse includes determining the
  A. rhythm and rate.
  C. rhythm and force.
  B. rate and force.
  D. presence and balance.

_____ 8. A patient described as having a "thready" pulse has a _____ pulse.
  A. strong
  C. weak
  B. irregular
  D. infrequent

_____ 9. The normal pulse rate for a school-age child (6–10 years) is
  A. 120 to 160.
  C. 70 to 110.
  B. 60 to 100.
  D. 80 to 120.

_____ 10. The normal pulse rate for an adult is
  A. 60 to 100.
  C. 80 to 120.
  B. 70 to 110.
  D. 90 to 140.

_____ 11. The pulse at the thumb side of the wrist is referred to as the _____ pulse.
  A. femoral
  C. carotid
  B. radial
  D. brachial

_____ 12. When assessing the carotid pulse, the EMT-B should
  A. palpate the artery as hard as he/she can.
  B. assess both sides at exactly the same time.
  C. be aware that excessive pressure can slow the heart.
  D. apply pressure until he/she feels the pulse rate rise.

_____ 13. The number of breaths a patient takes in one minute is called the
  A. minute volume.
  C. respiratory rate.
  B. minute pressure.
  D. quality of breathing.

_____ 14. The respiratory rate is classified as
  A. normal, slow, or rapid.
  C. labored, quick, or noisy.
  B. noisy, shallow, or normal.
  D. weak, thready, or full.

_____ 15. If the EMT-B is treating a patient with a sustained respiratory rate above
  _____ or below _____ breaths per minute, high-concentration oxygen must
  be administered.
  A. 20 : 10
  C. 24 : 8
  B. 20 : 12
  D. 24 : 10

_____ 16. The normal respiration rate for an adult at rest is
  A. 12 to 24.
  C. 20 to 30.
  B. 12 to 20.
  D. 20 to 40.

_____ 17. The normal respiration rate for a toddler (1–3 years) is
  A. 12 to 24.
  C. 20 to 30.
  B. 12 to 20.
  D. 20 to 40.

_____ 18. Shallow breathing occurs when
  A. there is only slight movement of the chest or abdomen.
  B. there is stridor or grunting on expiration.
  C. there is a complete obstruction.
  D. the chest muscles fully expand with each breath.

_____ 19. Many resting people breathe more with their _____ than with their _____
  muscles.
  A. diaphragm : pelvic
  C. chest : abdominal
  B. diaphragm : chest
  D. chest : pelvic

_____ 20. Signs of labored breathing include all of the following except:
  A. increase in the work of breathing.
  B. use of accessory muscles.
  C. retractions above the collarbones.
  D. delayed capillary refill.

_____ **21.** A harsh, high-pitched sound heard on inspiration when a patient has labored breathing is called
    A. nasal flaring.   **C.** stridor.
    B. grunting.   **D.** gurgling.

_____ **22.** When the quality of a patient's respirations are abnormal due to something blocking the flow of air, this is referred to as _____ breathing.
    A. normal   **C.** noisy
    B. shallow   **D.** labored

_____ **23.** A sound made by the patient that usually indicates the need to suction the airway is called
    A. gurgling.   **C.** stridor.
    B. crowing.   **D.** wheezing.

_____ **24.** The best places to assess skin color in adults are
    A. under the chin and the nostrils.
    B. the inside of the cheek and the nail beds.
    C. the nail beds and the upper chest.
    D. the toes and the earlobes.

_____ **25.** Blood loss, shock, hypotension, or emotional distress may result in skin that is
    A. flushed.   **C.** pale.
    B. gray.   **D.** jaundiced.

_____ **26.** A patient with a lack of oxygen in the red blood cells resulting from inadequate breathing or inadequate heart function will exhibit _____ skin.
    A. pink   **C.** flushed
    B. pale   **D.** cyanotic

_____ **27.** The skin of a patient who has liver abnormalities will appear
    A. flushed.   **C.** pale.
    B. mottled.   **D.** jaundiced.

_____ **28.** Cold, dry skin is frequently associated with
    A. high fever and/or heat exposure.
    B. exposure to cold.
    C. shock and anxiety.
    D. a body that is losing heat.

_____ **29.** Hot, dry skin is frequently associated with
    A. high fever, heat exposure.   **C.** shock and anxiety.
    B. exposure to cold.   **D.** heat loss.

_____ **30.** You notice that the patient's right arm is much cooler than the rest of the patient's body. This should lead you to consider a _____ system problem.
    A. nervous   **C.** circulatory
    B. respiratory   **D.** endocrine

_____ **31.** If you press on a child's nail bed and watch how long it takes for the normal pink color to return, you are testing for
    A. reflexes.   **C.** pain response.
    B. capillary refill.   **D.** nail bed temperature.

_____ **32.** If a patient is in direct sunlight or very bright conditions, the EMT-B should test the pupils by
    A. using a very bright light that is similar to the environmental light.
    B. covering the patient's eyes for a few moments, then uncovering one eye at a time.
    C. applying a cold towel to the patient's eyelids for ten seconds.
    D. moving the patient indoors to an area that has dimmer light.

_____ **33.** The pupils may be unequal due to any of the following conditions <u>except</u>

    A. stroke.
    C. eye injury.

    B. head injury.
    D. shock.

_____ **34.** Fright, blood loss, drugs, and treatment with eye drops may cause the patient's pupils to become

    A. constricted.
    C. unequal.

    B. dilated.
    D. unreactive.

_____ **35.** When the left ventricle of the heart relaxes and refills, the pressure in the arteries is called the _____ pressure.

    A. diastolic
    C. ventricular

    B. carotid
    D. systolic

_____ **36.** The pulse oximeter should be used with

    A. patients who have carbon monoxide poisoning.

    B. patients complaining of respiratory problems.

    C. any patient who is hypothermic.

    D. any patient suffering from severe shock.

_____ **37.** The pulse oximeter is helpful because it

    A. encourages you to be more aggressive with oxygen therapy.

    B. helps you decide when you should withhold oxygen.

    C. indicates when a patient is about to become hypothermic.

    D. gives an indication that the patient is a heavy smoker.

_____ **38.** The oximeter will produce falsely high readings in patients with

    A. hypoxia.
    C. carbon monoxide poisoning.

    B. barbiturate poisoning.
    D. croup.

_____ **39.** Chronic smokers may have a pulse oximeter reading that is

    A. lower than normal.
    C. 20% to 25% off.

    B. higher than normal.
    D. difficult to read.

_____ **40.** In a normal healthy person, one would expect the oximeter reading to be

    A. 86% to 90%.
    C. 95% to 99%.

    B. 91% to 94%.
    D. none of the above.

COMPLETE THE FOLLOWING

1. List five vital signs.

    A. _____

    B. _____

    C. _____

    D. _____

    E. _____

2. List the components of the SAMPLE history.

    S _____   **P** _____

    A _____   **L** _____

    M _____   **E** _____

LABEL THE DIAGRAM

Fill in the name of the pulse that can be found at each numbered location on the line provided.

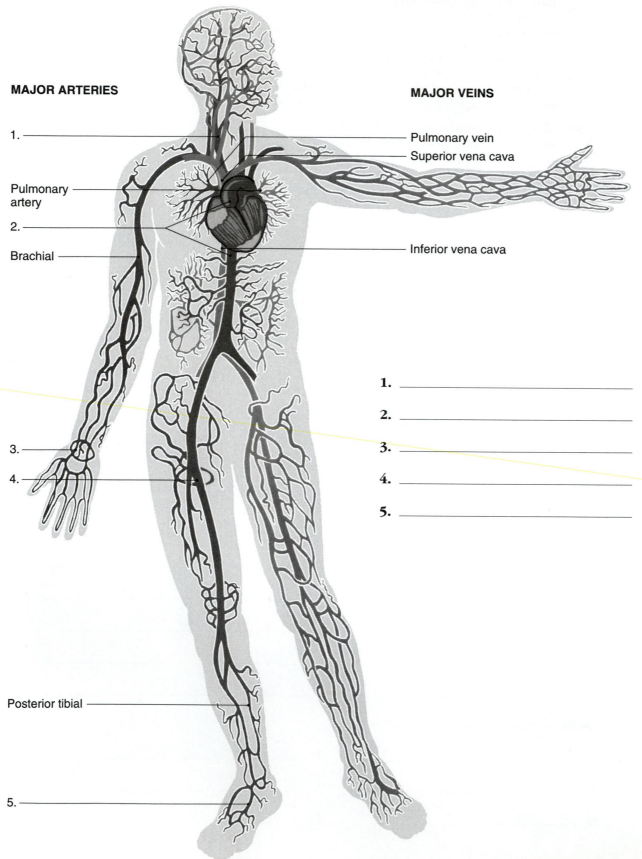

MAJOR ARTERIES

1. _____

Pulmonary artery _____

2. _____

Brachial _____

3. _____

4. _____

Posterior tibial _____

5. _____

MAJOR VEINS

Pulmonary vein

Superior vena cava

Inferior vena cava

1. _____

2. _____

3. _____

4. _____

5. _____

VIRTUAL STREET SCENES

(First review the Street Scenes on p. 192 of the textbook. Then answer the questions below.)

1. This patient's vital signs were not normal, which helped make it clear that she should go to the hospital. If her vital signs had been normal, would a refusal of transport have been acceptable?

2. What would be considered the "normal" range of vital signs for this patient?

3. Would you include in your prehospital care report the fact that the patient was having "black, tarry stools." Why or why not?

WEB SIMULATION

For interactive case studies that will help you review and practice basic skills, visit the *Emergency Care 9e Companion Website* at www.bradybooks.com/emergencycare.

EMT-BASIC SKILLS PERFORMANCE CHECKLISTS

▶ BLOOD PRESSURE BY AUSCULTATION

❑ Place the stethoscope around your neck.

❑ The patient should be seated or lying down.

❑ If the patient has not been injured, support his arm at the level of his heart.

❑ Place the cuff snugly around the upper arm so that the bottom of the cuff is about one inch above the crease of the elbow.

❑ With your fingertips, palpate the brachial artery at the crease of the elbow.

❑ Place the tips of the stethoscope arms in your ears.

❑ Position the diaphragm of the stethoscope directly over the brachial pulse or over the medial anterior elbow (front of the elbow) if no brachial pulse can be felt.

❑ Inflate the cuff with the bulb valve closed.

❑ Once you no longer hear the brachial pulse, continue to inflate the cuff until the gauge reads 30 mm Hg higher than the point where the sound pulse disappeared.

❑ Slowly release air from the cuff by opening the bulb valve, allowing the pressure to fall smoothly at the rate of approximately 10 mm per second.

❑ When you hear the first clicking or tapping sounds, note the reading on the gauge. This is the systolic pressure.

❑ Continue to deflate the cuff and listen for the point at which these distinctive sounds fade. When the sounds turn to dull, muffled thuds, the reading on the gauge is the diastolic pressure.

❑ After obtaining the diastolic pressure, let the cuff deflate rapidly.

▶ BLOOD PRESSURE BY PALPATION

❑ Find the radial pulse on the arm to which the blood pressure cuff is applied.

❑ With the bulb valve closed, inflate the cuff to a point where you can no longer feel the radial pulse.

❑ Note this point on the gauge and continue to inflate the cuff until the gauge reads 30 mm Hg higher than the point where the pulse disappeared.

❑ Slowly deflate the cuff, noting the reading at which the radial pulse returns. This reading is the systolic pressure.

❑ After obtaining the systolic reading, let the cuff deflate.

NOTE: You cannot determine a diastolic reading by palpation.

▶ USING THE PULSE OXIMETER

❑ Review the manufacturer's instruction manual for the specific unit you are using.

❑ Properly assemble finger-clip sensor and extension to pulse oximeter.

❑ Properly affix finger-clip sensor to index finger. (It may be necessary to quickly remove patient's fingernail polish.)

❑ Turn on pulse oximeter, and record heart and oxygen readings. Spot check mode and extended mode (30 minutes).

❑ When done using oximeter, shut off the unit. After each use, disassemble and store wiring and accessories in pouch provided.

❑ Review operation of all display indicators, pulse amplitude, low battery, pulse search, oxygen saturation, and pulse rate.

❑ Review all controls (i.e., measure button, battery check button, printer on/off, printer paper advance.)

❑ Change battery and paper printout as needed.

Chapter Ten

ASSESSMENT OF THE TRAUMA PATIENT

MATCH TERMINOLOGY/DEFINITIONS

A. Found upon palpation of a body part

B. Movement of part of the chest in the opposite direction from the rest of the chest during respiration

C. Persistent erection of the penis that can result from spinal-cord injury or certain medical problems

D. Quick assessment of the head, neck, chest, abdomen, pelvis, extremities, and posterior body to detect signs of injury

E. Surgical opening in the wall of the abdomen with a bag in place to collect excretions from the digestive system

F. Memory aid, the initials of which stand for deformities, contusions, abrasions, punctures/penetrations, burns, tenderness, lacerations, and swelling

G. Surgical incision in the neck held open by a metal or plastic tube

H. Bulging of the neck veins

I. Step of patient assessment that follows the initial assessment

J. A cut

K. Condition of being stretched, inflated, or larger than normal

L. An assessment of the head (including face, ears, eyes, nose, and mouth), neck, chest, abdomen, pelvis, extremities, and posterior of the body to detect signs and symptoms of injury

M. Permanent surgical opening in the neck through which the patient breathes

N. A bruise

O. Grating sensation or sound made when fractured bones rub against each other

_____ **1.** Colostomy

_____ **2.** Contusion

_____ **3.** Crepitation

_____ **4.** DCAP-BTLS

_____ **5.** Detailed physical exam

_____ **6.** Distention

_____ **7.** Focused history and physical exam

_____ **8.** Jugular vein distention

_____ **9.** Laceration

_____ **10.** Paradoxical motion

_____ **11.** Priapism

_____ **12.** Rapid trauma assessment

_____ **13.** Stoma

_____ **14.** Tenderness

_____ **15.** Tracheostomy

_____ 1. When evaluating a patient during the focused physical exam, the EMT-B needs to _____ each body part.
   A. auscultate and visualize
   B. percuss and palpate
   C. inspect and palpate
   D. visualize and percuss

_____ 2. The memory aid for remembering what to look for when conducting a physical exam is
   A. AVPU.
   B. PULSE.
   C. SAMPLE.
   D. DCAP-BTLS.

_____ 3. The "C" in DCAP-BTLS refers to
   A. compound.
   B. contusions.
   C. cardiac.
   D. circulation.

_____ 4. The "A" in DCAP-BTLS refers to
   A. alert.
   B. appearance
   C. asthma.
   D. abrasions.

_____ 5. The "P" in DCAP-BTLS refers to
   A. punctures/penetrations.
   B. palpation/pulse.
   C. priapism/penetrations.
   D. paradoxical motion/punctures.

_____ 6. The "S" in DCAP-BTLS refers to
   A. soft tissue.
   B. stable.
   C. swelling.
   D. stomach.

_____ 7. When a body part no longer has its normal shape, this is referred to as a
   A. hematoma.
   B. deformity.
   C. fracture.
   D. crepitation.

_____ 8. Reddened, blistered, or charred-looking areas are called
   A. abrasions.
   B. burns.
   C. lacerations.
   D. contusions.

_____ 9. The difference between pain and tenderness is
   A. pain only occurs when you squeeze an injury site, whereas tender areas hurt all the time.
   B. pain is considered unbearable, whereas tenderness is usually bearable.
   C. tenderness may not hurt unless the area is palpated, whereas pain is evident without palpation.
   D. pain only hurts for the first ten minutes, whereas tenderness doesn't go away.

_____ 10. A common result of injured capillaries bleeding under the skin is called
   A. swelling.
   B. puncture.
   C. laceration.
   D. abrasion.

_____ 11. When is it appropriate to apply a cervical collar?
   A. if the mechanism of injury exerts great force on the upper body
   B. if there is any pain in the abdomen
   C. if there is any burn injury to the neck
   D. if the patient has experienced any trauma

_____ 12. Any blow above the _____ may damage the cervical spine.
   A. clavicles
   B. diaphragm
   C. femur
   D. pelvis

_____ 13. The experienced EMT-B may refer to a soft cervical collar as a
  A. device of choice for a neck injury.
  B. "neck warmer."
  C. requirement for all auto collision patients.
  D. preferred extrication collar.

_____ 14. If a cervical collar is the wrong size, it may
  A. cause additional injury to the spine.
  B. make breathing more difficult or obstruct the airway.
  C. prevent the patient from moving her neck.
  D. take too much time to adjust and apply correctly.

_____ 15. The need for cervical immobilization should be based upon
  A. the trauma patient's level of responsiveness.
  B. the location of injuries to the patient.
  C. the mechanism of injury.
  D. all of the above.

_____ 16. Prior to applying the cervical collar, the EMT-B should
  A. complete the rapid trauma assessment.
  B. complete the detailed physical exam.
  C. assess the patient's neck.
  D. obtain the baseline vital signs.

_____ 17. When reconsidering the mechanism of injury, which of the following
  would not be considered a significant mechanism of injury?
  A. high speed motorcycle crash
  B. vehicle-pedestrian collision
  C. a ten-foot fall
  D. rollover vehicle collision

_____ 18. You are treating a patient who was in the front seat of an automobile
  involved in a collision. You observe that there is a spider-web crack in the
  windshield and the patient has facial lacerations. Most likely the patient
  A. will have a life-threatening head injury.
  B. did not wear a seat belt or three-point harness.
  C. will also complain of leg injuries.
  D. was involved in a rollover collision.

_____ 19. The EMT-B should "lift and look" under the airbag after the patient has
  been removed from the vehicle in order to
  A. obtain the serial number of the airbag.
  B. see if a hazardous chemical has been released.
  C. note any visible damage to the steering wheel.
  D. determine if it deployed properly.

_____ 20. When assessing the head of a critical trauma patient, in addition to
  DCAP-BTLS, the EMT-B should inspect/palpate for
  A. hematoma.   C. crepitation.
  B. scalp lacerations. D. abrasions.

_____ 21. When assessing the neck of a critical trauma patient, in addition to
  DCAP-BTLS, the EMT-B should inspect/palpate for
  A. jugular vein distention. C. lacerations.
  B. swelling.   D. burns.

_____ 22. The neck veins are usually not visible when the patient is
  A. lying flat. C. supine.
  B. sitting up. D. prone.

_____ 23. When assessing the chest of a critical trauma patient, in addition to DCAP-BTLS, the EMT-B should inspect/palpate for
A. hematoma.
B. paradoxical motion.
C. hemothorax.
D. jugular vein distention.

_____ 24. When assessing the abdomen of a critical trauma patient, in addition to DCAP-BTLS, the EMT-B should inspect/palpate for
A. distention of the kidneys.
B. colostomy and/or ileostomy.
C. crepitation.
D. paradoxical motion.

_____ 25. When assessing the pelvis of a critical trauma patient, in addition to DCAP-BTLS, the EMT-B should inspect/palpate for
A. paradoxical motion.
B. burns.
C. priapism.
D. bleeding.

_____ 26. The main difference between the rapid trauma assessment and the detailed physical exam is the
A. rapid trauma assessment is less detailed.
B. detailed physical exam is only done on medical patients.
C. rapid trauma exam is done in the ambulance.
D. detailed physical exam is done more quickly.

_____ 27. If you are treating a severely injured patient, it may be appropriate to skip the
A. initial physical exam.
B. detailed physical exam.
C. vital signs.
D. initial assessment.

_____ 28. Areas you will assess in the detailed physical exam that were not assessed in the rapid trauma assessment are
A. face, ears, eyes, nose, and mouth.
B. head, neck, chest, and abdomen.
C. chest, abdomen, pelvis, and extremities.
D. extremities and posterior of the body.

_____ 29. The final step of the detailed physical exam is to
A. complete the head-to-toe exam.
B. reassess the vital signs.
C. conduct a rapid trauma assessment.
D. examine the posterior of the body.

_____ 30. A bruise behind the ear is called
A. raccoon's eyes.
B. orbital hematoma.
C. Battle's sign.
D. Cushing reflex.

_____ 31. When performing the detailed physical exam, you note blood in the anterior chamber of the eye. This tells you the
A. patient was wearing contact lenses.
B. patient has a serious brain injury.
C. patient's eye is bleeding inside.
D. all of the above.

_____ 32. Clear fluid that may be draining from the ears and nose is called _____ fluid.
A. lymphatic
B. cerebrospinal
C. mucous
D. synovial

_____ 33. In addition to looking for DCAP-BTLS when examining the mouth, you should look for all of the following except
A. possible airway obstructions.
B. loose or broken teeth.
C. tongue lacerations or swelling.
D. crepitation.

_____ **34.** The detailed physical exam is <u>not</u> designed for the
  A. trauma patient with a significant mechanism of injury.
  B. patient with an unclear mechanism of injury.
  C. medical patient with few signs and symptoms.
  D. patient who could be either medical or trauma.

_____ **35.** If you are treating a patient who could be either medical or trauma, it is always best to assess for
  A. the medical problem first.   **C.** the trauma problem first.
  B. both problems at once.   **D.** loss of consciousness.

COMPLETE THE FOLLOWING

1. List the components of the focused history and physical exam for a trauma patient who is found with significant mechanism of injury.

  A. _____

  B. _____

  C. _____

  D. _____

  E. _____

  F. _____

  G. _____

  H. _____

2. List the components of the rapid trauma assessment.

  A. _____

  B. _____

  C. _____

  D. _____

  E. _____

  F. _____

  G. _____

LABEL THE PHOTOGRAPHS

Fill in the name of each injury assessed for in the focused physical exam of the trauma patient.

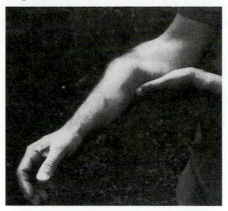

1. _____

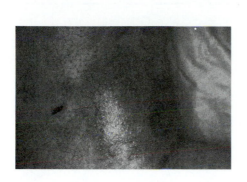

2. _____

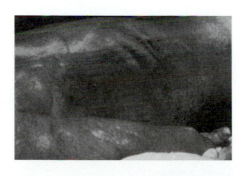

3. _____

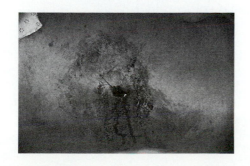

4. _____

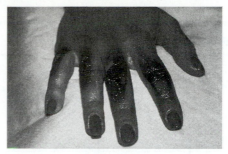

5. _____

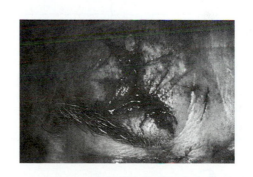

6. _____

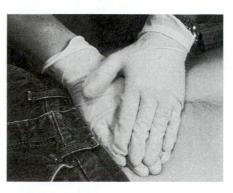

7. _____

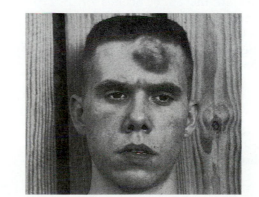

8. _____

Chapter 10 • *Assessment of the Trauma Patient* **85**

COMPLETE THE CHART

Fill in the additional things to assess in each area of the body during rapid trauma assessment.

Body Part	DCAP-BTLS	Plus
Head	Yes	1.
Neck	Yes	2. 3.
Chest	Yes	4. 5. 6.
Abdomen	Yes	7. 8. 9.
Pelvis	Yes	10. 11. 12.
Extremities	Yes	13. 14. 15.
Posterior	Yes	—

VIRTUAL STREET SCENES

(First review the Street Scenes on p. 229 of the textbook. Then answer the questions below.)

1. This patient has a wound to the chest. At what point should you consider ventilating him?

2. Should ALS be called?

3. If the patient had lost consciousness, what would have been your priorities for emergency care?

4. If the patient is injured on the left side of the chest at the mid-clavicular line at nipple level, what organs may be injured?

WEB SIMULATION

For interactive case studies that will help you review and practice basic skills, visit the *Emergency Care 9e Companion Website* at www.bradybooks.com/emergencycare.

EMT-BASIC SKILL PERFORMANCE CHECKLISTS

▶ FOCUSED HISTORY AND PHYSICAL EXAM—TRAUMA PATIENT WITH NO SIGNIFICANT MOI

❑ Take BSI precautions.

❑ Reconsider the MOI.

❑ Determine the patient's chief complaint.

❑ Perform a focused physical exam on the area the patient complains of plus areas of potential injury suggested by the MOI.

❑ Obtain baseline vital signs.

❑ Take a SAMPLE history.

❑ Perform interventions as needed.

❑ Transport.

▶ FOCUSED HISTORY AND PHYSICAL EXAM—TRAUMA PATIENT WITH SIGNIFICANT MOI

❑ Take BSI precautions.

❑ Reconsider the MOI.

❑ Continue manual stabalization of the head and neck.

❑ Consider requesting advanced life support.

❑ Reconsider your transport decision.

❑ Reassess mental status.

❑ Perform a rapid trauma assessment. After assessing the head and neck, apply a cervical collar and continue to maintain manual stabilization.

❑ Obtain baseline vital signs.

❑ Take a SAMPLE history.

(continued next page)

❑ Perform a detailed physical exam on scene, if there is time, or en route to the hospital.

❑ Perform an ongoing assessment, including vital signs.

❑ Transport.

▶ RAPID TRAUMA ASSESSMENT

❑ Take BSI precautions.

❑ Assess head: DCAP-BTLS + crepitation.

❑ Assess neck: DCAP-BTLS + jugular vein distention (JVD), crepitation.

❑ Assess chest: DCAP-BTLS + paradoxical motion, crepitation, breath sounds.

❑ Assess abdomen: DCAP-BTLS + firmness, softness, distention.

❑ Assess pelvis: DCAP-BTLS + pain, tenderness, distention.

❑ Assess extremities: DCAP-BTLS + distal pulse, motor function, sensation.

❑ Assess posterior: DCAP-BTLS.

▶ DETAILED PHYSICAL EXAM

❑ Take BSI precautions.

❑ Assess scalp and cranium: DCAP-BTLS + crepitation.

❑ Assess ears: DCAP-BTLS + drainage.

❑ Assess face: DCAP-BTLS.

❑ Assess eyes: DCAP-BTLS + discoloration, unequal pupils, foreign bodies, blood in anterior chamber.

❑ Assess nose: DCAP-BTLS + drainage, bleeding.

❑ Assess mouth: DCAP-BTLS + loose or broken teeth, objects that could cause obstruction, swelling or laceration of tongue, unusual breath odor, discoloration.

❑ Assess neck: DCAP-BTLS + jugular vein distention (JVD), crepitation.

❑ Assess chest: DCAP-BTLS + paradoxical motion, crepitation, breath sounds.

❑ Assess pelvis: DCAP-BTLS + pain, tenderness, motion.

❑ Assess extremities: DCAP-BTLS + distal pulse, motor function, sensation.

❑ Assess posterior: DCAP-BTLS.

❑ Reassess vital signs.

CASE STUDY

▶ MOTORCYCLE MISHAP

You are dispatched to a motorcycle collision in an intersection in your community. Apparently, a car made a right turn on red without stopping and the motorcycle, which had the green light, collided with the left side of the car. On arrival, you conduct a scene size-up. What four things should you be concerned about in the scene size-up of this collision?

You find out from a witness who was standing on the corner at the bus stop that the vehicles were probably traveling 40 mph and the cyclist crashed into the rear left door of the car. He was thrown off the motorcycle onto the roof of the car and then landed on his back in the street. The witness immediately rushed to aid the cyclist and at the same time motioned people in another vehicle to stop traffic and to call 9-1-1. The witness stated that the patient was in a lot of pain but never hit his head or lost consciousness. The cyclist was wearing a helmet, which he removed after the collision.

5. How does forming a general impression help you provide emergency care to the patient? On what is the general impression based?

Your general impression reveals a 20-year-old responsive male trauma patient with severe external blood loss. The patient is able to talk with you, although he is experiencing considerable pain in both his thighs and lower back. He is able to describe what happened in the collision, knows the day of the week, and is concerned about his new Sportster. His name is Tony, and he was on his way to the beach, which explains why he was wearing shorts and a T-shirt.

6. As you question Tony, what should one of your partners be doing?

7. What is Tony's mental status on the AVPU scale?

Tony keeps crying out, "It's my legs!" They are obviously broken but no longer seriously bleeding. You proceed with the initial assessment beginning with an assessment of Tony's airway.

8. Explain why it would be wrong to be distracted by Tony's pain and begin to treat his broken legs?

9. What should your initial assessment of Tony consist of?

Based upon your initial assessment of Tony, you have determined he is a high-priority patient, and an ALS unit should be requested if they are not en route already. You found his airway was open and clear, his breathing was present and adequate, he was moving air into both sides of his chest equally, but he has a weak, rapid radial pulse and his skin is pale, cool, and clammy to touch—possible signs of shock. One of your crew members has controlled the bleeding from Tony's thighs.

10. Why is Tony a high-priority patient?

11. How long should you wait for an ALS unit to arrive before transporting Tony?

As one of your crew members attends to Tony's injured legs and then places him onto a long backboard, you continue with the focused history and physical exam. Since you have reconsidered the mechanism of injury, you have decided to provide early transport for Tony as soon as he is packaged.

12. What would you be looking for with DCAP-BTLS?

13. What would you be asking about for the SAMPLE history?

14. What vital signs should you assess?

En route to the hospital, you have time to conduct a detailed physical exam. Tony is immobilized, receiving oxygen via nonrebreather mask, the backboard is in the Trendelenburg position, and you are keeping him warm with a blanket. His vitals are a respiration rate of 20—good quality, a pulse rate of 120—weak and regular, a blood pressure of 110/70, and pale, cool, and clammy skin.

15. What would the detailed physical exam include?

Chapter Eleven

ASSESSMENT OF THE MEDICAL PATIENT

MATCH TERMINOLOGY/DEFINITIONS

A. Description of where pain is located and where it spreads to

B. Description of the pain, such as stabbing, crampy, dull, or sharp

C. Description of what makes the pain worse, such as sitting, standing, eating certain foods

D. Description of how bad the pain is, often described on a scale of 1 to 10

E. Memory jogger designed to remind the EMT-B of what questions to ask the patient about his chief complaint

F. Necklace or bracelet designed to notify emergency personnel that a patient has a specific medical history or condition

G. Medicine-like bottle kept in the patient's refrigerator that contains a listing of his past medical history

H. Description of how fast or slow the pain came on and what the patient was doing when the pain started

I. The reason why EMS was called, usually in the patient's own words.

J. History relating to the patient's chief complaint

_____ 1. Chief complaint

_____ 2. Medical identification device

_____ 3. Onset of pain

_____ 4. OPQRST

_____ 5. Prior history

_____ 6. Provocation of pain

_____ 7. Quality of pain

_____ 8. Radiation of pain

_____ 9. Severity of pain

_____ 10. Vial of life

_____ **1.** The components of the focused history and physical exam for a responsive medical patient include all of the following except
   A. history of the present illness.   **C.** baseline vital signs.
   B. SAMPLE history.   **D.** rapid trauma exam.

_____ **2.** OPQRST is a memory aid to help the EMT-B remember the
   A. questions that ask about the past medical history.
   B. questions that expand on the history of the present illness.
   C. status of the patient's condition.
   D. mental status.

_____ **3.** When you ask a patient "Can you think of anything that might have triggered this pain?", you are questioning about
   A. onset.   **C.** quality.
   B. provokes.   **D.** radiation.

_____ **4.** When you ask a patient "How bad is the pain?", you are questioning about
   A. quality.   **C.** time.
   B. severity.   **D.** radiation.

_____ **5.** The "T" in "OPQRST" stands for
   A. temperature.   **C.** time.
   B. tibia.   **D.** trembling.

_____ **6.** When you ask a patient "Have you vomited?", you are questioning about
   A. signs and symptoms.   **C.** medication.
   B. allergies.   **D.** pertinent past history.

_____ **7.** The "P" in "SAMPLE" stands for
   A. perforation.   **C.** puncture wound.
   B. pertinent past history.   **D.** prehospital care report.

_____ **8.** When you ask a patient "How have you felt today?", you are asking about
   A. pertinent past history.   **C.** events leading to the illness.
   B. signs and symptoms.   **D.** last oral intake.

_____ **9.** A patient with a specific chief complaint and a known history may carry medication or other treatment with her. The EMT-B may need to request medical direction's permission to assist the patient with a(n)
   A. inhaler.   **C.** epinephrine.
   B. nitroglycerin.   **D.** any one of the above.

_____ **10.** When a medical patient complains of difficulty breathing, but does not take any prescribed medication for this condition, you should generally
   A. look for a medical identification device.
   B. consult with the patient's personal physician.
   C. transport the patient to the hospital.
   D. do all of the above.

_____ **11.** In terms of the initial approach to the focused history and physical exam, the biggest difference between a responsive and an unresponsive patient would be that
   A. the responsive patient gets the OPQRST questions last.
   B. the unresponsive patient will be given a rapid physical exam first.
   C. bystanders become more important if the patient is responsive.
   D. a rapid trauma exam is not done on an unconscious patient.

_____ **12.** In addition to DCAP-BTLS in the rapid physical exam on an unresponsive medical patient, you should include all of the following <u>except</u>
   A. look for jugular vein distention.
   B. determine firmness or rigidity of abdomen.
   C. check for incontinence of urine or feces.
   D. ask the SAMPLE history questions.

_____ **13.** When assessing a medical patient's extremities, be sure to check for
   A. central cyanosis.   **C.** pulmonary edema.
   B. sensation and motor function.   **D.** capillary refill.

_____ **14.** When conducting a physical exam, look for a necklace or bracelet. This is important because it may
   A. reveal the patient's name.
   B. give clues to the patient's residence.
   C. be a medical identification device.
   D. be the cause of the emergency.

_____ **15.** Why might it be important to check the refrigerator of a patient who is found unconscious at home?
   A. Last night's meal could be the cause.
   B. The patient may have a Vial-of-Life®.
   C. Most medications are kept in the refrigerator.
   D. The person's diet could be the cause of the problem.

COMPLETE THE FOLLOWING

1. List the components of a focused history and physical exam for an unresponsive medical patient.

   A. _____

   B. _____

   C. _____

   D. _____

2. List four questions to ask bystanders who witness a patient's medical emergency.

   A. _____

   B. _____

   C. _____

   D. _____

COMPLETE THE CHART

Complete the chart by writing the remainder of the word that follows each letter in the acronyms.

1.	S
2.	A
3.	M
4.	P
5.	L
6.	E
7.	O
8.	P
9.	Q
10.	R
11.	S
12.	T

VIRTUAL STREET SCENES

(First review the Street Scenes on pp. 242–243 of the textbook. Then answer the questions below.)

1. What would it have suggested to you if the patient had been talking in short, choppy sentences?

2. You found the patient's lung sounds "equal, but noisy, like a whistling sound." If you had found that this patient's chest was quiet, would that have been a good thing?

3. What is the term for the lung sounds heard in this patient's chest?

4. If the patient had her Albuterol inhaler with her, would it have been appropriate to contact medical direction for permission to assist in the administration of the medication?

WEB SIMULATION

For interactive case studies that will help you review and practice basic skills, visit the *Emergency Care 9e Companion Website* at www.bradybooks.com/emergencycare.

EMT-BASIC SKILLS PERFORMANCE CHECKLIST

▶ **FOCUSED HISTORY AND PHYSICAL EXAM—RESPONSIVE MEDICAL PATIENT**

❑ Take BSI precautions.

❑ Gather a history of the present illness.

❑ Gather a SAMPLE history.

❑ Perform a focused physical exam.

❑ Obtain baseline vital signs.

❑ Perform interventions. (Obtain medical direction as required locally.) Reassess vital signs.

❑ Transport.

▶ **FOCUSED HISTORY AND PHYSICAL EXAM—UNRESPONSIVE MEDICAL PATIENT**

❑ Take BSI precautions.

❑ Perform a rapid physical exam.

❑ Obtain baseline vital signs.

❑ Consider request for advanced life support.

❑ Gather a history of the present illness by asking family or bystanders OPQRST questions.

❑ Gather a SAMPLE history from family or bystanders.

❑ Perform interventions. (Obtain medical direction as required locally.) Reassess vital signs.

❑ Transport.

Chapter Twelve
ONGOING ASSESSMENT

MATCH TERMINOLOGY/DEFINITIONS

A. Changes in a patient's condition over time, that may show improvement or deterioration, and that can be shown by documenting repeated assessments

B. Actions taken to correct a patient's problems.

C. Four-step procedure for detecting changes in a patient's condition

_____ 1. Interventions

_____ 2. Ongoing assessment

_____ 3. Trending

MULTIPLE-CHOICE REVIEW

_____ 1. Which one of the following best describes the purpose of performing the ongoing assessment?
   A. To stabilze the patient's condition or to treat any life threats
   B. To detect and treat life threats and to evaluate the EMS system's effectiveness
   C. To evaluate the EMS system's effectiveness and to detect changes in patient condition
   D. To repeat key elements of assessment procedures already performed in order to detect changes in patient condition

_____ 2. The ongoing assessment may be omitted if
   A. the patient care report is not completed.
   B. you do not want to interrupt patient conversation.
   C. life-saving interventions prevent doing it.
   D. a short transport time prevents completion.

_____ 3. During the ongoing assessment of an infant or child patient,
   A. avoid eye contact at all times.   C. speak in a loud voice.
   B. stand above the patient.   D. use a reassuring voice.

_____ 4. The ongoing assessment includes all the following steps except
   A. reassess vital signs.
   B. repeat the initial assessment for life-threats.
   C. repeat the focused assessment.
   D. repeat all interventions.

_____ 5. Which of the following is the last step in the ongoing assessment?
   A. Reassess the vital signs.   C. Repeat the initial assessment.
   B. Check interventions.   D. Repeat the focused assessment.

6. Which of the following is <u>not</u> a step when repeating the initial assessment?
   A. Reestablish patient priorities.
   B. Monitor skin color and temperature.
   C. Maintain an open airway.
   D. Apply a cervical collar.

7. During your ongoing assessment, you note that the patient's pulse is rapid and his skin is cool and pale. This may indicate
   A. deterioration in mental status.
   B. heat exhaustion.
   C. an occluded airway.
   D. the onset of shock.

8. The mental status of an unresponsive child or infant can be checked by
   A. a sternal rub.
   B. assessing the capillaries for refill.
   C. shouting or by flicking the feet.
   D. asking the parent to stick a pin in the child's foot.

9. An example of checking interventions during the ongoing assessment of a medical patient is
   A. taking an initial blood pressure.
   B. bandaging a severe laceration.
   C. applying a tourniquet.
   D. assuring adequacy of oxygen delivery.

10. Frequently reassessing a patient establishes
    A. a paper trail.
    B. legal evidence.
    C. trends.
    D. a reason for treating the patient.

11. The best way to determine if the patient is improving or deteriorating is to
    A. ask the hospital.
    B. contact medical direction.
    C. do frequent ongoing assessments.
    D. keep repeating the initial assessment.

12. If the patient is considered stable, the recommended interval for reassessment is every _____ minutes.
    A. 5
    B. 10
    C. 15
    D. 20

13. You are treating a patient with a head injury who is breathing adequately, yet has an altered mental status. The recommended interval for reassessment is every _____ minutes.
    A. 5
    B. 10
    C. 15
    D. 20

14. You should repeat at least the initial assessment
    A. after you have noticed and documented trends.
    B. whenever you or your partner have the time and opportunity to do so.
    C. whenever you believe there may have been a change in the patient's condition.
    D. when directed to do so by medical direction.

15. During your ongoing assessment of an unresponsive patient, you hear gurgling sounds in her airway. What intervention should you take?
    A. Sit the patient up.
    B. Suction the patient.
    C. Check oxygen tubing.
    D. All of the above.

COMPLETE THE FOLLOWING

1. List the six steps involved in repeating the initial assessment.

   A. _____

   B. _____

   C. _____

   D. _____

   E. _____

   F. _____

2. List the three steps for checking interventions.

   A. _____

   B. _____

   C. _____

VIRTUAL STREET SCENES

(First review the Street Scenes on pp. 252–253 of the textbook. Then answer the questions below.)

1. Why do you think it is so important to monitor and maintain the airway of a stroke patient?

2. Many times a patient experiencing a stroke can hear but not speak. Why do you think this is something you should be aware of?

WEB SIMULATION

For interactive case studies that will help you review and practice basic skills, visit the *Emergency Care 9e Companion Website* at www.bradybooks.com/emergencycare.

EMT-BASIC SKILLS PERFORMANCE CHECKLIST

► **ONGOING ASSESSMENT**

❏ Take BSI precautions.

❏ Repeat the initial assessment for life-threats.

   ❏ Reassess mental status.

   ❏ Maintain an open airway.

   ❏ Monitor breathing for rate and quality.

   ❏ Reassess pulse for rate and quality.

   ❏ Monitor skin color, temperature, and condition.

   ❏ Reestablish patient treatment priorities.

❏ Reassess and record vital signs.

❏ Repeat focused assessment related to chief complaint or injuries.

❏ Check interventions performed for the patient.

   ❏ Assure adequacy of oxygen delivery and ventilation support.

   ❏ Assure management of bleeding.

   ❏ Assure adequacy of other interventions.

NOTE: Repeat the ongoing assessment every 15 minutes for a stable patient and every 5 minutes for an unstable patient.

Chapter Thirteen

PEDIATRIC, ADOLESCENT, AND GERIATRIC ASSESSMENT

MATCH TERMINOLOGY/DEFINITIONS

A. Child from 1 to 3 years of age

B. Child from 3 to 6 years of age

C. Elderly person, generally considered over 65 years of age or older

D. Child less than 1 year of age

E. Child from 12 to 18 years of age

F. "Soft spot" on an infant's skull

G. Child from 6 to 12 years of age

H. Abnormally low body temperature

I. Chin thrust forward to maintain an open airway

J. Newborns and infants, who do not know to open their mouths to breathe when the nose is obstructed

K. Tipping the head too far back

L. When a child under stress acts like a younger child

M. Chronic disorder resulting in dementia

N. Abnormal heart rhythm

O. When an elderly person replaces lost circumstances with imaginary ones

_____ **1.** Adolescent

_____ **2.** Alzheimer's disease

_____ **3.** Arrhythmia

_____ **4.** Confabulation

_____ **5.** Fontanelle

_____ **6.** Geriatric

_____ **7.** Hyperextension

_____ **8.** Hypothermia

_____ **9.** Infant

_____ **10.** Obligate nose breathers

_____ **11.** Preschooler

_____ **12.** Regression

_____ **13.** School age

_____ **14.** Sniffing position

_____ **15.** Toddler

MULTIPLE-CHOICE REVIEW

_____ **1.** For the purposes of rescue breathing and CPR, a child is any patient between the ages of
    A. 5 and 12.
    B. 1 and 6.
    C. 1 and 8.
    D. 6 months and 16 years.

_____ **2.** In general emergency care, more useful age groupings for children would include
    A. newborns and infants.
    B. toddlers and preschoolers.
    C. school age and adolescents.
    D. all of the above.

_____ 3. Infants up until about 18 months will have a soft spot called a(n)
  A. bulging puncture.
  B. sunken suture.
  C. fontanelle.
  D. intracranial pressure.

_____ 4. When an infant is crying, the fontanelle normally
  A. bulges out.
  B. sinks into the skull.
  C. remains the same in size.
  D. softens gradually.

_____ 5. Newborns usually breathe
  A. through their noses.
  B. through their mouths.
  C. very slowly.
  D. through their mouths and noses.

_____ 6. Hyperextension of the neck of an infant may result in
  A. swelling of the fontanelle.
  B. an airway obstruction.
  C. secretions that aid digestion.
  D. breathing from the diaphragm.

_____ 7. "Blind" finger sweeps are not performed on infants or children to clear an airway obstruction because the
  A. finger might force an obstruction down and wedge it in the narrow trachea.
  B. finger could cause hyperextension of the neck.
  C. adult finger is too large to insert in an infant's mouth.
  D. tongue takes up too much space to allow for finger insertion.

_____ 8. When faced with the stress of an emergency, some children will act like a younger child. This is called
  A. reflection.
  B. regression.
  C. transition.
  D. imitation.

_____ 9. It is always a good idea to _____ when assessing a child.
  A. speak loudly and rapidly
  B. stand and speak softly
  C. kneel down and talk at eye level
  D. stare directly into the child's eyes

_____ 10. If the parents are overreacting when you are caring for a child, you should
  A. ignore them.
  B. try to involve them in the child's care.
  C. let them help stabilize the child's head.
  D. ask the police to take them to the hospital in their vehicle.

_____ 11. When forming a general impression of a child, if the child talks in grunts only, you should assume the child
  A. has a digestive condition.
  B. has significant respiratory distress.
  C. doesn't want to talk to you.
  D. has poor language skills.

_____ 12. When forming a general impression, it is most likely that a withdrawn child or one who is emotionally flat is probably
  A. bored.
  B. sick.
  C. about to die.
  D. deaf.

_____ 13. To assess a child's breathing, observe all of the following except
  A. skin color.
  B. chest expansion.
  C. capillary refill.
  D. effort of breathing.

_____ 14. An infant's soft spot may bulge due to head trauma or
  A. meningitis.
  B. dehydration.
  C. excessive eating.
  D. anaphylaxis.

_____ **15.** Starting at age _____ , our organ systems lose about _____ percent function each year.
   A. 20 : 1
   B. 20 : 2
   C. 30 : 1
   D. 40 : 2

_____ **16.** Although older patients are at least twice as likely to use EMS as younger patients, older patients are less likely to
   A. accept care provided by EMS.
   B. have medical problems, rather than injuries.
   C. be involved in motor-vehicle collisions.
   D. do all of the above.

_____ **17.** Assessing the airway of an older patient is often difficult because of dentures and because
   A. large, poorly chewed pieces of food are often found.
   B. dysrhythmias occur frequently.
   C. an older person's trachea is usually narrower.
   D. of arthritic changes in the bones of the neck.

_____ **18.** Since older patients are less likely to show severe symptoms in certain conditions, it can be difficult to
   A. find a radial pulse.
   B. determine a patient's priority.
   C. assess for foreign body obstruction.
   D. note sudden onset of weakness.

_____ **19.** After interviewing an elderly patient, the family tells you that some of the patient's responses were wrong. This is sometimes the result of neurological problems as well as
   A. slurred speech.
   B. depression.
   C. medications.
   D. all of the above.

_____ **20.** When an elderly patient replaces lost circumstances with imaginary ones, this is known as
   A. depression.
   B. confabulation.
   C. flustering.
   D. dysrhythmia.

_____ **21.** Many older people have a _____ threshold for pain.
   A. high
   B. low
   C. zero
   D. None of the above.

_____ **22.** As a person ages, the systolic blood pressure has a tendency to
   A. decrease.
   B. increase.
   C. become erratic.
   D. stay constant.

_____ **23.** Hip fractures are common in elderly patients, especially women, due to
   A. women's shorter legs.
   B. motor-vehicle collisions.
   C. abnormal curvature of the hip.
   D. loss of calcium.

_____ **24.** An EMT-B should consider that any injury of an elderly person could be a sign of
   A. a severe fall.
   B. Alzheimer's disease.
   C. abuse or neglect.
   D. depression.

_____ **25.** The EMT-B can ease the fears of a geriatric patient by understanding the
   A. effect that loss of independence has on the patient.
   B. need to minimize the patient's fears.
   C. need to ignore the patient's concerns.
   D. proper treatment for all of the patient's diseases.

COMPLETE THE FOLLOWING

1. List six examples of patients who are high priority for immediate transport.

   A. _____

   B. _____

   C. _____

   D. _____

   E. _____

   F. _____

2. Explain how to deal with a geriatric patient's fears of loss of independence.

VIRTUAL STREET SCENES

(First review the Street Scenes on pp. 274–275 of the textbook. Then answer the questions below.)

1. Should an ALS unit be called for an intercept en route to the hospital?

2. Imagine you found that it was very cold in the apartment and the patient had on many layers of clothing. Why is it not uncommon for elderly people to do that? What might you expect as a consequence?

3. Unlike the patient in the Street Scene, some elderly patients become very anxious about going in the ambulance to the hospital. Why do you think that is true? What can you do about it?

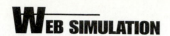

WEB SIMULATION

For interactive case studies that will help you review and practice basic skills, visit the *Emergency Care 9e Companion Website* at www.bradybooks.com/emergencycare.

EMT-BASIC SKILLS PERFORMANCE CHECKLIST

▶ **DEALING WITH THE PEDIATRIC PATIENT**

❑ Take BSI precautions.

❑ Identify yourself in a simple, informal way.

❑ Let the child know someone will call her parents.

❑ Determine if there are life-threatening problems and treat them immediately.

❑ Let the child have a nearby toy that she may want.

❑ Kneel or sit at the child's eye level.

❑ Smile.

❑ Touch the child or hold her hand or foot if appropriate.

❑ Explain all equipment that you plan to use in simple terms to the child.

❑ Make eye contact without staring at the child.

❑ Stop occasionally to confirm that the child understands your actions.

❑ Never lie to a child.

CASE STUDY

Abuser or loving parent?

You respond to a call for a motor-vehicle collision at an intersection. A police officer explains that two cars were involved and that car #1 did not stop at the stop sign and broad-sided car #2. The driver of car #1, a middle-aged man, is limping around outside of his vehicle. He says he has no injury but appears to be very anxious about the damage to the side of his new car. The driver of car #2 is sitting in the front seat of her car, consoling her toddler who is still crying. Both the mother, who appears to be approximately 20 years old, and her young son have lacerations to the front of their heads and blood stains on the front of their clothing. As you approach the vehicle, you note that there are two "spider-web" cracks in the windshield, one in front of the driver's seat and the other in front of the passenger seat.

1. At the scene of an automobile collision in an intersection, what is your greatest scene safety hazard?

2. Is there a need for another ambulance at the scene? Why or why not?

After taking BSI precautions, you approach car #2 and begin your assessment of the mother and child. You notice there is no car seat in the vehicle. After introducing yourself, you explain to the mother she should keep her head and neck still and that your partner would like to do the same for her child. She cooperates as she is concerned that her son has become a little "confused" since he mashed his head on the windshield.

3. Aside from manual stabilization of the head and neck, what are your initial concerns for the assessment of the child?

4. You note that the child is no longer crying and does not seem to care that you are evaluating him. Is this a significant finding? Explain.

5. Aside from AVPU, how else can you determine if the child's mental status is "normal" for this toddler?

6. What is the significance of the cracks in the car's windshield to the patient assessment process?

7. When you ask the mother if the child was restrained, she says, "He does not like the belt and there is no way I can keep him still enough to sit in a special seat." What is the significance of this statement in relation to the child's current mental status?

During your assessment, you note that the inside of the vehicle smells like "cheap wine" and the mother is acting as if she is intoxicated. When you assess the mother, you ask if she has eaten this afternoon or had anything to drink. She says she was upset today and had a few glasses of wine, but "Please don't tell the cops!" By this time, her child has been immobilized and is being placed into the ambulance by your partner and the First Responders. You proceed to immobilize the mother in the seated position with a vest-style immobilization device since her baseline vital signs are all normal and her other injuries are minor. The child, on the other hand, is being closely monitored since he has already vomited twice. You and your partner decide to go to the hospital as soon as the mother is loaded.

8. Should oxygen be administered to the child?

9. Would it be appropriate to set up an ALS intercept en route to the hospital?

10. After arrival at the hosptial, while you are cleaning up your equipment, the emergency department physician comes out to talk to you. He says that the child did not have a spine injury but the head trauma was serious. What should you say if he asks you how this incident and the child's injuries could have been prevented?

Chapter Fourteen

COMMUNICATIONS

MATCH TERMINOLOGY/DEFINITIONS

A. Federal agency that regulates radio communications

B. Device that picks up signals from lower-power radio units such as mobile and portable radios and retransmits them at a higher power

C. Unit used to measure the output power of a radio

D. Hand-held two-way radio

E. Two-way radio at a fixed site such as a hospital or dispatch center

F. Update on the patient's condition given to hospital personnel either face-to-face or over a radio

G. Two-way radio that is used or affixed in a vehicle

H. Phone that transmits through the air instead of over wires so that the phone can be transported and used over a wide area

I. Equipment that permits transmission of standard messages in condensed form by punching a key

J. "Press to talk" button on the EMS radio

_____ **1.** Base station

_____ **2.** Cellular phone

_____ **3.** Digital radio equipment

_____ **4.** FCC

_____ **5.** Mobile radio

_____ **6.** Portable radio

_____ **7.** PTT

_____ **8.** Repeater

_____ **9.** Verbal report

_____ **10.** Watt

MULTIPLE-CHOICE REVIEW

_____ **1.** The EMT-B's ability to communicate effectively is important because
   A. all EMTs are expected to be good public speakers.
   B. little information about a patient's condition is obtained by talking to the patient, bystanders, or family members.
   C. describing your assessment findings to the hospital may make a difference in the care the patient receives.
   D. none of the above.

_____ **2.** One of the key contributions to improvement in EMS over the years has been
   A. the type II, van-style ambulance vehicle.
   B. development of radio links among dispatcher, mobile units, and hospitals.
   C. the military anti-shock trousers.
   D. air conditioning in the transport vehicles.

_____ **3.** Components of a communications system include
   A. base stations.   **C.** portable radios.
   B. mobile units.   **D.** all of the above.

_____ 4. A device that picks up radio signals from lower-powered units and retransmits them at a higher power is called a
  A. mobile.   **C.** repeater.
  B. cellular.   **D.** portable.

_____ 5. The government agency that maintains order on the airwaves is called the
  A. FCC.   **C.** FEMA.
  B. FAA.   **D.** DOT.

_____ 6. The purposes of always following the general principles of radio transmission are to allow all persons to use the frequencies and to
  A. avoid having to repeat orders from medical direction.
  B. enable the EMT-B to talk in code language.
  C. prevent delays.
  D. do all of the above.

_____ 7. Of the following components of a radio report, which is the correct order?
  1) Major past illness
  2) Chief complaint
  3) Unit identification and level of provider
  4) Emergency medical care given
  A. 4, 1, 2, 3   **C.** 3, 2, 1, 4
  B. 3, 4, 1, 2   **D.** 1, 2, 4, 3

_____ 8. The reason why the ambulance was called is the
  A. major past illness.   **C.** presenting diagnosis.
  B. chief complaint.   **D.** call type.

_____ 9. During a radio report when the EMT-B says "The patient's abdomen does not feel rigid," he/she is attempting to advise the hospital of
  A. the baseline vital signs.
  B. the emergency medical care given.
  C. response of patient to the emergency medical care.
  D. pertinent findings of the physical exam.

_____ 10. During a radio report, when the EMT-B says "The patient's mental status has not changed during our care," he/she is attempting to advise the hospital of the
  A. baseline vital signs.
  B. emergency medical care given.
  C. response of patient to the emergency medical care.
  D. pertinent findings of the physical exam.

_____ 11. Whenever the EMT-B is requesting an order for medical direction over the radio, it is a good practice to
  A. repeat the physician's order word for word back to the physician.
  B. question all verbal orders that are given.
  C. speak quickly because the physician is busy.
  D. call the physician back again to verify.

_____ 12. If an order from the on-line physician appears to be inappropriate, then the EMT-B should
  A. switch to another frequency to find another physician.
  B. question the physician about the order.
  C. follow the physician's order as stated.
  D. ignore the order and do what he/she thinks is correct.

_____ 13. When an EMT-B stands with arms crossed looking down at the patient, the nonverbal message is,
  A. "I am here to help you."
  B. "I am not really interested."
  C. "I can empathize with your problem."
  D. "I am afraid of catching your disease."

_____ **14.** If it is obvious that a patient has a broken leg with a bone protruding, and the patient asks, "Is my leg broken?", what would be the most appropriate response?
   A. Relax and stay calm, you will be all right.
   B. I am not qualified to make that determination.
   C. No, it's a bad cut, and I'll control the bleeding with a bandage.
   D. Yes it is, and I will be as gentle as possible splinting it.

_____ **15.** When treating a toddler, the best approach is to
   A. kneel down so you are at the child's level.
   B. speak louder so the child can hear you above all the crying.
   C. stare directly into the child's eyes.
   D. tell the child you are a friend of his parents.

COMPLETE THE FOLLOWING

1. List five examples of components of a communications system.

   A. _____

   B. _____

   C. _____

   D. _____

   E. _____

2. List six interpersonal communications guidelines to use when dealing with patients, families, friends, and bystanders.

   A. _____

   B. _____

   C. _____

   D. _____

   E. _____

   F. _____

VIRTUAL STREET SCENES

(First review the Street Scenes on pp. 286–287 of the textbook, Then answer the questions below.)

1. Why was it important to call the hospital to alert them to a serious patient on the way?

2. If this call had occurred in your response area, who would have made the decision to call a helicopter?

3. In addition to radio communication, what other types of communication were involved in this call?

Web simulation

For interactive case studies that will help you review and practice basic skills, visit the *Emergency Care 9e Companion Website* at www.bradybooks.com/emergencycare.

EMT-BASIC SKILLS PERFORMANCE CHECKLIST

▶ RADIO REPORT

Pick an ambulance call on which you were recently an observer or a patient who you examined during the hospital observation portion of the EMT-B course. Without releasing any confidential information about the call, such as the patient's name and address, take a moment and organize your thoughts so you can provide a mock radio report to another crew member or your instructor.

❑ Unit identification (ambulance #_____).

❑ Level of provider.

❑ Estimated time of arrival (ETA).

❑ Patient's age and sex.

❑ Chief complaint (why they called EMS).

❑ Brief, pertinent history of the present illness or injury.

❑ Major past illnesses.

❑ Mental status (AVPU).

❑ Baseline vital signs.

❑ Pertinent findings of the physical exam.

❑ Emergency medical care given.

❑ Response to emergency medical care.

❑ Does medical direction have any questions or orders?

NOTE: There are a number of local formats for radio reports that may differ somewhat, yet they all adhere to the same principles. They should follow a logical order, be concise, and paint a picture of the patient's problem and the priorities for the hospital personnel.

Chapter Fifteen

DOCUMENTATION

MATCH TERMINOLOGY/DEFINITIONS

A. Information from an individual point of view

B. Report form used by EMS agencies to document prehospital assessment and care

C. Inaccurate entry or misrepresentation on a prehospital care report usually intended to cover up serious flaws in assessment or in care

D. Observable, measurable, and verifiable information

E. Exam finding that is not present or not true but is important to note (e.g., patient denies any shortness of breath)

F. Report on unusual, complex, or involved situations that is completed according to your service's standard operating procedures

G. Each individual box on a prehospital care report

H. Minimum elements that are recommended by the U.S. Department of Transportation be included in all prehospital care reports nationwide

I. Clipboard-format device that is able to recognize handwriting and convert it to computer text

J. Item affixed to a patient at a multiple-casualty incident used to record chief complaint and injuries, vital signs, and treatment given

_____ 1. Data element

_____ 2. Falsification

_____ 3. Minimum data set

_____ 4. Objective statement

_____ 5. PCR

_____ 6. Electronic clipboard

_____ 7. Pertinent negative

_____ 8. Special situation report

_____ 9. Subjective information

_____ 10. Triage tag

MULTIPLE-CHOICE REVIEW

_____ 1. The prehospital care report serves as a legal document as well as a(n)
A. press release form for your EMS agency.
B. receipt for the patient.
C. aid to research, education, and administrative efforts.
D. form to report all calls to the local police department.

_____ 2. Why is it necessary to complete a prehospital care report if on each call you give the emergency department staff a good oral report?
A. The QI committee needs something to hold you to.
B. It provides a means for the emergency department staff to review the patient's prehospital care.
C. They usually do not listen to oral reports.
D. Duplication is helpful in emergency call documentation.

_____ **3.** The copy of the prehospital care report left at the hospital
  A. is returned to the state for quality review and follow-up.
  B. is thrown out once it is key punched and added to computer file.
  C. should become part of the patient's permanent hospital record.
  D. is sent to the regional Emergency Medical Services agency.

_____ **4.** You are called to court to testify about a civil matter when a patient sues the city for an injury that occurred in a public place. Which of the following will best help you recall the events of the call?
  A. the questioning by the defense's attorney
  B. the questioning by the plaintiff's attorney
  C. a complete and accurate prehospital care report
  D. your tape recording of the call dispatch

_____ **5.** The person who completed a prehospital care report may be called to court to testify about
  A. the call in a criminal proceeding.   **C.** the call in a civil proceeding.
  B. the care provided to the patient.   **D.** all of the above.

_____ **6.** The routine review of prehospital care reports for conformity to current medical and organizational standards is a process called
  A. initial feedback.   **C.** stress debriefing.
  B. quality improvement.   **D.** system research.

_____ **7.** Each individual box on a prehospital care report is called a(n)
  A. narrative.   **C.** key punch.
  B. data element.   **D.** assessment.

_____ **8.** According to the U.S. Department of Transportation, in addition to other data elements, the minimum data set on a prehospital care report should include all of the following except
  A. respiratory rate and effort and skin color and temperature.
  B. times of incident, dispatch, and arrival at the patient.
  C. patient's social security number.
  D. capillary refill for patients less than 6 years old.

_____ **9.** The minimum data set includes all of the following except
  A. vital signs.   **C.** chief complaint.
  B. vehicle mileage.   **D.** times of the call.

_____ **10.** The time of dispatch is an example of _____ data on the prehospital care report.
  A. assessment   **C.** patient
  B. run   **D.** narrative

_____ **11.** Examples of patient data on a prehospital care report would be
  A. date of birth and age.
  B. time of arrival at the hospital.
  C. ambulance identification number.
  D. the hospital transported to.

_____ **12.** Experienced EMT-Bs consider a good prehospital care report as one that
  A. protects them against a QA review.
  B. is vague enough to prevent lawsuits.
  C. paints a picture of the patient.
  D. identifies symptoms overlooked by the patient.

_____ **13.** A statement such as "The patient has a swollen, deformed extremity" on the narrative portion of the prehospital care report is an example of
  A. subjective information.   **C.** pertinent negative information.
  B. objective information.   **D.** nonstandard abbreviations.

14. All of the following are examples of information that should be put in quotation marks on the prehospital care report <u>except</u>
    A. bystander statements.   C. objective information.
    B. chief complaint.   D. police officer's statements.

15. In the narrative section of a prehospital care report, the EMT-B should
    A. list his/her conclusions about the situation.
    B. include pertinent negatives.
    C. use the radio codes for each treatment.
    D. list the vital signs and times obtained.

16. Medical abbreviations should be used on a prehospital care report
    A. to save space in the narrative section.
    B. to replace all words you cannot spell.
    C. only if they are standardized.
    D. to ensure correct interpretation by physicians.

17. The prehospital care report form itself and the information on it should be considered
    A. the property of the ambulance service.
    B. confidential information.
    C. privileged information.
    D. the patient's property.

18. When a patient refuses transport, before the EMT-B leaves the scene, he/she should
    A. document assessment findings and care given.
    B. try again to persuade the patient to go to a hospital.
    C. ensure the patient is able to make a rational, informed decision.
    D. do all of the above.

19. When completing a prehospital care report on a patient refusal, the EMT-B should document all of the following <u>except</u>
    A. that he/she was willing to return if the patient changed his/her mind.
    B. the complete patient assessment.
    C. that alternative methods of care were offered.
    D. the patient's diagnosis.

20. If the EMT-B forgot to administer a treatment that is required by a state protocol, he/she should
    A. document on the PCR only treatment actually given.
    B. be sure to document an excuse for why the treatment was skipped.
    C. record that the patient was given the forgotten treatment.
    D. do none of the above.

21. Falsification of information on a prehospital care report may lead to
    A. suspension or revocation of your license or certification.
    B. better EMT-B education.
    C. longer response times.
    D. none of the above.

22. To correct an error discovered while writing the prehospital care report, the EMT-B should
    A. scribble out the error so it cannot be seen.
    B. draw a line through the error, initial it, and write the correct information.
    C. place his/her initials over the error.
    D. erase the error completely, and then write the correction.

_____ 23. If information was omitted on a prehospital care report, the EMT-B should
   A. prepare another report and substitute that for the earlier one.
   B. notify the service medical director immediately.
   C. add a note with the correct information, the date, and initial it.
   D. do nothing, as information should never be added after the call.

_____ 24. An example of an instance in which it would <u>not</u> be unusual for the EMT-B to obtain only a limited amount of information is
   A. during a multiple-casualty incident.
   B. during an interhospital transfer.
   C. while performing a non-emergency run.
   D. when encountering a child abuse case.

_____ 25. Special situation reports
   A. document events that should be reported to local regulatory authorities.
   B. can be submitted at any time after the call.
   C. need not be accurate and/or objective.
   D. are required on each call.

COMPLETE THE FOLLOWING

List ten examples of patient data on a prehospital care report.

A. _____

B. _____

C. _____

D. _____

E. _____

F. _____

G. _____

H. _____

I. _____

J. _____

VIRTUAL STREET SCENES

(First review the Street Scenes on p. 305 of the textbook. Then answer the questions below.)

1. What legal problem might be created if you had forgotten to record the patient's distal pulses, motor function, and sensation before and after immobilization?

2. What might it mean if the documentation had been sloppy and difficult to read?

3. Imagine that the patient had told you that he was drunk. Should you document that information? If so, how?

4. What will the emergency department staff do with your prehospital care report?

WEB SIMULATION

For interactive case studies that will help you review and practice basic skills, visit the *Emergency Care 9e Companion Website* at www.bradybooks.com/emergencycare.

Chapter Sixteen

GENERAL PHARMACOLOGY

MATCH TERMINOLOGY/DEFINITIONS

A. Specific signs or circumstances under which it is appropriate to administer a drug to a patient

B. Spray device with a mouthpiece that contains an aerosol form of a medication that a patient can spray directly into his/her airway

C. Semisolid paste form of a drug

D. Medication given by mouth to treat a conscious patient (one who is able to swallow) with an altered mental status and a history of diabetes

E. Brand name of a medication

F. Drug that helps to constrict the blood vessels and relax airway passages; it may be used to counter a severe allergic reaction.

G. Solid form of a drug; compressed powder

H. Powder, usually pre-mixed with water, that will adsorb some poisons and help prevent them from being absorbed by the body

I. This gas, in its pure form, is used as a drug to treat any patient whose medical or traumatic condition causes them to be hypoxic, or low in oxygen.

J. Liquid form of a drug in which a powder is mixed with a slurry or water

_____ 1. Activated charcoal

_____ 2. Epinephrine

_____ 3. Gel

_____ 4. Indications

_____ 5. Inhaler

_____ 6. Oral glucose

_____ 7. Oxygen

_____ 8. Suspension

_____ 9. Tablet

_____ 10. Trade name

MULTIPLE-CHOICE REVIEW

_____ 1. The study of drugs and their effects is called
   A. anatomy.
   B. physiology.
   C. medicinology.
   D. pharmacology.

_____ 2. Medications that are routinely carried on the EMS unit are
   A. activated charcoal, oral glucose, and oxygen.
   B. oxygen and nitroglycerin.
   C. epinephrine and prescribed inhalers.
   D. all of the above.

_____ **3.** Activated charcoal is an example of a
   A. powder, usually pre-mixed with water.
   B. prescribed inhaler.
   C. liquid for injection.
   D. fine powder for inhalation.

_____ **4.** Activated charcoal is given to a patient because it
   A. displaces poisons by surface tension.
   B. will bind some poisons to its surface.
   C. prevents the patient from vomiting.
   D. can be used in a patient without a gag reflex.

_____ **5.** Poorly managed diabetes can cause
   A. hypoxia, or low oxygen.   **C.** dilation of the coronary arteries.
   B. altered mental status.   **D.** absorption of poisons.

_____ **6.** Oral glucose is given between the patient's cheek and gum because
   A. this area contains blood vessels that allow easy absorption into
       the bloodstream.
   B. it will not be aspirated if the patient suddenly becomes unconscious.
   C. this area will cause the patient to regurgitate the stomach's contents.
   D. it will assist in dilating the coronary vessels as much as possible.

_____ **7.** Examples of medications a patient may have in his possession that
   the EMT-B may assist the patient in taking under the appropriate
   circumstances are
   A. activated charcoal, glucose injections, and anticonvulsants.
   B. home oxygen, antihypertensives, and anti-inflammatories.
   C. epinephrine auto-injector, a prescribed inhaler, and nitroglycerin.
   D. insulin, antihypertensives, and anticonvulsants.

_____ **8.** Patients who have a medical history of asthma, emphysema, and chronic
   bronchitis may carry _____ .
   A. nitroglycerin   **C.** a bronchodilator.
   B. an epinephrine auto-injector   **D.** a bronchoconstrictor.

_____ **9.** The drug nitroglycerin is used to _____ vessels.
   A. dilate the peripheral   **C.** dilate the coronary
   B. constrict the peripheral   **D.** constrict the coronary

_____ **10.** The government publication listing all drugs in the United States is called the
   A. *Physician's Desk Reference.*   **C.** *U.S. Pharmacopoeia.*
   B. *Hazmat Guidebook.*   **D.** *National Medicine Guidebook.*

_____ **11.** The name that the manufacturer uses in marketing a drug is called
   the _____ name.
   A. generic   **C.** official
   B. trade   **D.** original

_____ **12.** A circumstance in which a drug should not be used because it may cause
   harm to the patient or offer no effect in improving the patient's condition
   or illness is called a(n)
   A. indication.   **C.** adverse reaction.
   B. side effect.   **D.** contraindication.

_____ **13.** An action of a drug that is other than the desired action is called a(n)
   A. side effect.   **C.** contraindication.
   B. overdose.   **D.** systemic effect.

_____ **14.** Prior to administering a medication to a patient, you must know all of the following <u>except</u>
    A. the route of administration.
    B. the proper dose to administer.
    C. the actions the medication will take.
    D. both the generic and chemical names.

_____ **15.** Drugs prescribed for pain relief are called
    A. antiarrhythmics.   **C.** anticonvulsants.
    B. analgesics.   **D.** antihypertensives.

_____ **16.** Drugs prescribed to reduce high blood pressure are called
    A. antiarrhythmics.   **C.** anticonvulsants.
    B. analgesics.   **D.** antihypertensives.

_____ **17.** Drugs prescribed for heart rhythm disorders are called
    A. antidiabetics.   **C.** antiarrhythmics.
    B. bronchodilators.   **D.** anticonvulsants.

_____ **18.** Drugs prescribed to relax the smooth muscles of the bronchial tubes are called
    A. bronchospasms.   **C.** anticonvulsants.
    B. bronchodilators.   **D.** bronchoconstrictors.

_____ **19.** Drugs prescribed for prevention and control of seizures are called
    A. antidiabetics.   **C.** anticonvulsants.
    B. antihypertensives.   **D.** antidepressants.

_____ **20.** Drugs prescribed to help regulate the emotional activity of patients to minimize the psychological and emotional peaks and valleys are called
    A. antidepressants.   **C.** antiarrhythmics.
    B. analgesics.   **D.** anticonvulsants.

COMPLETE THE FOLLOWING

1. List six medications an EMT-B can administer or assist a patient in taking.

A. _____

B. _____

C. _____

D. _____

E. _____

F. _____

2. List the four "rights" to adhere to when administering a medication.

A. _____

B. _____

C. _____

D. _____

VIRTUAL STREET SCENES

(First review the Street Scenes on pp. 316–317 of the textbook. Then answer the questions below.)

1. Suppose the patient's wife had administered the nitroglycerin tablets before your arrival. What side effect should you be alert for?

2. What effect does a patient with chest pain expect from the nitroglycerin tablet? How does this effect occur?

3. Are there any "pertinent negatives" in the Sample Documentation? If so, what are they?

WEB SIMULATION

For interactive case studies that will help you review and practice basic skills, visit the *Emergency Care 9e Companion Website* at www.bradybooks.com/emergencycare.

Chapter Seventeen

RESPIRATORY EMERGENCIES

MATCH TERMINOLOGY/DEFINITIONS

A. Active process in which the intercostal muscles and the diaphragm contract, expanding the size of the chest cavity and causing air to flow into the lungs; also called inhalation

B. Sporadic, irregular breaths that are usually seen just before respiratory arrest

C. Blockage of the bronchi that lead from the trachea to the lungs

D. Pulling in of the accessory muscles to breathe

E. Passive process in which the intercostal muscles and the diaphragm relax, causing the chest cavity to decrease in size and forcing air from the lungs; also called exhalation

_____ **1.** Agonal respirations

_____ **2.** Bronchoconstriction

_____ **3.** Expiration

_____ **4.** Inspiration

_____ **5.** Retractions

MULTIPLE-CHOICE REVIEW

_____ **1.** The muscular structure that divides the chest cavity from the abdominal cavity is called the
   A. intercostal muscle.
   B. sternocleidomastoid.
   C. diaphragm.
   D. inguinal muscle.

_____ **2.** Expiration is a(n)
   A. active process that involves the relaxation of the intercostal muscles and the diaphragm.
   B. passive process that involves the relaxation of the intercostal muscles and the diaphragm.
   C. active process that involves the contraction of the intercostal muscles and the diaphragm.
   D. passive process that involves the contraction of the intercostal muscles and the diaphragm.

_____ **3.** To determine the quality of breathing, check for all of the following except
   A. presence of breath sounds.
   B. chest expansion.
   C. breathing rhythm.
   D. depth of respirations.

_____ **4.** An unresponsive patient with shallow, gasping breaths with only a few breaths per minute requires
   A. oxygen given via nasal cannula.
   B. immediate transport to a medical facility.
   C. immediate artificial ventilation with supplemental oxygen.
   D. oxygen given via nonrebreather mask.

_____ 5. The muscles in the neck and abdomen that sometimes assist in breathing are called _____ muscles.
A. extra
B. accessory
C. sub-diaphragmatic
D. smooth

_____ 6. Since oxygenation of the body's tissue is reduced in a patient with inadequate breathing, the skin may be _____ in color and feel _____ .
A. pale : dry and cool
B. red : clammy and hot
C. yellow : dry and warm
D. blue : clammy and cool

_____ 7. If an unresponsive adult patient makes _____ sounds, she may have a serious airway problem requiring immediate intervention.
A. snoring or gurgling
B. slight wheezing
C. sniffling
D. whistling or grunting

_____ 8. Statistically, a leading killer of infants and children is
A. motor-vehicle collisions.
B. heart attacks.
C. respiratory conditions.
D. infection.

_____ 9. The structure of an infant's or child's airway is different from an adult's in each of the following ways except
A. all airway structures are smaller and more easily obstructed.
B. their tongues are proportionately larger than an adult's.
C. the trachea is softer and more flexible.
D. the cricoid cartilage is more rigid.

_____ 10. Because the chest wall is softer in infants and children, they
A. must inhale twice the amount of air to breathe.
B. depend more heavily on the diaphragm for breathing.
C. grunt and gurgle whenever they breathe.
D. expend less energy than adults do when breathing.

_____ 11. The signs of inadequate breathing in infants and children include all of the following except
A. nasal flaring.
B. grunting.
C. "seesaw breathing."
D. quivering jaw.

_____ 12. Which one of the following would be most important to observe related to a patient's breathing?
A. presence of breathing and pulse rate
B. breathing pattern and adequacy of breathing
C. presence of breathing and adequacy of breathing
D. patient position and adequacy of breathing

_____ 13. The best method for providing artificial ventilation is the
A. pocket face mask without supplemental oxygen.
B. two-person bag-valve mask with supplemental oxygen.
C. flow-restricted, oxygen-powered ventilator.
D. one-person bag-valve mask with supplemental oxygen.

_____ 14. If you are unsure a patient requires artificial ventilation, you should
A. contact medical direction immediately.
B. move to the ambulance and transport rapidly.
C. increase the liter flow rate to the nonrebreather mask.
D. provide artificial ventilation.

_____ 15. The adequate rate of artificial ventilations for a nonbreathing adult patient is _____ breaths per minute.
A. 8
B. 12
C. 16
D. 20

_____ **16.** The adequate rate of artificial ventilations for a nonbreathing infant or child patient is _____ breaths per minute.
  A. 10   **C.** 20
  B. 15   **D.** 25

_____ **17.** If an infant or a child has _____ in the setting of a respiratory emergency, this usually indicates trouble.
  A. a fever   **C.** a low pulse
  B. cold skin   **D.** a rapid pulse

_____ **18.** You are artificially ventilating an adult patient in respiratory arrest. The chest does not rise and fall with each ventilation. The <u>first</u> action to take is to
  A. increase the oxygen flow rate.
  B. increase the force of ventilations.
  C. change the ventilatory device.
  D. recheck the airway.

_____ **19.** Why is it important to try to distinguish between a lower airway and an upper airway problem in an infant and a child?
  A. Suctioning can cause spasms with some lower respiratory diseases.
  B. You will need to give this information to the emergency department.
  C. Finger sweeps will not help to clear an upper airway obstruction.
  D. The lower airway may wheeze when treated with oxygen.

_____ **20.** The sign(s) of a lower airway problem include all of the following <u>except</u>
  A. wheezing.
  B. increased breathing effort upon exhalation.
  C. rapid breathing without stridor.
  D. yellow skin color.

_____ **21.** If your patient is able to speak only in short choppy sentences, this may mean she
  A. may have a language problem.
  B. is unable to hear you clearly.
  C. is experiencing breathing difficulty.
  D. is afraid of you.

_____ **22.** When an EMT-B states that the patient was in the tripod position due to respiratory distress, this means the patient was
  A. holding self up by two legs and one arm.
  B. leaning forward with hands resting on knees.
  C. in the recovery position.
  D. supine with knees flexed against the chest.

_____ **23.** Which pair of signs/symptoms is <u>not</u> commonly associated with breathing difficulty?
  A. crowing/restlessness
  B. retractions/shortness of breath
  C. increased pulse/tightness in chest
  D. vomiting/headache

_____ **24.** If a patient is suffering from breathing difficulty and is breathing adequately, administer oxygen via
  A. nasal cannula.
  B. nonrebreather mask.
  C. pocket face mask.
  D. bag-valve mask with supplemental oxygen.

_____ **25.** If a patient is experiencing breathing difficulty and is breathing adequately, it is usually best to place him in the _____ position.
  A. tripod   **C.** sitting-up
  B. supine   **D.** none of the above

_____ **26.** A patient with respiratory problems that cause bronchoconstriction may carry a(n)
    A. bronchoconstrictor.
    C. inhaler or puffer.
    B. metered dose aspirator.
    D. antihypertensive medication.

_____ **27.** Once you receive permission from medical direction to assist a patient with an inhaler, make sure you have all of the following <u>except</u>
    A. the right dose.
    B. an inhaler that is not expired.
    C. a large enough syringe.
    D. a patient who is alert enough to cooperate.

_____ **28.** Prior to coaching the patient in the use of an inhaler, the EMT-B should
    A. shake the inhaler vigorously.
    B. test the unit by spraying into the air.
    C. ensure that the patient is no longer alert.
    D. call the patient's personal physician.

_____ **29.** To ensure that the most medication is absorbed when using an inhaler, you should try to encourage the patient to
    A. take short, shallow breaths.
    B. hold the breath as long as possible.
    C. take a short nap.
    D. hyperventilate.

_____ **30.** The best way to document that a patient has a respiratory complaint is to
    A. describe your opinion of the patient's problem in detail.
    B. see if the patient can answer all the SAMPLE and OPQRST questions.
    C. ask the patient to describe the difficulty in his own words.
    D. carefully count the patient's breathing rate for at least two minutes.

COMPLETE THE FOLLOWING

1. List nine conditions of inadequate breathing.

    A. _____

    B. _____

    C. _____

    D. _____

    E. _____

    F. _____

    G. _____

    H. _____

    I. _____

2. List four signs of inadequate breathing in infants and children.

    A. _____

    B. _____

    C. _____

    D. _____

3. List eight signs of breathing difficulty.

A. _____

B. _____

C. _____

D. _____

E. _____

F. _____

G. _____

H. _____

LABEL THE DIAGRAMS

Fill in each phase of respiration on the line provided.

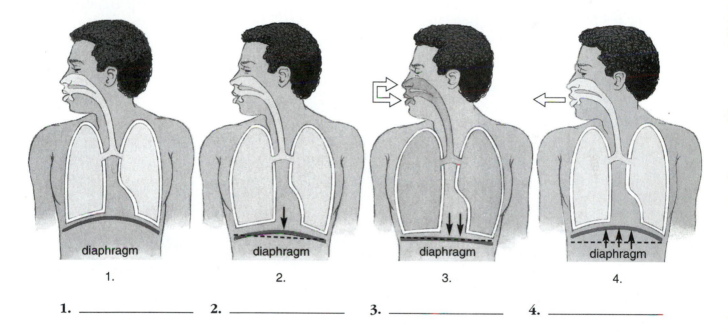

diaphragm 1. diaphragm 2. diaphragm 3. diaphragm 4.

1. _____ 2. _____ 3. _____ 4. _____

VIRTUAL STREET SCENES

(First review the Street Scenes on pp. 332–333 of the textbook. Then answer the questions below.)

1. You have already reported that the patient has emphysema. Imagine that you were also told the patient was coughing earlier in the day. Would it be worth documenting the cough on your PCR? Why or why not?

2. If advanced life support (ALS) had been available, would it have been appropriate to request their assisstance?

3. Is it possible to assist the ventilations of a patient who is in a semi-sitting position?

WEB SIMULATION

For interactive case studies that will help you review and practice basic skills, visit the *Emergency Care 9e Companion Website* at www.bradybooks.com/emergencycare.

EMT-BASIC SKILLS PERFORMANCE CHECKLIST

▶ PRESCRIBED INHALER

❑ Conduct a scene size-up.

❑ Take BSI precautions.

❑ Perform initial assessment.

❑ Perform focused history and physical exam.

❑ Confirm indications for inhaler use.

❑ Obtain medical direction for prescribed patient-assisted inhaler. (generics: albuterol, isoetharine, metaproterenol, etc.)

❑ Check contraindications for inhaler use.

❑ Assure right patient, right medication, right dose, right route, and patient is alert enough to use inhaler.

❑ Check expiration date of inhaler.

❑ Check if patient has already taken any doses.

❑ Assure inhaler is at room temperature or warmer.

❑ Shake inhaler vigorously several times.

❑ Have patient exhale deeply.

❑ Have patient put lips around the opening of inhaler.

❑ Have patient depress the hand-held inhaler as he begins to inhale deeply.

❑ Instruct patient to hold breath for as long as comfortable so medication can be absorbed.

❑ Put oxygen back on patient.

❑ Allow patient to breathe a few times, and repeat dose if so ordered by medical direction.

❑ If patient has a spacer device for inhaler, it should be used.

Chapter Eighteen

CARDIAC EMERGENCIES

MATCH TERMINOLOGY/DEFINITIONS

▶ **PART A**

A. Buildup of fatty deposits on the inner walls of arteries

B. Dilation, or ballooning, of a weakened section in the wall of an artery

C. Condition of excessive fluid buildup in the lungs and/or other organs and body parts because of the inadequate pumping of the heart

D. Condition in which artery walls become hard and stiff due to calcium deposits

E. When the heart has ceased generating electrical impulses

F. Blanket term for any kind of heart problem

G. Irregular, or absent, heart rhythm

H. Diseases that affect the arteries of the heart

I. Condition in which a portion of the myocardium dies as a result of oxygen starvation; often called a heart attack by laypersons

J. Pain in the chest that occurs when the blood supply to the heart is reduced and a portion of the heart muscle is not receiving enough oxygen

_____ 1. Acute myocardial infarction

_____ 2. Aneurysm

_____ 3. Angina pectoris

_____ 4. Arrhythmia

_____ 5. Arteriosclerosis

_____ 6. Asystole

_____ 7. Atherosclerosis

_____ 8. Cardiac compromise

_____ 9. Congestive heart failure

_____ 10. Coronary artery disease

A. Condition in which the heart's electrical impulses are disorganized, preventing the heart muscle from contracting normally

B. Blockage

C. Accumulation of fluid in the feet or ankles

D. Cardiac arrest that occurs within two hours of the onset of symptoms

E. Accumulation of fluid in the lungs

F. Condition in which the heartbeat is quite rapid; if rapid enough, it will not allow the heart's chambers to fill with enough blood between beats to produce blood flow sufficient to meet the body's needs

G. Clot of blood and plaque that has broken loose from the wall of an artery and then moves to smaller arteries and blocks blood flow

H. Clot formed of blood and plaque attached to the inner wall of an artery

I. Condition in which the heart's electrical rhythm remains relatively normal, yet the mechanical pumping activity fails to follow the electrical activity, causing cardiac arrest

J. Swelling resulting from a buildup of fluid in tissues

_____ 1. Edema

_____ 2. Embolism

_____ 3. Occlusion

_____ 4. Pedal edema

_____ 5. Pulmonary edema

_____ 6. Pulseless electrical activity

_____ 7. Sudden death

_____ 8. Thrombus

_____ 9. Ventricular fibrillation

_____ 10. Ventricular tachycardia

MULTIPLE-CHOICE REVIEW

_____ 1. Cardiac compromise is a term that refers to
   A. a heart attack.
   B. sudden death.
   C. any kind of problem with the heart.
   D. a period of time when the heart stops.

_____ 2. Chest pain from the heart is typically described by the patient as any of the following except
   A. dull.
   B. squeezing.
   C. tearing.
   D. crushing.

_____ 3. The pain or discomfort from a heart problem commonly radiates to the
   A. arms and jaw.
   B. feet and head.
   C. stomach and lower abdomen.
   D. right arm and lower abdomen.

_____ 4. In addition to chest pain or discomfort, the patient with cardiac compromise will also complain of
   A. diarrhea.
   B. shivering.
   C. dyspnea.
   D. headache.

_____ 5. Patients with heart problems may complain of any of the following except
   A. pain in the center of the chest.
   B. mild chest discomfort.
   C. sudden onset of sharp abdominal pain.
   D. difficulty breathing.

_____ 6. If the heart is beating too fast or too slow, the patient with cardiac compromise may also
    A. have stomach pain.   C. have a seizure or convulsion.
    B. lose consciousness.   D. have right-side weakness.

_____ 7. The signs and symptoms of cardiac compromise include all of the following except
    A. difficulty breathing and abnormal pulse rate.
    B. sudden onset of sweating with nausea or vomiting.
    C. sharp lower abdominal pain and a fever.
    D. pain in the chest or upper abdomen.

_____ 8. The emergency medical care of the patient with cardiac compromise should include all of the following except
    A. placing the patient in the position of comfort.
    B. administering high-concentration oxygen by nonrebreather mask.
    C. administering high-flow oxygen by a nasal cannula.
    D. assisting the patient with nitroglycerin administration if medical direction authorizes.

_____ 9. What is the typical "position of comfort" for a conscious patient who is having chest pain and difficulty breathing?
    A. Fowler's   C. sitting up
    B. supine   D. lying down with knees bent

_____ 10. All of the following cardiac compromise patients are candidates for immediate transport except a patient with
    A. no history of cardiac problems.
    B. a history of cardiac problems, who does not have nitroglycerin.
    C. prescribed nitroglycerin.
    D. with a systolic blood pressure of less than 100.

_____ 11. You should consider using nitroglycerin when the patient
    A. is hypertensive and has a headache.
    B. has his own nitroglycerin and has crushing chest pain.
    C. loses consciousness after feeling dizzy.
    D. has chest pain for over five minutes and is hypotensive.

_____ 12. Which of the following is the best description of the role of medical direction in the treatment of a cardiac compromise patient?
    A. authorizing the EMT-B to administer oxygen via nonrebreather mask
    B. prescribing nitroglycerin that the EMT-B can then assist the patient in taking
    C. authorizing the EMT-B to assist the patient in taking his prescribed nitroglycerin
    D. contacting the patient's physician to ensure the patient's nitroglycerin prescription is not out-of-date

_____ 13. A patient is complaining of chest pain. In order for the EMT-B to administer nitroglycerin, all of the following conditions must be met except
    A. medical direction should authorize its administration.
    B. the patient's physician should have prescribed the medication.
    C. the patient's blood pressure is lower than 100 systolic.
    D. the patient's blood pressure is greater than 100 systolic.

_____ 14. The maximum number of doses of nitroglycerin routinely given in the field is
    A. one.   C. three.
    B. two.   D. four.

_____ 15. After administering three doses of nitroglycerin, if the patient's blood pressure falls below 100 systolic, you should
   A. administer another dose of nitroglycerin.
   B. reassess the patient's vital signs.
   C. treat for shock and transport promptly.
   D. do all of the above.

_____ 16. Nitroglycerin is contraindicated for the patient who has
   A. a head injury.
   B. a systolic blood pressure of 110.
   C. not yet taken the maximum dose.
   D. been complaining of the pain for at least twenty minutes.

_____ 17. Which of the following is not a common side effect of nitroglycerin?
   A. hypotension   C. pulse rate changes
   B. headache   D. palpitations

_____ 18. After administering nitroglycerin, it is important to
   A. immediately administer the next dose.
   B. discontinue the oxygen therapy.
   C. reassess the vital signs.
   D. lay the patient down.

_____ 19. Cardiovascular emergencies are caused, directly or indirectly, by all of the following except
   A. changes in the inner walls of arteries.
   B. problems with the heart's electrical function.
   C. problems with the heart's mechanical function.
   D. complications resulting from cardiovascular surgery.

_____ 20. When the body is subjected to exertion or stress, the heart rate will normally
   A. increase.   C. become irregular.
   B. decrease.   D. stop temporarily.

_____ 21. Two conditions commonly cause narrowing or blocking of the arteries. One condition is atherosclerosis, and the other is
   A. aneurysm.   C. arteriosclerosis.
   B. dysrhythmia.   D. congestive heart failure.

_____ 22. Factor(s) that put a person at risk for developing coronary artery disease include
   A. lack of exercise.   C. obesity.
   B. cigarette smoking.   D. all of the above.

_____ 23. Which of the following risk factors can be modified to reduce the risk of coronary artery disease?
   A. age   C. hypertension
   B. heredity   D. none of the above

_____ 24. The reason an emergency occurs in most cardiac-related medical emergencies is due to
   A. reduced blood flow to the myocardium.
   B. cardiac arrest.
   C. loss of consciousness.
   D. breathing difficulty.

_____ 25. Angina pectoris means, literally,
   A. a small heart attack.   C. paralyzed chest muscles.
   B. a pain in the chest.   D. breathing difficulty.

_____ 26. Why is nitroglycerin administered to the patient with chest pain?
   A. It increases blood flow to the brain.
   B. It dilates the blood vessels and decreases the work of the heart.
   C. It constricts the blood vessels and raises the blood pressure.
   D. It is easy to administer in unconscious patients.

_____ 27. A condition in which a portion of the myocardium dies as a result of oxygen starvation is known as
   A. coronary occlusion.
   B. acute myocardial infarction.
   C. myocardial starvation.
   D. acute angina attack.

_____ 28. When a cardiac arrest occurs within two hours of the onset of cardiac symptoms, this is referred to as
   A. prehospital death.
   B. prehospital arrest.
   C. sudden death.
   D. ventricular tachycardia.

_____ 29. Unfortunately, nearly _____ of the patients who experience a cardiac arrest within two hours of the onset of symptoms have no previous history of cardiac problems.
   A. 10%   **C.** 60%
   B. 25%   **D.** 80%

_____ 30. Changes in the field care of the acute myocardial infarction (AMI) have made _____ and _____ two of the most important treatment methods.
   A. oxygen : PASG   **C.** thrombolytics : defibrillation
   B. rapid transport : surgery **D.** none of the above

_____ 31. Congestive heart failure is a(n)
   A. clotting of the coronary artery.
   B. condition in which excessive fluids build up in the lungs and/or other organs.
   C. infection in the heart that makes it difficult to oxygenate the blood.
   D. chronic lung condition that requires a low concentration of oxygen administration.

_____ 32. When there is damage to the left ventricle and blood backs up into the lungs, this usually presents in the form of
   A. pedal edema.   **C.** thrombolytics.
   B. pulmonary edema.   **D.** diaphoresis.

_____ 33. The elements of the chain of survival include early access to all of the following except
   A. CPR.   **C.** advanced care.
   B. defibrillation.   **D.** diagnosis.

_____ 34. Ways to decrease the EMS access time include
   A. installing a 9-1-1 system.
   B. placing 9-1-1 stickers on telephones.
   C. providing public information workshops.
   D. all of the above.

_____ 35. Which of the following steps is not necessary to ensure that CPR can be delivered earlier to cardiac arrest victims?
   A. Send CPR-trained professionals to patients faster.
   B. Ensure that heart specialists are involved in CPR training.
   C. Train laypeople in CPR.
   D. Have dispatchers instruct callers in how to perform CPR.

_____ **36.** Who is the typical cardiac arrest victim?
  A. a male in his sixties
  B. a female in her forties
  C. a male in his seventies
  D. There is no pattern to cardiac arrests.

_____ **37.** The most common witness to a cardiac arrest is a
  A. male in his forties.   **C.** man in his sixties.
  B. female in her forties.   **D.** female in her sixties.

_____ **38.** The single most important factor in determining survival from cardiac arrest is
  A. nitroglycerin administration.
  B. training middle-aged and older people in CPR.
  C. early CPR.
  D. early defibrillation.

_____ **39.** If the response time from the moment a call is received to arrival of the defibrillator is longer than _____ minutes, virtually no one survives a cardiac arrest.
  A. 6   **C.** 10
  B. 8   **D.** 12

_____ **40.** When treating a cardiac arrest patient and there is no ACLS unit in the community, the EMT-B should
  A. discontinue resuscitative efforts and pronounce the patient.
  B. package quickly and transport to the closest medical facility.
  C. call for ACLS from another town and wait for their arrival.
  D. continue to provide CPR at the scene until the patient regains a pulse.

_____ **41.** In order to manage a patient in cardiac arrest, the EMT-B should be able to do all of the following <u>except</u>
  A. use a bag-valve-mask device with oxygen.
  B. use an automated external defibrillator.
  C. request advanced life support backup (when available).
  D. administer epinephrine via IV or ET tube.

_____ **42.** Which of the following is an unnecessary step for the EMT-B to take when using a fully automated defibrillator?
  A. Assess the patient.
  B. Turn on the power.
  C. Put the pads on the patient's chest.
  D. Press the button to deliver the shock.

_____ **43.** The primary electrical disturbance resulting in cardiac arrest is
  A. asystole.   **C.** ventricular tachycardia.
  B. ventricular fibrillation. **D.** pulseless electrical activity.

_____ **44.** The shockable rhythms include all of the following <u>except</u>
  A. asystole and PEA.   **C.** pulseless ventricular tachycardia.
  B. ventricular fibrillation. **D.** ventricular tachycardia.

_____ **45.** A nonshockable rhythm that can be the result of a terminally sick heart or severe blood loss is called
  A. pulseless electrical activity.   **C.** pulseless ventricular tachycardia.
  B. ventricular tachycardia.   **D.** ventricular fibrillation.

_____ **46.** A nonshockable rhythm that is commonly called "flatline" is named
  A. pulseless electrical activity.   **C.** asystole.
  B. ventricular tachycardia.   **D.** ventricular fibrillation.

_____ **47.** When the AED is analyzing the patient's heart rhythm, the EMT-B must
    A. continue the CPR compressions.   **C.** hyperventilate the patient.
    B. avoid touching the patient.   **D.** reassess for a carotid pulse.

_____ **48.** The AED should routinely be used on
    A. trauma victims.   **C.** patients under 8 years of age.
    B. patients under 55 pounds.   **D.** patients with a shockable rhythm.

_____ **49.** The AED pads are first attached to the cables. Then the pad attached to the _____ cable goes on the _____ lower ribs.
    A. white : left
    B. white : right
    C. red : left
    D. red : right

_____ **50.** After the first set of three stacked shocks, you check the patient's carotid pulse. The patient has a pulse and is breathing adequately. You should then _____ and transport.
    A. give high-concentration oxygen via bag-valve mask
    B. provide artificial ventilations with high-concentration oxygen
    C. give high-concentration oxygen via nonrebreather mask
    D. repeat the cycle of three stacked shocks

_____ **51.** After six shocks, the EMT-B should _____ unless local protocol says otherwise.
    A. give two more in a row   **C.** terminate the arrest
    B. transport the patient   **D.** increase the rate of ventilation

_____ **52.** Which of the following is not a general principle of AED use?
    A. Hook up oxygen before beginning defibrillation.
    B. Avoid contact with patient during rhythm analysis.
    C. Be sure everyone is "clear" before delivering each shock.
    D. Avoid defibrillation in a moving ambulance.

_____ **53.** Of the cardiac arrest patients listed below, which one can be defibrillated immediately?
    A. soaking wet patient lying in the rain
    B. trauma patient with severe blood loss
    C. patient on a metal deck being cradled by another person
    D. patient with an implanted defibrillator

_____ **54.** If it is necessary to remove a nitroglycerin patch to defibrillate a patient, you should
    A. wear gloves.
    B. wear goggles.
    C. ensure you have a replacement patch.
    D. cleanse the patient's skin with alcohol.

_____ **55.** If a patient has a cardiac pacemaker and needs to be defibrillated, the EMT-B should
    A. perform the procedure as he/she would for other cardiac patients.
    B. remove the pacemaker before defibrillation.
    C. place the pad several inches away from the pacemaker battery.
    D. double the power setting on the AED.

COMPLETE THE FOLLOWING

1. List the four elements of the chain of survival.

A. _____

B. _____

C. _____

D. _____

LABEL THE DIAGRAM

Fill in the name of each component of the cardiovascular system on the line provided.

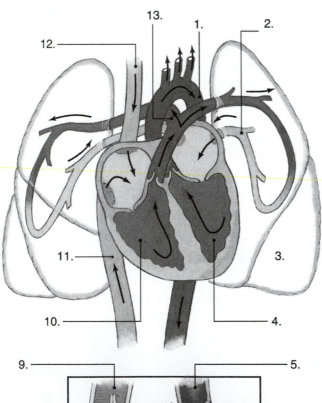

1. _____

2. _____

3. _____

4. _____

5. _____

6. _____

7. _____

8. _____

9. _____

10. _____

11. _____

12. _____

13. _____

VIRTUAL STREET SCENES

(First review the Street Scenes on pp. 364–365 of the textbook. Then answer the questions below.)

1. It was decided very quickly that ALS should be dispatched. This was an appropriate decision. Why is ALS needed in this type of call?

2. If the patient had prescribed nitroglycerin, would it have been appropriate to assist her in the administration of it? (Assume that you have a standing order to assist with nitroglycerin.)

3. If you had applied the AED and it did not shock the patient, what would that have meant?

4. How often should vital signs be taken on this patient? What is her priority?

WEB SIMULATION

For interactive case studies that will help you review and practice basic skills, visit the *Emergency Care 9e Companion Website* at www.bradybooks.com/emergencycare.

EMT-BASIC SKILLS PERFORMANCE CHECKLISTS

▶ **NITROGLYCERIN ASSIST**

❑ Take BSI precautions.

❑ Perform focused assessment for cardiac patient.

❑ Take BP (systolic pressure must be above 100 mm Hg).

❑ Contact medical direction for authorization to administer.

❑ Assure patient is alert.

❑ Assure right patient, right medication, right dose, and right route.

❑ Check expiration date.

❑ Assist patient with nitroglycerin administration.

❑ Reassess vital signs and chest pain after each dose. Document findings.

NOTE: If the blood pressure falls below 100 systolic, treat the patient for shock (hypoperfusion). Transport promptly.

▶ **CARDIAC ARREST MANAGEMENT AND THE AED**

❑ Take BSI precautions.

❑ Assess patient for breathing and pulses.

❑ If no pulse is present, direct CPR while attaching AED to patient.

❑ Direct rescuer to stop CPR.

❑ Verify absence of spontaneous pulse.

❑ Turn on defibrillator power.

❑ Ensure all individuals are standing clear of patient.

❑ Initiate analysis of rhythm.

❑ Deliver shock (up to three successive shocks).

❑ Verify presence or absence of spontaneous pulse. If absent:

　　–Direct resumption of CPR for one minute.
　　–Gather additional information on arrest event.
　　–Confirm effectiveness of CPR (ventilation and compressions).
　　–Direct insertion of an airway adjunct (oropharyngeal/nasopharyngeal).
　　–Direct ventilation of patient with high-concentration oxygen.
　　–Assure CPR continues without unnecessary/prolonged interruption.

❑ After one minute of CPR, re-evaluate patient.

❑ Repeat defibrillator sequence.

❑ Check carotid pulse.

❑ If there is a spontaneous pulse, check patient's breathing.

❑ If breathing is adequate, provide high-concentration oxygen by nonrebreather mask. If breathing is inadequate, ventilate patient with high-concentration oxygen.

❑ Transport patient without delay.

Chapter Nineteen

DIABETIC EMERGENCIES AND ALTERED MENTAL STATUS

MATCH TERMINOLOGY/DEFINITIONS

A. Form of sugar that provides the body's basic source of energy

B. Condition brought about by decreased insulin production; also called "sugar diabetes" or simply "diabetes"

C. Hormone produced by the pancreas or taken as a medication by many diabetics that aids cells in utilizing glucose

D. Uncontrolled muscular movements

E. Prolonged seizure, or when a person suffers two or more convulsive seizures without regaining full consciousness

F. Low blood sugar

G. Medical condition that sometimes causes seizures

H. High blood sugar

I. Sudden change in sensation, behavior, or movement that can, in its most severe form, produce convulsions

J. Blockage or bursting of a major blood vessel supplying the brain; also called a cerebrovascular accident (CVA)

_____ **1.** Convulsions

_____ **2.** Diabetes mellitus

_____ **3.** Epilepsy

_____ **4.** Glucose

_____ **5.** Hyperglycemia

_____ **6.** Hypoglycemia

_____ **7.** Insulin

_____ **8.** Seizure

_____ **9.** Status epilepticus

_____ **10.** Stroke

MULTIPLE-CHOICE REVIEW

_____ **1.** The relationship of glucose to insulin is often described as
   A. oppositional.
   B. synergistic.
   C. a lock and key mechanism.
   D. antagonistic.

_____ **2.** The condition brought about by decreased insulin production is known as
   A. diabetes mellitus.
   B. hypotension.
   C. hypoglycemia.
   D. cerebrovascular accident.

_____ **3.** The most common medical emergency for the diabetic patient is called
   A. diabetes mellitus.
   B. hypotension.
   C. hypoglycemia.
   D. cerebrovascular accident.

_____ **4.** When a diabetic overexercises or overexerts, a medical condition called _____ can develop.
   A. hypoglycemia
   B. hyperglycemia
   C. diabetes mellitus
   D. acute pulmonary edema.

135

_____ 5. Which of the following is <u>not</u> a cause of hypoglycemia?
 A. The patient may have taken too much insulin by mistake.
 B. The patient ate a box of candy too fast.
 C. The patient has been vomiting.
 D. The patient has been fasting.

_____ 6. If sugar is not replenished quickly for the hypoglycemic patient, the
 A. patient may have permanent brain damage.
 B. patient may go into pulmonary edema.
 C. patient will have chest pain.
 D. body can live off its internal sugar supply for up to two weeks.

_____ 7. The clues that a patient is a diabetic include all of the following <u>except</u>
 A. a medical identification bracelet.
 B. the presence of insulin in the refrigerator.
 C. low-fat food in the freezer.
 D. information provided by family members.

_____ 8. Which one of the following is <u>not</u> a common oral medication used to treat diabetes?
 A. Humulin   C. Glucotrol
 B. Sugunoil   D. Micronase

_____ 9. An intoxicated appearance and uncharacteristic behavior are typical of
 A. shock.   C. cardiac arrest.
 B. dehydration.   D. diabetic emergency.

_____ 10. Diabetics often present the EMT-B with all of the following signs and symptoms <u>except</u>
 A. cold, clammy skin.   C. anxiety.
 B. decreased heart rate.   D. combativeness.

_____ 11. In order for the EMT-B to consider administering oral glucose, the patient must have an altered mental status, a
 A. history of diabetes, and be awake enough to swallow.
 B. prescribed medication, and an absent gag reflex.
 C. history of seizures, and be awake.
 D. Medic Alert tag that says "diabetic," and a head injury.

_____ 12. When reassessing a patient to whom you have administered oral glucose, you note the patient's condition has not improved. What action should you take?
 A. Call the patient's personal physician.
 B. Give glucose in orange juice.
 C. Consult medical direction about whether to administer more glucose.
 D. Administer oxygen by nasal cannula.

_____ 13. Which position is most appropriate for transport of the diabetic patient who is not awake enough to swallow and does not need ventilation?
 A. supine   C. recovery
 B. prone   D. Fowler's

_____ 14. Which statement is most correct related to children with diabetes?
 A. Children are more likely than adults to eat correctly.
 B. Children are less likely than adults to exhaust blood sugar levels.
 C. Children are more at risk than adults for developing hypoglycemia.
 D. Children have a greater risk for medical emergencies than adults.

_____ 15. Which of the following would <u>most</u> likely indicate an alteration in the patient's blood sugar level?
 A. right lower abdominal pain   C. change in mental status
 B. nausea and vomiting   D. rigid abdomen on palpation

_____ **16.** Before and after administering oral glucose, make sure you
   A. check for distal pulses in both arms.
   B. document the mental status of the patient.
   C. increase the oxygen flow rate by 5 liters per minute.
   D. have the patient drink a glass of water.

_____ **17.** A trade name for oral glucose is
   A. D_5W.   **C.** Insulin.
   B. Lactose.   **D.** Insta-glucose.

_____ **18.** A patient is very confused and disoriented. Before deciding the patient has
   a behavioral problem, the EMT-B should consider all of the following <u>except</u>
   A. a potential head injury.   **C.** hypoxia.
   B. a brain tumor.   **D.** glucose allergy.

_____ **19.** People with diabetes routinely test the level of sugar in their blood using a
   A. capnograph.   **C.** urinal.
   B. glucose meter.   **D.** oximeter.

_____ **20.** Complications of diabetes include
   A. kidney failure.   **C.** blindness.
   B. heart disease.   **D.** any of the above.

_____ **21.** The reading on the device described in question #19 is reported in
   A. grams of sugar per liter of blood.
   B. centimeters of blood per decimeter of sugar.
   C. milligrams of glucose per deciliter of blood.
   D. none of the above.

_____ **22.** If the diabetic is symptomatic and has a sugar level below _____, he is
   considered hypoglycemic.
   A. 140   **C.** 100
   B. 120   **D.** 80

_____ **23.** If the diabetic is symptomatic and has a sugar level above _____, he is
   considered hyperglycemic.
   A. 120   **C.** 80
   B. 100   **D.** 60

_____ **24.** The <u>most</u> common cause of seizures in adults is
   A. taking a double dose of anti-seizure medication.
   B. taking a small dose of anti-seizure medication.
   C. not taking anti-seizure medication.
   D. use of illicit street drugs.

_____ **25.** Seizures are commonly caused by all of the following <u>except</u>
   A. cold exposure.   **C.** a brain tumor.
   B. a high fever.   **D.** an infection.

_____ **26.** Which of the following is <u>not</u> a characteristic of an idiopathic seizure?
   A. lasts longer than 10 minutes **C.** has an unknown cause
   B. occurs spontaneously   **D.** often starts in childhood

_____ **27.** Convulsive seizures may be seen with
   A. epilepsy or hypoglycemia.
   B. hyperventilation or AMI.
   C. anaphylaxis or pulmonary embolism.
   D. hyperglycemia or asthma.

_____ **28.** The best-known condition that results in seizures is
   A. a stroke.   **C.** measles.
   B. epilepsy.   **D.** eclampsia.

_____ 29. Most people associate a _____ seizure with epilepsy.
   A. generalized tonic-clonic   C. simple partial
   B. complex partial   D. idiopathic

_____ 30. When obtaining the medical history of a seizure patient, find out from
          bystanders all of the following except
   A. how long the seizure lasted.
   B. what the patient did after the seizure.
   C. what the patient was doing prior to the seizure.
   D. what the family's reaction was to the seizure.

_____ 31. A seizure patient becomes cyanotic. After convulsions have ended, what
          action should you take?
   A. Wait for the patient's color to return to normal.
   B. Place a nonrebreather mask with oxygen on the patient.
   C. Provide artificial ventilations with supplemental oxygen.
   D. Monitor the pulse closely for 2 minutes.

_____ 32. You notice that a bystander has placed a tongue blade in the corner of a seizure
          patient's mouth. What should you do?
   A. Begin oxygen therapy with a nonrebreather mask.
   B. Carefully remove the object from the patient's mouth.
   C. Immobilize the patient on a long spine board.
   D. Immediately transport to the hospital.

_____ 33. A seizure will normally last about _____ minutes.
   A. 1 to 3   C. 7 to 10
   B. 4 to 6   D. 30

_____ 34. A patient has two or more back-to-back seizures without regaining full
          consciousness. This is called
   A. repeating seizure.   C. status asthmaticus.
   B. status epilepticus.   D. convulsions.

_____ 35. If you suspect a conscious patient has had a stroke, you should transport
          her in the _____ position.
   A. recovery   C. prone
   B. supine   D. semi-sitting

_____ 36. A stroke patient has difficulty saying what he is thinking even
          though he clearly understands you. This is called
   A. receptive aphasia.   C. miscommunication.
   B. expressive aphasia.   D. confusion.

_____ 37. The patient can speak clearly but cannot understand what you are
          saying. This is called
   A. expressive aphasia.   C. receptive aphasia.
   B. hyperactivity.   D. petit mal seizure.

_____ 38. A common sign of a cerebrovascular accident is
   A. tingling in both legs.   C. low blood pressure.
   B. diminished urine flow.   D. headache.

_____ 39. Signs and symptoms of a stroke include
   A. vomiting.   C. loss of bladder control.
   B. seizures.   D. all of the above.

_____ 40. When a patient has many of the signs and symptoms of a stroke,
          which completely resolve in less than 24 hours, this is called a(n)
   A. altered mental status (AMS).   C. acute myocardial infarction (AMI).
   B. transient ischemic attack (TIA). D. cerebrovascular accident (CVA).

COMPLETE THE FOLLOWING

1. List six of the signs and symptoms associated with a diabetic emergency.

   A. _____

   B. _____

   C. _____

   D. _____

   E. _____

   F. _____

2. Give four reasons a diabetic may develop hyperglycemia.

   A. _____

   B. _____

   C. _____

   D. _____

VIRTUAL STREET SCENES

(First review the Street Scenes on pp. 384–385 of the textbook. Then answer the questions below.)

1. What advice should be given to this patient and his friend before they walk away?

2. Aside from not eating all day, what are other possible causes of hypoglycemia?

3. If you did not have oral glucose with you, what else could you have used to help bring up this patient's sugar level?

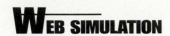

WEB SIMULATION

For interactive case studies that will help you review and practice basic skills, visit the *Emergency Care 9e Companion Website* at www.bradybooks.com/emergencycare.

EMT-BASIC SKILLS PERFORMANCE CHECKLIST

▶ **ORAL GLUCOSE ADMINISTRATION**

❑ Conduct a scene size-up.

❑ Take BSI precautions.

❑ Perform initial assessment.

❑ Perform focused history and physical exam and take vital signs.

❑ Consult medical direction.

❑ Assure signs and symptoms of altered mental status with a history of diabetes.

❑ Assure patient is awake with a gag reflex.

❑ Place glucose on tongue depressor between cheek and gum.

❑ Perform ongoing assessment.

Chapter Twenty
ALLERGIC REACTIONS

MATCH TERMINOLOGY/DEFINITIONS

A. Red, itchy, possibly raised blotches on the skin that often result from an allergic reaction

B. Severe or life-threatening allergic reaction in which the blood vessels dilate, causing a drop in blood pressure, and the tissues lining the respiratory system swell, interfering with the airway

C. Something that causes an allergic reaction

D. Hormone produced by the body; as a medication, it constricts blood vessels and dilates respiratory passages and is used to relieve severe allergic reactions.

E. Syringe (pre-loaded with medication) that has a spring-loaded device that pushes the needle through the skin when the tip of the device is pressed firmly against the body

_____ 1. Allergen

_____ 2. Anaphylaxis

_____ 3. Auto-injector

_____ 4. Epinephrine

_____ 5. Hives

MULTIPLE-CHOICE REVIEW

_____ 1. An exaggerated response of the body's immune system to any substance is called a(n) _____ reaction.
   A. vasoconstricting
   B. immune
   C. allergic
   D. syncopal

_____ 2. Why are allergic reactions sometimes treated as a high priority?
   A. The patient can vomit.
   B. The patient can become covered with hives.
   C. They can speed up the heart rate.
   D. They can cause airway obstruction.

_____ 3. The first time a patient is exposed to an allergen, the person's immune system
   A. reacts violently.
   B. shuts down.
   C. forms antibodies.
   D. ignores the allergen.

_____ 4. The second time a patient is exposed to an allergen, the body reactions include all of the following except
   A. destruction of antibodies.
   B. difficulty breathing.
   C. massive swelling.
   D. dilation of the blood vessels.

_____ 5. Common causes of allergic reactions include all of the following except
   A. hornet stings.
   B. eggs and milk.
   C. poison ivy and penicillin.
   D. red fruits and vegetables.

6. Why is it important to find out if a patient is allergic to latex?
   A. so you do not wear gloves that could cause an allergic reaction
   B. because the patient will also be allergic to milk
   C. because latex allergy can produce antitoxins
   D. because a latex allergy causes immediate cardiac arrest

7. The respiratory signs and symptoms of anaphylactic shock include all of the following <u>except</u>
   A. rapid breathing.   C. cough.
   B. hives.   D. stridor.

8. The effects on the cardiac system of an allergic reaction could include _____ heart rate and _____ blood pressure.
   A. decreased : decreased
   B. increased : increased
   C. decreased : increased
   D. increased : decreased

9. To be considered a severe allergic reaction, a patient must have signs and symptoms of shock or
   A. a history of allergies.   C. respiratory distress.
   B. massive swelling.   D. increased blood pressure.

10. After administering epinephrine, the EMT-B should
    A. prepare another dose.
    B. reassess the patient after 2 minutes.
    C. decrease the oxygen being administered.
    D. allow the patient to remain at home.

11. If you see a patient who has no history of allergies and is having her first allergic reaction, you should
    A. consult with medical direction.
    B. treat for shock and transport immediately.
    C. administer epinephrine via auto-injector.
    D. attempt to determine the cause immediately.

12. If a patient has an epinephrine auto-injector, besides helping him take the medication, you should always
    A. ask if the patient has any spare auto-injectors for the trip to the hospital.
    B. call the patient's physician and request another dosage of the medication.
    C. determine if other family members have a history of allergic reactions.
    D. take the insect or substance that caused the reaction to the hospital.

13. The recommended location for injection with the auto-injector is the
    A. center of the back.   C. buttocks.
    B. lateral mid thigh.   D. biceps.

14. Epinephrine auto-injectors come in two different sizes. The child size contains
    A. 0.05 mg.   C. 0.5 mg.
    B. 0.15 mg.   D. 1.0 mg.

15. Which statement is true related to anaphylactic reactions in infants and children?
    A. Infants frequently experience anaphylactic reactions.
    B. Children "outgrow" allergies as they mature.
    C. Anaphylactic reactions are common in younger children.
    D. Parents seldom can provide useful information about the child's medical history.

COMPLETE THE FOLLOWING

1. List ten signs and symptoms of allergic reaction or anaphylactic shock.

   A. _____

   B. _____

   C. _____

   D. _____

   E. _____

   F. _____

   G. _____

   H. _____

   I. _____

   J. _____

2. For a patient to be considered in anaphylaxis, list two signs either of
   which must be evident.

   A. _____

   B. _____

LABEL THE DIAGRAMS

Fill in the name of each substance that may cause an allergic reaction on the
line provided.

1. _____

2. _____

3. _____

4. _____

VIRTUAL STREET SCENES

(First review the Street Scenes on pp. 398–399 of the textbook. Then answer the questions below.)

1. If the patient had an epinephrine auto-injector, would it be appropriate to use it in this situation? If so, where would you inject it?

2. Would it be appropriate to call for an estimated time of arrival (ETA) on the ALS unit? Why or why not?

3. If the patient went into cardiac arrest, what would be your patient care priorities?

WEB SIMULATION

For interactive case studies that will help you review and practice basic skills, visit the *Emergency Care 9e Companion Website* at www.bradybooks.com/emergencycare.

EMT-BASIC SKILLS PERFORMANCE CHECKLIST

▶ **EPINEPHRINE AUTO-INJECTOR ASSIST**

❑ Take BSI precautions.

❑ Perform an initial assessment. Provide high-concentration oxygen by nonrebreather mask.

❑ Obtain SAMPLE history.

❑ Take patient's vital signs.

❑ Contact medical direction for authorization.

❑ Obtain patient's prescribed auto-injector.

❑ Check medication for expiration date.

❑ Check medication for cloudiness or discoloration.

❑ Remove safety cap from the injector.

❑ Assure injector is prescribed for patient.

❑ Remove cap from auto-injector. Place tip of auto-injector against patient's thigh (lateral portion, midway between waist and knee).

(continued next page)

❑ Push injector firmly against thigh until injector activates.

❑ Hold injector in place until medication is injected (at least 10 seconds).

❑ Properly discard auto-injector in biohazard container.

❑ Document patient's response to medication and time.

❑ Perform ongoing assessment, paying special attention to the patient's ABCs and vital signs, while transporting.

CASE STUDY

▶ THE LAKEFRONT EMERGENCY

You respond to a camp on the lake for a call from a woman having difficulty breathing. Upon your arrival, after ensuring the scene is safe, you find a woman in her forties who is clutching her chest and is having obvious breathing difficulty.

1. Is there a need for another ambulance?

2. Should you call for an ALS unit to respond?

After taking BSI precautions, you begin your initial assessment. There is no reason to suspect trauma, and the patient has an open airway. She is responsive, although she talks in short, choppy sentences. She knows her name, where she is, and the day of the week.

3. Why is she talking in short, choppy sentences?

4. What would be your assessment of her level of responsiveness?

A high-pitched musical tone is heard as she breathes. She shows other signs of respiratory distress.

5. What is the name of her breathing sound, and what are some of the potential causes of this sound?

6. What are some additional signs of breathing difficulty that you may observe in this patient?

You decide that beginning oxygen administration is an appropriate thing to do at this time.

7. How would you deliver the oxygen, and how many liters per minute would you administer?

You note the patient has a weak and rapid radial pulse. There is no reason to suspect any life-threatening external bleeding in this instance. The patient is very pale and is sweating profusely. She also complains of chest tightness and dizziness, which she denies she has ever had before.

8. Would you prioritize this patient as a low or high priority? Why?

9. What would be the best position in which to transport the patient and why?

As you begin to prepare the patient for transport, you start the focused history and physical exam. The patient has chest tightness and breathing difficulty, which came on suddenly. The pain is across the upper chest, doesn't radiate, and is constant. Nothing the patient does makes the pain go away; she states it is a 7 on a scale of 1 to 10 with 10 being the worst pain she ever had. The pain has been present for approximately 15 minutes. You assign a crew member to obtain a complete set of vital signs as you quickly listen to her lungs. She has a weak and rapid pulse at 110, respirations are labored at 26 per minute, and her blood pressure is 88/50.

10. As you load the patient into the ambulance, what additional history should you obtain?

Your patient states she was cleaning out the gutter and may have been stung by a bee. She previously reacted severely to a bee sting and carries a "bee-sting kit."

11. **A)** What medicine is usually in these kits? **B)** Should you help her take the medicine?

12. **A)** Is it necessary to call a doctor? **B)** What must be checked prior to administering the medicine?

As you leave the scene, the driver arranges for an ALS intercept on the way to the hospital. Other than reassessing the patient after administering the medication, you continue to monitor the patient. About five minutes en route, your driver pulls the ambulance to the side of the road momentarily as the ALS paramedic jumps in with his equipment. Then you proceed to the hospital.

13. What would be your quick report to the paramedic on **A)** the patient's chief complaint, **B)** your assessment of the situation, and **C)** the treatment you have given?

14. What care would you expect to see the paramedic give en route to the hospital?

Chapter Twenty-One

POISONING AND OVERDOSE EMERGENCIES

MATCH TERMINOLOGY/DEFINITIONS

A. Any substance that can harm the body by altering cell structure or functions

B. Stimulants, such as amphetamines, that affect the central nervous system to excite the user

C. State in which a patient's body reacts severely when deprived of an abused substance

D. Poisons that are taken into the body through unbroken skin

E. Depressants, such as barbiturates, that depress the central nervous system

F. Poisons that are swallowed

G. Class of drugs that affect the nervous system and change many normal body activities; their legal use is for relief of pain

H. Substance that absorbs many poisons and prevents them from being absorbed by the body

I. Thinning down or weakening by mixing with something else

J. Severe reaction that can be part of alcohol withdrawal, characterized by sweating, trembling, anxiety, and hallucinations

K. Poisons that are breathed in

L. Mind-affecting or mind-altering drugs that act on the central nervous system to produce excitement and distortion of perceptions

M. Poisonous substance secreted by bacteria, plants, or animals

N. Vaporizing compounds, such as cleaning fluid, that are breathed in by an abuser to produce a "high"

O. Substance that will neutralize a poison or its effects

_____ **1.** Absorbed poisons

_____ **2.** Activated charcoal

_____ **3.** Antidote

_____ **4.** Delirium tremens

_____ **5.** Dilution

_____ **6.** Downers

_____ **7.** Hallucinogens

_____ **8.** Ingested poisons

_____ **9.** Inhaled poisons

_____ **10.** Narcotics

_____ **11.** Poison

_____ **12.** Toxin

_____ **13.** Uppers

_____ **14.** Volatile chemicals

_____ **15.** Withdrawal

MULTIPLE-CHOICE REVIEW

_____ 1. Which of the following is an environmental clue at the scene that can be used to help you determine that your patient may have been poisoned?
A. The patient appears to have been vomiting.
B. There is an empty pill bottle on the night table.
C. The patient has an altered mental status.
D. The patient states he/she has a headache.

_____ 2. Which of the following is the most accurate definition of a poison? A poison is any
A. substance that can harm the body, sometimes seriously enough to create a medical emergency
B. foreign substance swallowed by the patient
C. substance that could kill the patient if it is injected into the body
D. substance labeled with a hazardous material placard or label

_____ 3. Most of the over one million poisonings in the United States yearly are due to
A. suicide attempts by adults.
B. attempts to murder someone.
C. accidents involving young children.
D. teenagers on illicit drugs.

_____ 4. A substance secreted by plants, animals, or bacteria that is poisonous to humans is called a
A. chemical.
B. toxin.
C. narcotic.
D. drug.

_____ 5. Due to the poisons they produce, plants such as _____ can be dangerous to humans or pets.
A. mistletoe
B. mushrooms
C. rubber plants
D. all of the above

_____ 6. Bacteria may produce toxins that cause deadly diseases such as
A. HIV.
B. botulism.
C. penicillin.
D. steroids.

_____ 7. For most poisonous substances, the reaction is more serious in
A. the evening hours.
B. the elderly and the ill.
C. smaller concentrations.
D. summer.

_____ 8. Which one of the following is not a way that poisons damage the body?
A. destroying skin and other tissues
B. enhancing normal biochemical processes
C. overstimulating the central nervous system
D. displacing oxygen on the hemoglobin

_____ 9. Poisons may enter the body through any of the following routes except
A. inhalation.
B. ingestion.
C. injection.
D. excretion.

_____ 10. Carbon monoxide, chlorine, and ammonia are examples of _____ poisons.
A. ingested
B. injected
C. inhaled
D. swallowed

_____ 11. Examples of absorbed poisons include
A. insecticides and agricultural chemicals.
B. carbon monoxide and ammonia.
C. insect stings and snake bites.
D. aspirin and LSD.

_____ 12. The venom of a snake bite is an example of an _____ poison.
A. ingested
B. injected
C. inhaled
D. absorbed

_____ 13. Why is it important to determine when the ingestion of a poison occurred?
   A. Different poisons act on the body at different rates.
   B. Those who ingest poison in the evening tend to vomit more.
   C. Dilution of the poison is not effective after ten minutes.
   D. The antidote will work more effectively once the poison is in the intestines.

_____ 14. If you suspect poisoning by ingestion, after assuring a child has a patent airway, ask the parent for the child's
   A. name.
   B. weight.
   C. last visit to a physician.
   D. favorite drink.

_____ 15. The most common results of poison ingestion are
   A. altered mental status and diarrhea.
   B. nausea and vomiting.
   C. abdominal pain and diarrhea.
   D. chemical burns around the mouth and stomach pain.

_____ 16. Activated charcoal is used to
   A. act as an antidote.
   B. dilute the poisonous substance.
   C. reduce the amount of poison absorbed by the body.
   D. speed up the digestion of most chemicals in the body.

_____ 17. The difference between activated charcoal and regular charcoal is that
   A. activated charcoal is manufactured to have many cracks and crevices.
   B. regular charcoal is too large to swallow.
   C. activated charcoal is mixed with a substance to cause vomiting.
   D. regular charcoal is not diluted when used.

_____ 18. The decision on when to use activated charcoal is best made
   A. en route to the hospital.
   B. upon arrival at the emergency department.
   C. with medical direction or poison-control center consultation.
   D. in consultation with the patient's family physician.

_____ 19. Activated charcoal is not routinely used with ingestion of
   A. caustic substances.
   B. strong acids.
   C. strong alkalis.
   D. all of the above.

_____ 20. Examples of caustic substances include all of the following except
   A. lye.
   B. venom.
   C. toilet bowl cleaner.
   D. oven cleaner.

_____ 21. A patient who continues to cough violently after a gasoline ingestion should
   A. not be given activated charcoal.
   B. not be given oxygen.
   C. be transported immediately.
   D. be treated like a patient with an airway obstruction.

_____ 22. When a physician orders dilution of an ingested substance, you can use either water or
   A. a cola drink.
   B. coffee.
   C. milk.
   D. apple juice.

_____ 23. The most common inhaled poison is
   A. carbon dioxide.
   B. nitrogen.
   C. carbon monoxide.
   D. phosgene.

_____ 24. As you approach a patient who has passed out while cleaning a large tank, you smell an unusual odor. What should you do?
   A. Stand back and attempt to learn more about the chemical involved.
   B. Rapidly remove the patient from the area using a drag maneuver.
   C. Ignore the smell; it is probably a normal odor around industrial sites.
   D. Ask his coworkers to bring the patient to your ambulance.

_____ **25.** The principal prehospital treatment of a patient who has inhaled poison is
  A. administering activated charcoal to the patient.
  B. administering high-concentration oxygen.
  C. providing full spinal immobilization.
  D. administering an antidote.

_____ **26.** Besides motor-vehicle exhaust, where else might you find carbon monoxide?
  A. in the patient compartment of your ambulance
  B. wherever you can smell its odor
  C. around an improperly vented wood-burning stove
  D. around the foundation of a house

_____ **27.** How does carbon monoxide affect the body?
  A. It causes severe respiratory burns.
  B. It prevents the normal carrying of oxygen by the red blood cells.
  C. It causes the tissues in the airway to swell, making breathing difficult.
  D. It stimulates the central nervous system to decrease oxygen consumption.

_____ **28.** A conscious patient who you suspect has carbon monoxide poisoning may exhibit any of the following <u>except</u>
  A. cyanosis.
  C. dizziness.
  B. altered mental status.
  D. cherry red lips.

_____ **29.** If a patient has been contaminated by a poisonous powder, how should she be treated?
  A. Brush off as much powder as possible, then irrigate.
  B. Immediately start irrigation with very cold water.
  C. Leave the powder in place and transport immediately.
  D. Irrigate with water for 20 minutes.

_____ **30.** If you smell alcohol on the breath or clothes of a patient, you should
  A. call for police immediately.
  B. not let this sidetrack you from doing a complete assessment.
  C. ask the patient how much he has had to drink today.
  D. assume that the patient will not give you the entire truth about his condition.

_____ **31.** Of the following signs and symptoms, which one is <u>not</u> seen with alcohol abuse but is with a diabetic emergency?
  A. acetone breath
  B. hallucinations
  C. slurred speech
  D. swaying and unsteadiness of movement

_____ **32.** The sweating, trembling, anxiety, and hallucinations found in the alcohol withdrawal patient are called
  A. withdrawal signs.
  C. delirium tremens.
  B. seizures.
  D. Parkinson's tremors.

_____ **33.** A patient who has mixed alcohol and drugs will exhibit
  A. uncontrolled shivering.
  C. extreme calmness.
  B. depressed vital signs.
  D. all of the above.

_____ **34.** When interviewing an intoxicated patient, do not begin by asking if he has taken any drugs. The reason for this statement is that
  A. the presence of drugs will negate the presence of the alcohol.
  B. the patient may feel you are accusing him of a crime.
  C. alcoholics generally do not take drugs.
  D. the patient would probably not tell the truth.

_____ **35.** Drugs that stimulate the nervous system to excite the user are called
  A. uppers.
  C. narcotics.
  B. downers.
  D. antihypertensives.

_____ 36. Tranquilizers or sleeping pills are examples of
A. uppers.   C. narcotics.
B. downers.   D. hallucinogens.

_____ 37. Drugs that have a depressant effect on the central nervous system are called
A. uppers.   C. narcotics.
B. downers.   D. hallucinogens.

_____ 38. Drugs capable of producing stupor or sleep that are often used to relieve pain are called
A. uppers.   C. narcotics.
B. downers.   D. hallucinogens.

_____ 39. Mind-altering drugs that act on the nervous system to produce an intense state of excitement or distortion of the user's perceptions are called
A. uppers.   C. narcotics.
B. downers.   D. hallucinogens.

_____ 40. A class of drugs that have few legal uses and are dissolved in the mouth are called
A. narcotics.   C. hallucinogens.
B. uppers.   D. downers.

_____ 41. Cleaning fluid, glue, and model cement are examples of
A. hallucinogens.   C. diuretics.
B. volatile chemicals.   D. narcotics.

_____ 42. A patient who has overdosed on an upper may have signs and symptoms such as
A. excitement, increased pulse and breathing rates, dilated pupils, and rapid speech.
B. sluggishness, sleepiness, and lack of coordination of body and speech.
C. fast pulse rate, dilated pupils, flushed face, and "see" or "hear" things.
D. reduced pulse rate and rate and depth of breathing, constricted pupils, and sweating.

_____ 43. A patient who has overdosed on a downer may have signs and symptoms such as
A. excitement, increased pulse and breathing rates, dilated pupils, and rapid speech.
B. sluggishness, sleepiness, and lack of coordination of body and speech.
C. fast pulse rate, dilated pupils, flushed face, and "see" or "hear" things.
D. reduced pulse rate and rate and depth of breathing, constricted pupils, and sweating.

_____ 44. A patient who has overdosed on a hallucinogen may have signs and symptoms such as
A. excitement, increased pulse and breathing rates, dilated pupils, and rapid speech.
B. sluggishness, sleepiness, and lack of coordination of body and speech.
C. fast pulse rate, dilated pupils, flushed face, and "see" or "hear" things.
D. reduced pulse rate and rate and depth of breathing, constricted pupils, and sweating.

_____ 45. A patient who has overdosed on a narcotic may have signs and symptoms such as
A. excitement, increased pulse and breathing rates, dilated pupils, and rapid speech.
B. sluggishness, sleepiness, and lack of coordination of body and speech.
C. fast pulse rate, dilated pupils, flushed face, and "see" or "hear" things.
D. reduced pulse rate and rate and depth of breathing, constricted pupils, and sweating.

COMPLETE THE FOLLOWING

1. What information should the EMT-B document for medical direction when treating a patient you suspect was poisoned?

   A. _____   E. _____

   B. _____   F. _____

   C. _____   G. _____

   D. _____   H. _____

2. List at least six signs and symptoms of alcohol abuse.

   A. _____

   B. _____

   C. _____

   D. _____

   E. _____

   F. _____

LABEL THE DIAGRAMS

Fill in the way that each type of poison enters the body.

1. _____

2. _____

3. _____

4. _____

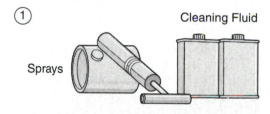
① Sprays   Cleaning Fluid

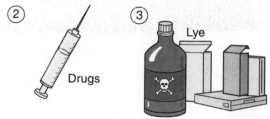
② Drugs

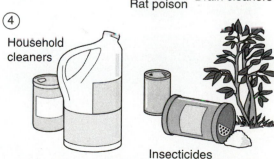
③ Lye   Rat poison   Drain cleaners

④ Household cleaners   Insecticides

COMPLETE THE CHART

Fill in the type of commonly abused drug on the line provided. Indicate on the chart whether each drug is an upper, downer, narcotic, mind-altering, or volatile chemical.

AMPHETAMINE   1. _____

CODEINE   2. _____

LSD   3. _____

PSILOCYBIN   4. _____

GASOLINE   5. _____

SECOBARBITAL   6. _____

METHAQUALONE   7. _____

COCAINE   8. _____

DEXTROAMPHETAMINE   9. _____

CHLORAL HYDRATE   10. _____

MESCALINE   11. _____

MORNING GLORY SEEDS   12. _____

STP   13. _____

HEROIN   14. _____

BUTYL NITRATE   15. _____

PCP   16. _____

PRELUDIN   17. _____

METHADONE   18. _____

BARBITURATES   19. _____

DEMEROL   20. _____

VIRTUAL STREET SCENES

(First review the Street Scenes on pp. 420–421 of the textbook. Then answer the questions below.)

1. Imagine you were confronted with an infant who had an altered mental status, as well as evidence of ingested poison. Would you quickly administer activated charcoal to the patient? Why or why not?

2. If the infant continues to vomit, what emergency care should be your highest priority?

3. Why is it necessary to take the oil to the hospital?

WEB SIMULATION

For interactive case studies that will help you review and practice basic skills, visit the *Emergency Care 9e Companion Website* at www.bradybooks.com/emergencycare.

EMT-BASIC SKILL PERFORMANCE CHECKLISTS

▶ **MANAGEMENT OF INGESTED POISONS**

❑ Take BSI precautions.

❑ Conduct an initial assessment.

❑ Maintain an open airway.

❑ Perform a focused history and physical exam.

❑ Assess baseline vital signs and gather a SAMPLE history.

❑ Quickly gather information about the substance.

❑ Call medical direction on the scene or en route.

❑ If directed, administer activated charcoal.

❑ Position patient for vomiting and save all vomitus. Have suction ready.

❑ Perform an ongoing assessment.

❑ Transport as soon as possible.

▶ MANAGEMENT OF INHALED POISONS

❑ Size-up the situation to prevent injury to yourself and your crew.

❑ Take BSI precautions.

❑ Remove patient from the source.

❑ Avoid contaminating yourself with poison.

❑ Maintain an open airway. Stay alert for vomiting. Properly position patient and have suction equipment ready.

❑ Conduct an initial assessment.

❑ Administer high-concentration oxygen by nonrebreather mask.

❑ Perform a focused history and physical exam, including SAMPLE history.

❑ Remove contaminated clothing and jewelry.

❑ Assess baseline vital signs.

❑ Quickly gather information about the product (containers, bottles, and labels).

❑ Call medical direction on the scene or en route.

❑ Transport as soon as possible.

❑ Perform ongoing assessment en route.

NOTE: In the presence of hazardous fumes or gases, wear protective clothing and self-contained breathing apparatus or wait for those who are properly trained and equipped to enter the scene and bring the patient out to a safe area.

▶ MANAGEMENT OF ABSORBED POISONS

❑ Size-up the situation, and take the necessary precautions to prevent injury to yourself and your crew.

❑ Take BSI precautions.

❑ Remove the patient from the source. Avoid contaminating yourself with the poison.

❑ Conduct an initial assessment.

❑ Maintain an open airway.

❑ Administer high-concentration oxygen.

❑ Perform a focused history and physical exam, including SAMPLE history and vital signs.

❑ Brush powders from the patient. Be careful not to abrade the patient's skin.

❑ Remove contaminated clothing and other articles such as shoes and jewelry.

❑ Quickly gather information about the product.

❑ If appropriate, irrigate with a large amount of clear water for at least 20 minutes. Call medical direction.

❑ Perform an ongoing assessment.

❑ Be alert for shock, and transport as soon as possible.

Chapter Twenty-Two

ENVIRONMENTAL EMERGENCIES

MATCH TERMINOLOGY/DEFINITIONS

▶ **PART A**

A. Change from liquid to gas; as perspiration on the skin vaporizes, the body experiences a cooling effect.

B. Abbreviation that stands for arterial gas embolism

C. Application of an external heat source to rewarm the body of a hypothermic patient

D. Carrying away of heat by currents of air or water or other gases or liquids

E. Death caused by changes in the lungs resulting from immersion in water

F. Direct transfer of heat from one material to another through direct contact

G. Condition resulting from nitrogen trapped in the body's tissues caused by coming up too quickly from a deep, prolonged dive

H. Application of heat to the lateral chest, neck, armpits, and groin of a hypothermic patient

I. Increase in body temperature above normal; life-threatening in its extreme

J. Gas bubble in the bloodstream; more accurately called an arterial gas embolism

_____ 1. Active rewarming

_____ 2. AGE

_____ 3. Air embolism

_____ 4. Central rewarming

_____ 5. Conduction

_____ 6. Convection

_____ 7. Decompression sickness

_____ 8. Drowning

_____ 9. Evaporation

_____ 10. Hyperthermia

A. Condition of having begun to drown; the patient may be conscious, unconscious with heartbeat and pulse, or with no heartbeat or pulse but still able to be resuscitated.

B. Covering a hypothermic patient and taking other steps to prevent further heat loss and help the body rewarm itself

C. Sending out energy, such as heat, in waves into space

D. Breathing; during this process, the body loses heat as warm air is exhaled from the body.

E. Cooling or freezing of particular parts of the body

F. Generalized cooling that reduces body temperature below normal; life-threatening in its extreme

G. Substances produced by animals or plants that are poisonous to humans

H. Chilling caused by conduction of heat from the body when the body or clothing is wet

I. Toxin produced by certain animals such as snakes, spiders, and some marine life-forms

J. Chilling caused by convection of heat from the body in the presence of air currents

_____ 1. Hypothermia

_____ 2. Local cooling

_____ 3. Near-drowning

_____ 4. Passive rewarming

_____ 5. Radiation

_____ 6. Respiration

_____ 7. Toxins

_____ 8. Venom

_____ 9. Water chill

_____ 10. Wind chill

MULTIPLE-CHOICE REVIEW

_____ 1. Water conducts heat away from the body _____ than still air.
   A. 25 times faster
   B. 25 times slower
   C. 50 times faster
   D. 50 times slower

_____ 2. The body loses heat from respiration, radiation, conduction, convection, and
   A. excretion.
   B. induction.
   C. evaporation.
   D. condensation.

_____ 3. When there is _____ wind, there is _____ heat loss.
   A. more : less
   B. less : greater
   C. more : greater
   D. no : maximum

_____ 4. Most radiant heat loss occurs from a person's
   A. arms and legs.
   B. chest and back.
   C. head and neck.
   D. feet and hands.

_____ 5. Predisposing factors to hypothermia include all of the following except
   A. burns.
   B. diabetes.
   C. spinal-cord injuries.
   D. headache.

_____ 6. Which one of the following is not a reason infants and children are more prone to hypothermia?
   A. They have small muscle mass.
   B. They have large skin surface in relation to their total body mass.
   C. They are unable to shiver effectively.
   D. They have more body fat than adults do.

_____ 7. You are treating an elderly patient with a possible leg fracture who was found lying on his cold garage floor where he had been all night. You should also consider
   A. a cerebrovascular accident.
   B. hypothermia.
   C. pulmonary edema.
   D. hyperperfusion.

_____ **8.** When a patient's core body temperature drops below 90°F, the patient
   A. may be shivering uncontrollably.
   B. may no longer be shivering.
   C. will be pulseless.
   D. will suddenly become alert.

_____ **9.** All of the following are signs and symptoms of hypothermia <u>except</u>
   A. high blood pressure and low pulse.
   B. stiff or rigid posture.
   C. cool abdominal skin temperature.
   D. loss of motor coordination.

_____ **10.** Passive rewarming involves
   A. applying heat packs to the patient.
   B. covering the patient.
   C. administering heated oxygen to the patient.
   D. massaging the patient's limbs.

_____ **11.** The treatment of the hypothermic patient who is alert and responding may include all of the following <u>except</u>
   A. removal of all of the patient's wet clothing.
   B. actively rewarming the patient during transport.
   C. rapidly giving the patient plenty of hot liquids.
   D. providing care for shock and providing oxygen.

_____ **12.** When actively rewarming a patient,
   A. apply heat to the chest, neck, armpits, and groin.
   B. quickly rewarm the patient.
   C. give the patient stimulants to drink.
   D. immerse the arms and feet in hot water.

_____ **13.** The reason why you should rewarm the body's core first is to
   A. prevent blood from collecting in the extremities due to vasodilation.
   B. quickly circulate cold blood throughout the body.
   C. speed up the blood flow to the extremities.
   D. increase blood flow to the brain to prevent unconsciousness.

_____ **14.** When transporting an alert patient with mild hypothermia, it is recommended that you
   A. transport in Fowler's position.
   B. massage the legs so the patient can walk.
   C. keep the patient at rest.
   D. leave the wet clothes in place.

_____ **15.** In a heat emergency, EMT-B care of a patient with moist, pale, normal-to-cool skin includes all of the following <u>except</u>
   A. place the patient in an air-conditioned ambulance.
   B. fan the patient so he begins to shiver.
   C. elevate the patient's legs.
   D. administer oxygen.

_____ **16.** In a heat emergency, if a patient with moist, pale, normal-to cool skin is responsive and not nauseated, the EMT-B should
   A. skip the oxygen.
   B. place cold packs in the patient's armpits.
   C. have the patient drink water.
   D. do all of the above.

_____ 17. When treating the unresponsive patient with severe hypothermia,
  A. keep the patient's head raised above the feet for the transport to the hospital.
  B. place the patient in a warm bathtub for at least twenty minutes.
  C. provide high-concentration oxygen that has been passed through a warm humidifier.
  D. massage the extremities for 35–45 seconds.

_____ 18. Because patients with extreme hypothermia may not reach biological death for over 30 minutes, the medical philosophy is
  A. if there is a pulse, start CPR.
  B. they are not dead until they're warm and dead.
  C. resuscitate for no longer than 30 minutes.
  D. always resuscitate very aggressively.

_____ 19. A cold injury usually occurring to exposed areas of the body that is brought about by direct contact with a cold object or exposure to cold air is called
  A. an early local cold injury.   C. frostbite.
  B. a superficial late cold injury.   D. a deep local cold injury.

_____ 20. The skin color of a patient with a superficial local cold injury will change from _____ to _____ .
  A. red : white   C. red : blue
  B. white : red   D. white : blue

_____ 21. If a superficial local cold injury is on an extremity, the EMT-B should
  A. splint and leave uncovered.
  B. rub the extremity briskly.
  C. not re-expose the injury to cold.
  D. immerse the extremity in hot water.

_____ 22. When muscles, bones, deep blood vessels, and organ membranes become frozen, this type of injury is called
  A. a superficial local cold injury.   C. a deep local cold injury.
  B. frostnip.   D. local cooling.

_____ 23. In frostbite, the affected area first appears
  A. black and stiff.   C. red and blotchy.
  B. white and waxy.   D. blue and abraded.

_____ 24. Do not allow the frostbite patient to smoke or drink alcohol because
  A. the patient may suffer altered mental status or fall asleep.
  B. these would stimulate the patient to move, which could cause further injury.
  C. constriction of blood vessels and decreased circulation to the injured tissues may result.
  D. either could contaminate the frostbitten area.

_____ 25. Active rewarming of a frozen part
  A. is seldom recommended in the field.
  B. includes using very hot water.
  C. is performed without removing the patient's clothing.
  D. includes covering the patient's face.

_____ 26. When assessing a patient you suspect is in extreme hypothermia, check the carotid pulse for _____ seconds.
  A. 5–10   C. 30–45
  B. 15–25   D. 50–60

_____ 27. The environment associated with hyperthermia includes
  A. heat and high winds.   C. heat and high humidity.
  B. heat and light rain.   D. heat and low humidity.

_____ **28.** The higher the humidity is, the
   A. less you perspire.
   B. less your perspiration evaporates.
   C. less you radiate heat.
   D. more you lose heat from your body.

_____ **29.** The medical problems resulting from dry heat are often worse than those from moist heat because
   A. dry heat is more common.
   B. moist heat tires people quickly.
   C. dry heat causes more sunburn.
   D. dry heat affects the respiratory system more quickly.

_____ **30.** When salts are lost by the body through sweating, the patient may have all of the following <u>except</u>
   A. muscle cramps.
   B. weakness or exhaustion.
   C. dizziness or periods of faintness.
   D. fluid buildup in the lungs.

_____ **31.** A patient with heat exhaustion will present with
   A. dry, hot skin.
   B. moist, pale, normal-to-cool skin.
   C. a lack of sweating.
   D. rapid strong pulse.

_____ **32.** The signs and symptoms of a heat emergency in patients who have hot, dry or moist skin include
   A. slow and shallow breathing.
   B. seizures.
   C. constricted pupils.
   D. muscle cramps.

_____ **33.** The signs and symptoms of a heat emergency in patients who have hot, dry or moist skin include all of the following <u>except</u>
   A. generalized weakness.
   B. loss of consciousness or altered mental status.
   C. profuse perspiration.
   D. full and rapid pulse.

_____ **34.** Which of the following is a large contributor to adolescent and adult drownings?
   A. inexperience with equipment
   B. substance abuse
   C. stomach cramps
   D. car crash immersions

_____ **35.** During a drowning incident, water flowing past the epiglottis causes
   A. a reflex to close the mouth.
   B. the victim to gasp for more air.
   C. a reflex spasm of the larynx.
   D. the victim to begin hyperventilating.

_____ **36.** About 10% of drowning victims die from
   A. too much fluid in their lungs.
   B. lack of air.
   C. cervical-spine injuries.
   D. crushing chest injury.

_____ **37.** If you are not an experienced swimmer, you should
   A. never attempt to go into the water to do a rescue.
   B. don a floatation device prior to going into the water.
   C. use a boat as your first approach to conduct the rescue.
   D. coach the patient in floating techniques.

_____ **38.** If you suspect that a patient still in the pool has a possible spine injury,
   A. spineboard the patient as you pull him from the water.
   B. immobilize and spineboard the patient while still in the water.
   C. quickly remove the patient from the water to prevent hypothermia.
   D. encourage the patient to swim to the side of the pool.

_____ **39.** Two special medical problems seen in scuba-diving accidents are decompression sickness and
   A. carbon monoxide poisoning.
   C. air embolism.
   B. oxygen toxicity.
   D. arthritis.

_____ **40.** The risk of decompression sickness is increased by
   A. air travel within 12 hours of a dive.
   B. breathing 100% oxygen immediately after the dive.
   C. drinking fluids before and after the dive.
   D. none of the above.

_____ **41.** A toxin produced by some animals that is harmful to humans is called
   A. poison.
   C. venom.
   B. lymph.
   D. allergen.

_____ **42.** Typical sources of injected poisons include _____ bites and stings.
   A. spider
   C. snake
   B. scorpion
   D. all of the above

_____ **43.** While cleaning out the crawl space below the house, you experience blotchy skin, redness in your arm, weakness, and nausea. It is possible that you
   A. are developing heat stroke.
   B. were bitten by a poisonous spider.
   C. are having a diabetic reaction.
   D. are allergic to something in the air.

_____ **44.** Signs and symptoms of injected poisoning include all of the following <u>except</u>
   A. lack of sensation in one side of the body.
   B. puncture marks.
   C. muscle cramps, chest tightening, and joint pains.
   D. excessive saliva formation and profuse sweating.

_____ **45.** If you suspect that your patient has been bitten by a snake, you should do all of the following <u>except</u>
   A. call for medical direction.
   B. clean the injection site with soap and water.
   C. remove rings, bracelets, or other constricting items on the bitten limb.
   D. capture the live snake and bring it in the ambulance to the emergency department.

COMPLETE THE FOLLOWING

1. List six of the signs and symptoms of heat exhaustion.

   A. _____

   B. _____

   C. _____

   D. _____

   E. _____

   F. _____

2. List six of the signs and symptoms of heat stroke.

A. _____

B. _____

C. _____

D. _____

E. _____

F. _____

3. List ten of the signs and symptoms of an insect bite or sting.

A. _____

B. _____

C. _____

D. _____

E. _____

F. _____

G. _____

H. _____

I. _____

J. _____

VIRTUAL STREET SCENES

(First review the Street Scenes on pp. 446–447 of the textbook. Then answer the questions below.)

1. If the condition of the patient requires that you actively rewarm him, what should you do?

2. At the scene, if the patient goes into cardiac arrest, should CPR be performed?

3. Usually patients in hypothermia have a slow pulse. In this case, the vital signs showed tachycardia. What might this indicate in a patient?

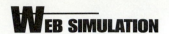

WEB SIMULATION

For interactive case studies that will help you review and practice basic skills, visit the **Emergency Care 9e Companion Website** at www.bradybooks.com/emergencycare.

EMT-BASIC SKILL PERFORMANCE CHECKLISTS

▶ ACTIVE RAPID REWARMING OF FROZEN PARTS

❑ Take BSI precautions.

❑ Conduct an initial assessment.

❑ Conduct focused history and physical exam, including baseline vital signs.

❑ Consider administering oxygen by nonrebreather mask.

❑ Heat water to a temperature between 100°F and 105°F.

❑ Fill the container with the heated water and prepare the injured part by removing clothing, jewelry, bands, or straps.

❑ Fully immerse the injured part. Do not allow the injured area to touch the sides or bottom of the container. Do not place any pressure on the affected part. Continuously stir the water. When the water cools below 100°F, remove the affected part and add more warm water. The patient may complain of moderate pain as the affected area rewarms or may experience some period of intense pain.

❑ If you complete rewarming of the part, gently dry the affected area and apply a dry sterile dressing.

❑ Place dry sterile dressings between fingers and toes before dressing hands and feet.

❑ Cover the site with blankets or whatever is available to keep the affected area warm. Do not allow these coverings to come in contact with the injured area or to put pressure on the site.

❑ Keep the patient at rest. Do not allow the patient to walk if a lower extremity has been frostbitten or frozen.

❑ Keep the entire patient warm.

❑ Continue to monitor the patient.

❑ Assist circulation according to local protocol. (Some systems recommend rhythmically and carefully raising and lowering the affected limb.)

❑ Do not allow the limb to refreeze.

❑ Transport patient as soon as possible with the affected limb slightly elevated.

WATER RESCUE—POSSIBLE SPINAL INJURY

❑ Take BSI precautions.

❑ Conduct an initial assessment.

❑ Splint head and neck with arms.

❑ Roll patient over into supine position.

❑ Ensure airway and breathing. (Note: If patient is not breathing, remove him from the water on a backboard as soon as possible.)

❑ Provide manual stabilization of the head and neck.

❑ Assess pulses, motor function, and sensation in all four extremities.

❑ Slide backboard under patient.

❑ Apply properly sized rigid extrication collar.

❑ Tie down torso, then the head and neck with straps.

❑ Float board to the edge of the water.

❑ Remove patient from water with as much assistance as needed.

❑ Obtain baseline vital signs.

❑ Conduct focused history and physical exam.

❑ Reassess pulses, motor function, and sensation in all four extremities.

❑ Administer oxygen, and prepare to transport patient.

CASE STUDY

▶ TOO COLD FOR COMFORT

You respond to a call for a child with an altered mental status in the backyard of a private residence. It is late in the afternoon on a windy day, so you grab your uniform jacket as you jump into the ambulance. On arrival, you are met by three children, ages approximately 9 to 12, who state that their little sister has been acting "funny." Their parent is at the store, and they called her on the cell phone. She was the one who called 9-1-1 and should be home momentarily.

Apparently the children have been practicing diving in the pool for the past four hours. The youngest child, Robin—a very thin, small seven year old—is sitting by the edge of the pool shivering.

1. What are your initial assessment concerns with the patient?

2. Is it necessary for you to wait until the parent arrives to question the children?

3. Besides obtaining a set of baseline vital signs, what additional history may be helpful to obtain?

Upon questioning, you find that Robin has not been playing as a part of the group for at least the last hour. When you ask the children if they were cold, they say they did not notice the temperature, just the wind, until a few minutes ago when the sun went down. They also are able to confirm that Robin has no medical history, takes no meds, has no allergies, and has not eaten since lunchtime. When you question Robin, it is clear that she is confused and shivering, cool to the touch, and breathing rapidly.

4. After ruling out trauma, you place the child on your stretcher. What would be the best position?

5. When the mother arrives, you advise her of your findings. She is in agreement that the child should be checked in the hospital. What do you suspect may be wrong with this child?

6. Would it be appropriate to administer oxygen to Robin?

7. If you took her temperature, what do you suspect you would find?

8. Why might this child be prone to hypothermia?

The parent tells you that the children are all very good swimmers and they are practicing for a diving competition. She only ran out for a half hour to go to the store. The children are quick to call her on the cell phone whenever there is a problem. She also says that she told them to get out of the pool before she left for the store.

9. When she asks you how a similar incident could be prevented in the future, what should you say?

Chapter Twenty-Three
BEHAVIORAL EMERGENCIES

MATCH TERMINOLOGY/DEFINITIONS

A. Humane device made of leather used to hold a patient still to prevent the patient from injuring himself or others

B. Display of emotions, such as fear, grief, or anger, in response to an accident, serious illness, or death

C. Death of a person due to a body position that restricts breathing for a prolonged time

D. When a patient's behavior is not typical for the situation; when the patient's behavior is unacceptable or intolerable to the patient, his family, or the community; or when the patient may harm himself or others

E. Manner in which a person acts

_____ 1. Behavioral emergency

_____ 2. Behavior

_____ 3. Positional asphyxia

_____ 4. Soft restraint

_____ 5. Stress reaction

MULTIPLE-CHOICE REVIEW

_____ 1. Physical causes of altered behavior include all of the following except
   A. inadequate blood flow to the brain.
   B. mind-altering substances.
   C. excessive heat or cold.
   D. differing lifestyles.

_____ 2. Altered behavior ranging from irritability to altered mental status can be due to any of the following except
   A. lack of oxygen.   C. hypoactivity.
   B. head trauma.   D. hypoglycemia.

_____ 3. To calm a patient who is experiencing a stress reaction, you should
   A. complete your assessment as quickly as possible.
   B. allow the patient to control the situation.
   C. explain things to the patient honestly.
   D. restrain the patient quickly.

_____ 4. Which one of the following is not usually a common presentation of a patient experiencing a behavioral emergency?
   A. panic or anxiety   C. repetitive motions
   B. neat appearance   D. pressured-sounding speech

_____ 5. When you are called to care for a patient who has attempted suicide or is about to attempt suicide, your first concern should be
   A. how you will restrain the patient.
   B. your personal safety.
   C. determining the patient's method for suicide.
   D. the patient's and family's safety.

_____ 6. High suicide rates occur at ages
  A. 15–25.   **C.** 30–35.
  B. 25–30.   **D.** 35–40.

_____ 7. Which one of the following is <u>not</u> an example of a self-destructive activity?
  A. a defined lethal plan of action that has been verbalized
  B. giving away personal possessions
  C. denial of suicidal thoughts
  D. previous suicide threats

_____ 8. When a suicidal patient exhibits sudden improvement from depression, the EMT-B should consider that the patient is
  A. no longer suicidal.   **C.** still at risk for suicide.
  B. is now ready to accept care.   **D.** none of the above.

_____ 9. When assessing an aggressive patient for a possible threat to you or your crew, take all of the following actions <u>except</u>
  A. try to determine the patient's history of aggressive behavior.
  B. pay attention to the patient's vocal activity.
  C. take note of the patient's posturing.
  D. assess the patient in the kitchen.

_____ 10. If a patient stands in a corner of the room with fists clenched and screaming obscenities, you should
  A. request police backup and keep the doorway in sight.
  B. raise your voice to a higher level than the patient's.
  C. challenge the patient in an attempt to calm him.
  D. explain that you would respond in the same way.

_____ 11. Use of reasonable force to restrain a patient should involve an evaluation of all of the following <u>except</u> the
  A. patient's size and strength.
  B. family's ability to pay for your services.
  C. patient's mental status.
  D. available methods of restraint.

_____ 12. The use of force by an EMT-B is allowed
  A. to defend against an attack by an emotionally disturbed patient.
  B. only when the police are present.
  C. whenever a patient refuses any of your treatments.
  D. whenever you suspect the patient has been drinking.

_____ 13. Once the decision has been made to restrain a patient, which one of the following steps should be avoided?
  A. Use multiple straps to restrain the patient.
  B. Reassure the patient throughout the procedure.
  C. Reassess the patient's distal circulation frequently.
  D. Use two rescuers to secure the patient.

_____ 14. A restrained patient who is spitting on rescuers can best be managed by
  A. placing in a prone position on the stretcher.
  B. wrapping the patient's mouth with roller gauze.
  C. placing 3-inch tape across the patient's mouth.
  D. placing a surgical mask on the patient's face.

_____ 15. When a patient is a danger to himself or others and needs to be transported against his will, the EMT-B should
  A. restrain the patient immediately.
  B. transport the patient with the family's assistance.
  C. contact the police for assistance.
  D. contact the patient's physician.

COMPLETE THE FOLLOWING

1. List nine potential risk factors for suicide.

   A. _____

   B. _____

   C. _____

   D. _____

   E. _____

   F. _____

   G. _____

   H. _____

   I. _____

2. List four precautions for your safety and that of your crew when you feel your patient may hurt himself or others.

   A. _____

   B. _____

   C. _____

   D. _____

VIRTUAL STREET SCENES

(First review the Street Scenes on pp. 458–459 of the textbook. Then answer the questions below.)

1. Suppose that the patient had suddenly become violent, flailing his arms and screaming obscenities. Should you help the police hold him down?

2. Once the patient is down, how should he be restrained?

3. Since the patient is having a behavioral emergency, is it acceptable to skip taking vital signs?

WEB SIMULATION

For interactive case studies that will help you review and practice basic skills, visit the *Emergency Care 9e Companion Website* at www.bradybooks.com/emergencycare.

Chapter Twenty-Four
OBSTETRICS AND GYNECOLOGICAL EMERGENCIES

MATCH TERMINOLOGY/DEFINITIONS

▶ **PART A**

A. Normal head-first birth

B. Neck of the uterus at the entrance to the birth canal

C. Implantation of the fertilized egg in an oviduct, the cervix of the uterus, or in the abdominopelvic cavity

D. Placenta, part of the umbilical cord, and some tissues from the lining of the uterus that are delivered after the birth of the baby

E. Baby developing in the womb

F. Condition in which the placenta separates from the uterine wall

G. Deliberate actions taken to stop a pregnancy

H. When more than one baby is born during a single delivery

I. Spontaneous (miscarriage) or induced termination of pregnancy

J. Three stages of the delivery of a baby that begin with the contractions of the uterus and end with the expulsion of the placenta

K. Thin, membranous "bag of waters" that surrounds the developing fetus

L. Amniotic fluid that is greenish or brownish-yellow rather than clear; an indication of possible maternal or fetal distress during labor

M. When the buttocks or both legs of a baby deliver first during birth

N. Skin between the vagina and the anus

O. When the presenting part of the baby first appears through the vaginal opening

_____ **1.** Abortion

_____ **2.** Abruptio placentae

_____ **3.** Afterbirth

_____ **4.** Amniotic sac

_____ **5.** Breech presentation

_____ **6.** Cephalic presentation

_____ **7.** Cervix

_____ **8.** Crowning

_____ **9.** Ectopic pregnancy

_____ **10.** Fetus

_____ **11.** Induced abortion

_____ **12.** Labor

_____ **13.** Meconium staining

_____ **14.** Multiple birth

_____ **15.** Perineum

PART B

A. When the umbilical cord presents first and is squeezed between the vaginal wall and the baby's head

B. Dizziness and a drop in blood pressure caused when the mother is in a supine position and the weight of the uterus, infant, placenta, and amniotic fluid compress the inferior vena cava, reducing return of blood to the heart and cardiac output

C. When the fetus and placenta deliver before the 28th week of pregnancy, commonly called a miscarriage

D. Muscular abdominal organ where the fetus develops; also called the womb

E. Born dead

F. Any newborn weighing less than 5½ pounds or one that is born before the 37th week of pregnancy

G. Fetal structure containing the blood vessels that carry blood to and from the placenta

H. Organ of pregnancy where exchange of oxygen, foods, and wastes occurs between a mother and fetus

I. Condition in which the placenta is formed in an abnormal location (usually low in the uterus and close to or over the cervical opening) that will not allow for a normal delivery of the fetus

J. Birth canal

_____ 1. Placenta

_____ 2. Placenta previa

_____ 3. Premature infant

_____ 4. Prolapsed umbilical cord

_____ 5. Spontaneous abortion

_____ 6. Stillborn

_____ 7. Supine hypotensive syndrome

_____ 8. Umbilical cord

_____ 9. Uterus

_____ 10. Vagina

MULTIPLE-CHOICE REVIEW

_____ 1. The nine months of pregnancy are divided into three-month trimesters. During the second trimester, the
  A. fetus is being formed and there is little uterine growth during this period.
  B. uterus grows very rapidly while the woman's blood volume, cardiac output, and heart rate increase.
  C. uterus is often seen reaching up to the epigastrium by this time.
  D. uterus develops to full size.

_____ 2. The normal birth position is _____ and is called a _____ birth.
  A. head first : breech   C. feet first : breech
  B. head first : cephalic   D. feet first : cephalic

_____ 3. The first stage of labor starts
  A. with conception.
  B. at the nine-month point.
  C. with regular contractions of the uterus.
  D. when the cervix is dilated.

_____ 4. The second stage of labor starts with
  A. the birth of the baby.
  B. regular contractions of the uterus.
  C. the delivery of the afterbirth.
  D. the entry of the baby into the birth canal.

_____ 5. The third stage of labor begins with
A. the birth of the baby.   C. dilation of the cervix.
B. delivery of the afterbirth.   D. full growth of the uterus.

_____ 6. The third stage of labor is complete when
A. the baby is born.
B. the afterbirth is expelled.
C. twenty minutes have passed since the delivery.
D. the uterus is firm again.

_____ 7. The process by which the cervix gradually widens and thins out is called
A. delivery.   C. staining.
B. dilation.   D. contraction.

_____ 8. As the fetus moves downward and the cervix dilates, normally the amniotic
sac breaks and fluid leaks out. If this fluid is greenish or brownish-yellow
in color, this may indicate
A. fetal or maternal distress.
B. the fetus is dead.
C. the mother is pushing too hard.
D. the amniotic sac broke too early.

_____ 9. The greenish or brownish-yellow fluid expelled from the amniotic sac is
called
A. a bloody show.   C. meconium staining.
B. vena cava syndrome.   D. amniotic bile.

_____ 10. When a mother in labor states she feels the need to move her bowels, this
means the
A. birth will be delayed.   C. birth moment is nearing.
B. uterus is almost dilated.   D. baby is in distress.

_____ 11. The contraction duration is timed from the
A. start of the pain until the delivery of the infant.
B. beginning of the contraction to when the uterus relaxes.
C. end of a contraction to the beginning of the next one.
D. peak of the contraction to the end of the contraction.

_____ 12. The contraction interval, or frequency, is timed from the
A. start of one contraction to the start of the next.
B. beginning of the contraction to when the uterus relaxes.
C. peak of the contraction to the end of the contraction.
D. start of the pain until the delivery of the infant.

_____ 13. Delivery is imminent when the contractions last _____ seconds and
are _____ minutes apart.
A. 15 : 5 to 8   C. 45 : 8 to 10
B. 30 : 2 to 3   D. 90 : 5 to 8

_____ 14. The EMT-B's primary roles at a normal childbirth scene are to determine
whether the delivery will occur at the scene and, if so, to
A. determine if the delivery can be delayed.
B. assist the mother as she delivers the infant.
C. carefully deliver the infant.
D. immobilize the patient.

_____ 15. The sterile obstetrical kit does not contain
A. a rubber bulb syringe for suctioning.
B. several individually wrapped sanitary napkins.
C. heavy flat twine to tie the cord.
D. cord clamps or hemostats.

_____ **16.** When evaluating the mother for a possible home delivery, the EMT-B should ask
  A. if pregnancy problems run in the family.
  B. the frequency and duration of contractions.
  C. if the mother feels she needs to urinate.
  D. the father's blood type and medical history.

_____ **17.** It is important to ask the mother if you can examine for crowning if the mother
  A. is straining during contractions
  B. is in her ninth month of pregnancy
  C. is pregnant for the first time
  D. It is not important to ask permission to examine the mother.

_____ **18.** You are treating a 25-year-old female who is 8 months pregnant. She states she has contractions every 15 minutes or so, which last for about 20 seconds. She is not exactly sure what labor pain is like because this is her first pregnancy. Her vitals are pulse of 96, blood pressure of 130/70, and respirations of 22. What should you do next?
  A. Administer oxygen and transport immediately.
  B. Prepare for a home delivery immediately.
  C. Ask if her water broke and prepare for a quiet ride to the hospital.
  D. Tell her to call you back when the contractions are more frequent.

_____ **19.** If you determine that the delivery is imminent based on the presence of crowning and other signs, you should
  A. contact medical direction.
  B. transport as quickly as possible.
  C. ask the mother to go the bathroom first.
  D. ask the mother to hold her legs closed.

_____ **20.** When a full-term pregnant woman in a supine position complains of dizziness and you note a drop in blood pressure, this could be due to a condition called _____ syndrome.
  A. diabetes mellitus
  B. supine hypotension
  C. Cushing's reflex
  D. fluid retention

_____ **21.** To counteract the pressure of the uterus on the inferior vena cava, you should
  A. raise the patient's legs.
  B. transport the patient on her left side.
  C. raise the patient's head.
  D. apply the PASG.

_____ **22.** During a delivery, the EMT-B will need all of the following infection control gear <u>except</u>
  A. surgical gloves.
  B. a mask.
  C. eye protection.
  D. a Tyvek suit.

_____ **23.** During delivery, encourage the mother to
  A. breathe rapidly and deeply.
  B. hold her breath every 2 minutes.
  C. close her mouth and breathe through her nose.
  D. breathe deeply through her mouth.

_____ **24.** When supporting the baby's head during a delivery, the EMT-B should do all of the following <u>except</u>
  A. pull on the baby's shoulders when they appear.
  B. apply gentle pressure to control the delivery.
  C. place one hand below the baby's head.
  D. spread fingers evenly around the baby's head.

_____ **25.** If the amniotic sac has not broken by the time the baby's head is delivered, you should
  A. stop the delivery and transport immediately.
  B. use your finger to puncture the membrane.
  C. contact medical control immediately.
  D. delay the delivery until it breaks.

_____ **26.** If you cannot loosen or unwrap the umbilical cord from around the infant's neck, you should
  A. stop the delivery and transport immediately.
  B. tell the mother to push more forcefully.
  C. clamp the cord in two places and cut between the clamps.
  D. contact medical direction for advice.

_____ **27.** Most babies are born
  A. face down and then rotate to either side.
  B. face up and then rotate to either side.
  C. feet and buttocks first and do not rotate.
  D. face up and do not rotate.

_____ **28.** When suctioning a newborn,
  A. compress the bulb syringe when inside the baby's mouth.
  B. compress the bulb syringe before placing it in the baby's mouth.
  C. suction the nose and then the mouth.
  D. insert the syringe about 22 inches into the baby's mouth.

_____ **29.** Once the baby's feet are delivered,
  A. pick the baby up by the feet using a firm grasp.
  B. lay the baby on her side with head slightly lower than her torso.
  C. lay the baby on her side and massage her back.
  D. pick the baby up by the feet and massage her back.

_____ **30.** To assess the newborn, the EMT-B should do all of the following except
  A. note ease of breathing.
  B. check movement in the extremities.
  C. note skin coloration.
  D. check the response to a sternal rub.

_____ **31.** Why is it necessary to suction the baby's mouth before the nose?
  A. so the baby can gasp and begin breathing
  B. so the baby is stimulated to cry
  C. to prevent aspiration of materials from her mouth
  D. because this will open the nasopharynx passageway.

_____ **32.** If assessment of the infant's breathing reveals shallow, slow, or absent respirations, the EMT-B should
  A. provide oxygen by nonrebreather mask.
  B. use a gentle but vigorous rubbing of the infant's back.
  C. provide artificial ventilations at 40 to 60 per minute.
  D. provide artificial ventilations at 20 to 30 per minute.

_____ **33.** In a normal birth, the infant must be breathing on her own
  A. before you clamp and cut the cord.
  B. prior to transportation to the hospital.
  C. prior to considering ventilation.
  D. in order to use an oral airway.

_____ **34.** The first umbilical cord clamp should be placed about _____ inches from the baby.
  A. 4   **C.** 8
  B. 6   **D.** 10

_____ **35.** The second umbilical cord clamp should be placed about _____ inches from the baby.
   A. 3   **C.** 7
   B. 5   **D.** 9

_____ **36.** If the placenta does not deliver within _____ minutes of the baby's birth, transport the mother and baby to a medical facility without delay.
   A. 5   **C.** 15
   B. 10   **D.** 20

_____ **37.** It is not uncommon for the mother to tear part of the perineum during a delivery. If this occurs,
   A. massage the uterus for at least 15 minutes.
   B. apply a sanitary napkin and gentle pressure.
   C. transport the patient on her left side immediately.
   D. contact medical direction immediately.

_____ **38.** Which of the following is an appropriate action to take for a breech presentation?
   A. Place the mother on her left side.
   B. Provide low-concentration oxygen.
   C. Pull on the baby's legs to deliver.
   D. Initiate rapid transport upon recognition.

_____ **39.** If you see the umbilical cord presenting first,
   A. gently push up on the baby's head or buttocks to take pressure off of the cord.
   B. use two gloved fingers to check the cord for a pulse and keep the cord cool.
   C. raise the mother's head and lower buttocks to lessen pressure on the birth canal.
   D. attempt to push the cord back if it is not wrapped around the baby's neck.

_____ **40.** When a baby's limb presents first, the EMT-B should
   A. push gently on the extremity to prevent it from advancing.
   B. pull gently on the limb to encourage delivery.
   C. administer low-concentration oxygen to the mother.
   D. begin rapid transport of the patient immediately.

_____ **41.** When assisting with the delivery of twins,
   A. the afterbirth will be delivered after each individual infant.
   B. clamp the cord of the first baby before the second baby is born.
   C. labor contractions will stop after the first delivery.
   D. transport the mother immediately.

_____ **42.** Premature infants are at high risk for hypothermia because
   A. they are smaller than most babies.
   B. their brains are less developed than full-term baby.
   C. they lack fat deposits that would normally keep them warm.
   D. their temperature-regulating structures are not fully developed.

_____ **43.** When oxygen is administered to an infant, it should be given by
   A. a nonrebreather mask.   **C.** a pediatric nasal cannula.
   B. flowing it past the baby's face. **D.** a demand valve unit.

_____ **44.** If you suspect meconium staining when the infant is born,
   A. contact medical control for advice.
   B. avoid stimulating the infant before suctioning the oropharynx.
   C. suction the nose, then the mouth.
   D. provide oxygen to the mother.

_____ **45.** A condition in which the placenta is formed low in the uterus and close to the cervical opening preventing the normal delivery of the fetus is called
  A. abruptio placentae.
  B. stillborn birth.
  C. placenta toxemia.
  D. placenta previa.

_____ **46.** Which one of the following is true of seizures in pregnancy?
  A. They are usually associated with low blood pressure.
  B. They tend to occur early in pregnancy.
  C. They pose a threat to the mother but not the unborn baby.
  D. They are usually associated with extreme swelling of the extremities.

_____ **47.** The greatest danger associated with blunt trauma to the pregnant woman's abdomen and pelvis is
  A. cramping abdominal pains.
  B. spontaneous abortion.
  C. massive bleeding and shock.
  D. elevated blood pressure.

_____ **48.** Which one of the following is true about the physiology of a pregnant woman?
  A. Vital signs may be interpreted as suggestive of shock when they are actually normal.
  B. The pregnant woman has a pulse rate that is 10–15 beats per minute slower than the nonpregnant female.
  C. A woman in later pregnancy may have a blood volume that is up to 48% lower than her nonpregnant state.
  D. Assessing for shock is easier in the pregnant patient than for a nonpregnant patient.

_____ **49.** Unless a back or neck injury is suspected, all pregnant women who have suffered blunt trauma injury should be transported in the _____ position.
  A. supine
  B. left lateral recumbent
  C. Trendelenburg
  D. Fowler's

_____ **50.** Which of the following is true of the treatment necessary for a woman with vaginal bleeding associated with abdominal pain?
  A. Massage the abdomen vigorously.
  B. Assume the woman is pregnant and transport.
  C. Treat as if she has potentially life-threatening injury.
  D. Determine the cause before treatment is begun.

COMPLETE THE FOLLOWING

1. List seven things you should do when evaluating the expectant mother.

A. _____

B. _____

C. _____

D. _____

E. _____

F. _____

G. _____

2. List eight steps you should take when providing care for the premature infant.

A. _____

B. _____

C. _____

D. _____

E. _____

F. _____

G. _____

H. _____

LABEL THE DIAGRAMS

Fill in the name of each structure of pregnancy on the line provided.

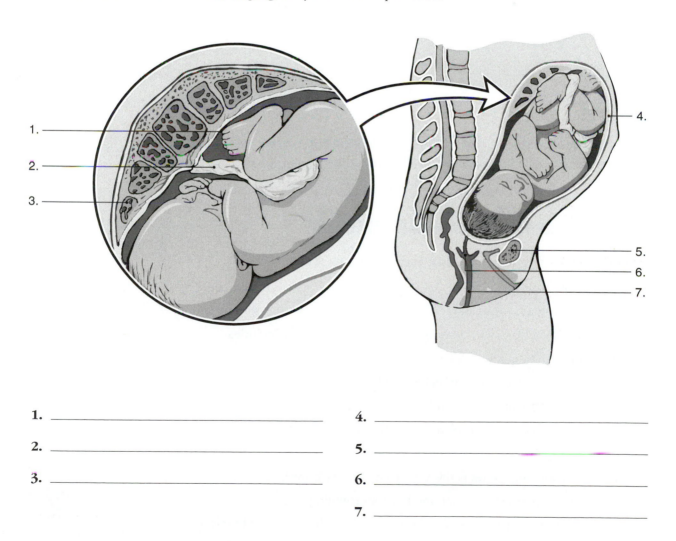

1. _____   4. _____

2. _____   5. _____

3. _____   6. _____

     7. _____

VIRTUAL STREET SCENES

(First review the Street Scenes on pp. 486–487 of the textbook. Then answer the questions below.)

1. Imagine that when you observe crowning, you also observe that the amniotic sac is intact. What should you do?

2. When the amniotic fluid is expelled from the bag, you notice that it is dark green. What is this called? What does it indicate? What should you do about it?

3. Suppose that after delivery of the placenta, you observe that the mother is continuing to bleed excessively. Is there anything you can do to help her?

WEB SIMULATION

For interactive case studies that will help you review and practice basic skills, visit the *Emergency Care 9e Companion Website* at www.bradybooks.com/emergencycare.

EMT-BASIC SKILLS PERFORMANCE CHECKLIST

▶ **EVALUATING THE MOTHER FOR IMMINENT DELIVERY**

❏ Take BSI precautions.

❏ Conduct an initial assessment.

❏ Obtain mother's history to determine active labor. History includes:

–Length of pregnancy.

–Number of previous pregnancies and births.

–If the "bag of waters" has broken.

–Frequency and duration of uterine contractions.

–Recent vaginal discharge or hemorrhage.

–If she is straining or feels the urge to move her bowels.

❏ With mother's permission, examine her for crowning.

❏ Feel for uterine contractions when she says she is having a contraction.

❏ Take another set of vitals and make the decision to prepare for a delivery or to begin transport.

Chapter Twenty-Five

PUTTING IT ALL TOGETHER FOR THE MEDICAL PATIENT

MATCH TERMINOLOGY/DEFINITIONS

A. Passageway by which air enters or leaves the body

B. Respiration, or process by which a person inhales and exhales air

C. Movement of blood throughout the body

D. Form of sugar, the body's basic source of energy

E. Action taken to correct a patient's problem

F. Pain in the chest, occurring when blood supply to the heart is reduced and a portion of the heart muscle is not receiving enough oxygen

G. Orders from the on-duty physician given directly to an EMT-B in the field by radio or telephone

H. Decision on the seriousness of the patient's condition

_____ 1. Intervention

_____ 2. Circulation

_____ 3. Airway

_____ 4. Priority determination

_____ 5. On-line medical direction

_____ 6. Breathing

_____ 7. Angina pectoris

_____ 8. Glucose

MULTIPLE-CHOICE REVIEW

_____ 1. The limited number of interventions an EMT-B can provide include all of the following except
   A. administration of intravenous fluids.
   B. application of an AED.
   C. application of oxygen.
   D. insertion of oral or nasal airways.

_____ 2. When a patient presents with more than one condition or a familiar condition but under unusual circumstances, the EMT-B should
   A. call medical control right away
   B. call for an ALS unit right away.
   C. assess the patient as usual.
   D. assign a higher priority to the patient.

_____ 3. When a patient tells you he has a disease with which you are not familiar, it is best to respond by saying
   A. I'm not familiar with that disease. Could you tell me about it?
   B. That doesn't concern me. My job is to treat emergencies.
   C. Interesting disease. I studied it during EMS training.
   D. I'm not a physician. Just tell me what's wrong today.

_____ 4. When a patient has two or more medical conditions that are presenting symptoms at the same time, it is good to
   A. treat them all at once.
   B. treat them one at a time.
   C. consult with medical direction for advice.
   D. just manage the ABCs and forget the rest.

_____ 5. The patient with slurred speech may have had
   A. a cardiovascular accident.   C. a seizure.
   B. an overdose.   D. any one of the above.

_____ 6. The patient with chest pain may have any of the following conditions except
   A. angina.   C. seizure.
   B. acute myocardial infarction.   D. rib fracture.

_____ 7. A patient who is vomiting coffee-ground colored material probably has
   A. internal bleeding   C. gall bladder problems.
   B. a seizure history.   D. ingested a strong acid.

_____ 8. A wheeze is a common breathing sound found in a patient having
   A. an asthma attack.   C. bronchospasm.
   B. an allergic reaction   D. any one of the above.

_____ 9. There is no specific EMT-B intervention for the patient with
   A. chest pain.   C. a fractured leg.
   B. abdominal pain.   D. a serious laceration.

_____ 10. Each one of the following is an example of patient problems that have no specific EMT-B intervention except
   A. headache.   C. hyperthermia.
   B. sickle-cell crisis.   D. post-surgical complications.

COMPLETE THE FOLLOWING

List six examples of EMT-B interventions for medical patients.

A. _____

B. _____

C. _____

D. _____

E. _____

F. _____

VIRTUAL STREET SCENES

(First review the Street Scenes on pp. 496–497 of the textbook. Then answer the questions below.)

1. Imagine that in addition to his fever, the patient had vomiting and a rash. What BSI precautions should you take?

2. If the patient also complains of dizziness when he stands up, how might it change your emergency care?

3. Suppose this patient had a history of diabetes and also has cool, clammy skin. Would this change your management of the patient?

WEB SIMULATION

For interactive case studies that will help you review and practice basic skills, visit the *Emergency Care 9e Companion Website* at www.bradybooks.com/emergencycare.

Interim Exam Two

Use the answer sheet on pages 191–192 to complete this exam. It is perforated so it can be easily removed from this book.

1. During the initial assessment, all of the following are assessed <u>except</u>
   - A. airway.
   - B. mental status.
   - C. circulation.
   - D. blood pressure.

2. Which is <u>not</u> a component of the initial assessment?
   - A. determining patient priority
   - B. evaluating extremity mobility
   - C. forming a general impression
   - D. assessing breathing

3. When forming your general impression of a child's condition, the environment can provide clues. An example would be a child
   - A. complaining of nausea or vomiting.
   - B. holding pieces of a toy in his/her hand.
   - C. with a blood pressure of 120/80.
   - D. with a rapid heart beat.

4. When forming a general impression, the EMT-B takes into consideration all of the following <u>except</u> the patient's
   - A. position.
   - B. age and sex.
   - C. blood pressure.
   - D. sounds.

5. After forming a general impression, the next step of the initial assessment is
   - A. assessing breathing.
   - B. assessing mental status.
   - C. determining the priority of the patient.
   - D. assessing airway.

6. The "V" in "AVPU" stands for
   - A. virtual.
   - B. visible.
   - C. verbal.
   - D. vertex.

7. The "P" in "AVPU" stands for
   - A. pulse.
   - B. painful.
   - C. paralysis.
   - D. paraesthesia.

8. The lowest and the most serious mental status is
   - A. A.
   - B. V.
   - C. P.
   - D. U.

9. If a patient's level of responsiveness is lower than Alert, you should
   - A. apply a cervical collar.
   - B. administer high-concentration oxygen.
   - C. place him in a recovery position.
   - D. bandage all bleeding wounds.

10. If a patient is talking or crying, assume the patient
    - A. is in little pain.
    - B. has no life-threatening bleeding.
    - C. has an open airway.
    - D. has an "A" mental status.

11. If the patient is not alert and her breathing rate is slower than 8 breaths per minute, the EMT-B should
    - A. insert an oral airway.
    - B. place the patient in a prone position.
    - C. assist ventilations with a bag-valve mask.
    - D. apply the PASG.

12. If the skin is pale and clammy, this indicates
    - A. nervous system damage.
    - B. poor circulation.
    - C. extremely high temperature.
    - D. an airway problem.

13. A patient who gives a poor general impression should be considered a _____ priority.
    - A. high
    - B. low
    - C. delayed
    - D. stable

14. Which one of the following is <u>not</u> an example of a high-priority condition?
    - A. difficulty breathing
    - B. nausea and vomiting
    - C. a severed artery
    - D. a mental status of "U"

15. The initial assessment takes different forms, which depend on the age of the patient and whether or not he
    - A. has a medical problem or a trauma problem.
    - B. is alert or conscious.
    - C. has a history of diabetes.
    - D. has a history of head injury.

16. When evaluating circulation in infants, the EMT-B should use
    - A. the femoral pulse.
    - B. the distal pulse check.
    - C. capillary refill.
    - D. the radial pulse.

17. The mental status of an unconscious infant is typically checked by
    A. splashing cold water on him.
    B. shouting and flicking his feet.
    C. performing a pin prick on the feet.
    D. applying a sternal rub.

18. Which one is not a high-priority condition?
    A. shock
    B. a fever and rash
    C. a complicated childbirth
    D. severe pain anywhere

19. The difference between the general impression steps for a medical patient and those for a trauma patient is
    A. manual stabilization of the head for a trauma patient.
    B. no SAMPLE is taken for a trauma patient.
    C. the medical patient is treated faster.
    D. the AVPU is not used for a medical patient.

20. When the EMT-B documents that the chest pain patient denies shortness of breath, this is most appropriately termed
    A. an informative objective.
    B. advisory information.
    C. a pertinent negative.
    D. run data information.

21. When writing the narrative section of a prehospital care report, the EMT-B should do all of the following except
    A. use medical terminology correctly.
    B. avoid nonstandard abbreviations.
    C. write legibly and use correct spelling.
    D. state one's personal opinion of the patient's condition.

22. Which statement best describes an important concept of documentation?
    A. Always fill out a continuation sheet.
    B. If it's not written down, you didn't do it.
    C. It should include plenty of medical terms.
    D. Document everything you see.

23. If the patient does not wish to go to the hospital, you should
    A. document with a refusal-of-care form.
    B. take the patient to the hospital anyway.
    C. end your assessment immediately.
    D. call for another crew to subdue him.

24. When an important part of the assessment or care was not performed, this is called
    A. submission.   C. inhibition.
    B. omission.   D. commission.

25. When an EMT-B makes up a set of vitals for inclusion on the prehospital care report, this is called
    A. assault.   C. falsification.
    B. libel.   D. battery.

26. An objective statement is
    A. one that is made from a particular point of view.
    B. one that is made by the patient or a family member.
    C. one that describes observable or measurable information.
    D. one's own assessment of what is wrong with the patient.

27. When the EMT-B writes "The patient is alert and oriented" on the prehospital care report, this is an example of
    A. objective information.
    B. a statement beyond his/her training.
    C. subjective information.
    D. nonfactual information.

28. When you are documenting exactly what a patient told you on the prehospital care report, you should
    A. paraphrase for brevity.
    B. summarize the key points.
    C. use medical terminology.
    D. use quotes around the statement.

29. Writing a statement such as "The patient's daughter was rude to us" on a prehospital care report is
    A. not relevant.
    B. objective information.
    C. run data information.
    D. an example of what should be included in quotes.

30. The next step in the initial assessment after establishing unresponsiveness is to
    A. ensure an open airway.
    B. check for adequate breathing.
    C. check for circulation.
    D. look for profuse bleeding.

31. The term "sixth sense" is used to describe
    A. an EMT-B's clinical judgment.
    B. the six steps in an initial assessment.
    C. a patient's sensory functions.
    D. the ability to hear.

32. Which one of the following is a true vital sign?
    A. nausea
    B. skin temperature
    C. level of responsiveness
    D. age

33. The normal pulse rate for an adult at rest is between _____ beats per minute.
    A. 50 and 70
    B. 60 and 100
    C. 65 and 95
    D. 80 and 100

34. During the determination of vital signs, the initial pulse rate for patients 1 year and older is normally taken at the _____ pulse.
    A. carotid
    B. femoral
    C. pedal
    D. radial

35. When the pulse force is weak and thin, it is described as
    A. shallow.
    B. full.
    C. partial.
    D. thready.

36. Normal at-rest respiration rates for adults vary from _____ breaths per minute.
    A. 5 to 10
    B. 12 to 20
    C. 15 to 30
    D. 20 to 32

37. A noisy, harsh sound heard during inhalation that indicates a partial airway obstruction is
    A. gurgling.
    B. snorting.
    C. stertorous respirations.
    D. crowing.

38. Systolic blood pressure indicates the arterial pressure created as the
    A. artery contracts.
    B. artery relaxes.
    C. heart contracts.
    D. heart relaxes.

39. Diastolic blood pressure indicates the arterial pressure created as the
    A. heart contracts.
    B. heart refills.
    C. artery contracts.
    D. artery relaxes.

40. The technique of measuring blood pressure with a sphygmomanometer and a stethoscope is called
    A. palpation.
    B. auscultation.
    C. oscillation.
    D. priapism.

41. Determining blood pressure by palpation is
    A. not as accurate as the auscultation method.
    B. used when there is no noise around a patient.
    C. is documented as the "palp/diastolic"
    D. used whenever the patient is hypertensive.

42. Information that you can see, hear, feel, and smell are called
    A. signs.
    B. sensations.
    C. symptoms.
    D. assessments.

43. When the EMT-B asks the patient "Have you recently had any surgery or injuries?" he is inquiring about the
    A. patient's medications.
    B. patient's pertinent past history.
    C. events leading up to the illness.
    D. allergies that the patient may have.

44. When the EMT-B asks the patient "Are you on birth control pills?" she is inquiring about the
    A. patient's medications.
    B. patient's pertinent past history.
    C. events leading up to the illness.
    D. allergies that the patient may have.

45. An acronym used to remember what questions to ask about the patient's present problem and past history is
    A. AVPU.
    B. CUPS.
    C. SAMPLE.
    D. PEARL.

46. When conducting a patient interview on an adult patient, the EMT-B should do all of the following except
    A. position oneself close to the patient.
    B. identify oneself and reassure the patient.
    C. gently touch the patient's shoulder or rest a hand over the patient's hand.
    D. avoid asking the patient's age.

47. Normal diastolic pressures range from _____ mm Hg.
    A. 50 to 80
    B. 50 to 90
    C. 60 to 80
    D. 60 to 90

48. Using the formula presented in the text, a 36-year-old man would have an estimated systolic blood pressure of
    A. 116 mm Hg.
    B. 126 mm Hg.
    C. 136 mm Hg.
    D. 146 mm Hg.

49. Using the formula presented in the text, a 26-year-old woman would have an estimated systolic blood pressure of
    A. 106 mm Hg.
    B. 116 mm Hg.
    C. 126 mm Hg.
    D. 136 mm Hg.

50. Why should the stethoscope not be placed under the cuff and then inflated when evaluating the blood pressure?
    A. It may give a false reading.
    B. It can dent the stethoscope.
    C. The patient will not like the feeling.
    D. It will prevent pumping the cuff to the proper pressure.

51. When taking a patient's blood pressure, the stethoscope is placed over the _____ artery.
    A. carotid
    B. radial
    C. brachial
    D. femoral

52. The best indication of potential injury is the
    A. type of accident.
    B. type of injury.
    C. mechanism of injury.
    D. position of the patient.

53. When there are no apparent hazards at the scene of a collision, the danger zone should extend _____ feet in all directions from the wreckage.
    A. 25   C. 75
    B. 50   D. 100

54. In the up-and-over injury pattern, the patient is most likely to sustain _____ injuries.
    A. knee   C. head
    B. hip   D. leg

55. A keen awareness that there may be injuries based on the mechanism of injury is called
    A. sixth sense.
    B. general impression.
    C. index of suspicion.
    D. kinesthetic sense.

56. The purpose of the initial assessment is to
    A. take the patient's vital signs.
    B. gather information about the accident.
    C. discover and treat life-threatening conditions.
    D. obtain the patient's history.

57. The first step in the focused history and physical exam for any trauma patient is to
    A. make a status decision.
    B. check for an open airway.
    C. reconsider the mechanism of injury.
    D. treat life-threatening conditions.

58. The "A" in DCAP-BTLS stands for
    A. allergies.   C. abrasions.
    B. alert.   D. arrhythmia.

59. All of the following are clues that help an EMT-B determine the need for cervical immobilization except
    A. mechanism of injury.
    B. level of responsiveness.
    C. location of injuries.
    D. breathing rate.

60. Which of the following is true of the rapid trauma assessment?
    A. It begins with examination of the posterior body and ends with examination of the head.
    B. It evaluates areas of the body where the greatest threats to the patient may be.
    C. It is performed on a trauma patient without significant mechanism of injury.
    D. It includes careful examination of the face, eyes, ears, nose, and mouth.

61. On which type of patient is the detailed physical exam most often performed?
    A. trauma patient with a significant mechanism of injury
    B. trauma patient with no significant mechanism of injury
    C. a responsive medical patient
    D. an unresponsive medical patient

62. To obtain a history of a patient's present illness,
    A. ask the OPQRST questions.
    B. conduct the subjective interview.
    C. ask the SAMPLE questions.
    D. use the look, listen, feel, and smell method.

63. The "P" in OPQRST stands for
    A. punctures.   C. provokes.
    B. penetrations.   D. pulses.

64. The steps in the focused history and physical exam of the unresponsive medical patient include the following:
    1. Obtain baseline vital signs.
    2. Gather the history of the present illness from bystanders and family.
    3. Conduct a rapid physical exam.
    4. Gather a SAMPLE history from bystanders and family.

    Which is the correct order in which the above steps should be performed?
    A. 3, 1, 2, 4   C. 3, 2, 4, 1
    B. 2, 3, 4, 1   D. 1, 2, 3, 4

65. For a stable patient, the EMT-B should perform the ongoing assessment every _____ minutes.
    A. 5   C. 15
    B. 10   D. 20

66. During the ongoing assessment, whenever you believe there may have been a change in the patient's condition, you should immediately
    A. repeat the initial assessment.
    B. transport the patient immediately.
    C. document trends in vital signs.
    D. repeat the rapid trauma assessment.

67. Cool, clammy skin most likely indicates
    A. high fever.
    B. exposure to cold.
    C. mild fever.
    D. hypoperfusion (shock).

68. As an EMT-B, your overriding concern at all times is
A. the patient's safety.
B. the safety of patients and bystanders.
C. the patient's life.
D. your own safety.

69. During the detailed physical exam of the head of a trauma patient, inspect the
A. ears and nose for blood or clear fluids.
B. inner surface of the eyelids.
C. skin color of the cheeks.
D. mouth for blood and clear fluids.

70. Meningitis and _____ trauma can cause the fontanelle to bulge in an infant.
A. multiple   C. extremity
B. head   D. abdominal

71. Infants and young children under the age of _____ are abdominal breathers.
A. 2   C. 8
B. 4   D. 16

72. Children in this age group generally feel that they are indestructible but may have fears of permanent injury or disfigurement.
A. toddlers   C. adolescent
B. preschool   D. school age

73. Geriatric patients usually have decreased elasticity of the lungs and decreased activity of cilia that results in
A. increased risk of heart attack.
B. diminished activity and tolerance of physical stress.
C. decreased ability to clear foreign substances from the lungs.
D. decreased energy and tolerance of hot and cold.

74. Loss of skin elasticity and shrinking of sweat glands in a geriatric patient causes
A. diminished activity and tolerance of physical stress.
B. decreased ability to clear foreign substances from the lungs.
C. decreased energy and tolerance of hot and cold.
D. thin, dry, wrinkled skin.

75. Diminished function of the thyroid gland is one of the effects of aging. This results in
A. thin, dry, wrinkled skin.
B. decreased energy and tolerance of heat and cold.
C. depression and loss of social support.
D. decreased strength.

76. When an elderly patient falls, this may be an indication of a more serious problem such as
A. viral pneumonia.
B. acute alcoholism.
C. abnormal heart rhythm.
D. severe depression.

77. Repeaters are
A. phones that transmit radio signals over air waves instead of wires.
B. devices used to transmit radio signals over long distances.
C. patients who consistently call 9-1-1.
D. a type of cellular phone used in EMS.

78. Which one of the following is an appropriate interpersonal communication technique?
A. standing above a patient
B. avoiding eye contact
C. directly facing a patient
D. standing, arms crossed

79. What is the <u>first</u> item given to the hospital in your medical radio report to the receiving facility?
A. the patient's age and sex
B. unit identification/level of provider
C. estimated time of arrival
D. emergency medical care given

80. Which of the following is <u>not</u> considered an essential component of the verbal report to the receiving facility?
A. patient's chief complaint
B. additional treatment given en route
C. additional vital signs taken en route
D. patient's attitude.

81. Which of the following is true of the medical radio report?
A. Use codes to communicate patient information.
B. Ensure that you give the hospital your patient diagnosis.
C. Paint a picture of the patient's problem in words.
D. Speak rapidly to limit transmission time.

82. To avoid misunderstanding and miscommunication when speaking with medical direction, you should do all of the following <u>except</u>
A. Give information clearly and accurately.
B. Repeat back the order you are given word for word.
C. Ask the physician to repeat the order if it is unclear.
D. Avoid questioning the physician about the order.

83. Medications that are carried on the ambulance and that EMT-Bs can administer include activated charcoal, oxygen, and
A. oral glucose.   C. epinephrine.
B. nitroglycerin.   D. all of the above.

84. Any action of a drug other than the desired action is called a
    A. contraindication.   C. reflex.
    B. indication.   D. side effect.

85. When a drug is administered subcutaneously, this means the drug is
    A. dissolved under the tongue.
    B. injected into a vein.
    C. rubbed into a muscle.
    D. injected under the skin.

86. Which of the following is true of the structure of infants' and children's airways?
    A. The trachea is more rigid and less flexible than an adult's.
    B. The tongue is proportionately smaller than an adult's.
    C. The cricoid cartilage is more rigid than an adult's.
    D. They depend more on the diaphragm for respiration than adults do.

87. The means of providing artificial ventilation are
    1. Pocket face mask without supplemental oxygen.
    2. Two-person bag-valve mask with supplemental oxygen.
    3. Flow-restricted, oxygen-powered ventilator
    4. One-person bag-valve mask with supplemental oxygen

    What is the best method to use?
    A. 1   C. 3
    B. 2   D. 4

88. The adequate rate of artificial ventilations for a nonbreathing adult patient is _____ breaths per minute.
    A. 8   C. 16
    B. 12   D. 20

89. The adequate rate of artificial ventilations for a nonbreathing infant or child patient is _____ breaths per minute.
    A. 10   C. 20
    B. 15   D. 25

90. Which of the following respiratory sounds made by an unresponsive adult most likely indicates a serious airway problem requiring immediate intervention?
    A. snoring or gurgling
    B. slight wheezing
    C. sniffling
    D. whistling or grunting

91. The skin of a patient with inadequate breathing will most likely be
    A. pale, cool, and dry
    B. red, hot, and clammy
    C. yellow, warm, and dry
    D. blue, cool, and clammy

92. If a patient is experiencing breathing difficulty, but is breathing adequately, it is usually best to place him in the _____ position.
    A. tripod   C. sitting-up
    B. supine   D. recovery

93. Which one of the following is a cause of adult chest pain due to a decreased blood supply to the heart muscle?
    A. cerebral vascular accident
    B. arrhythmia
    C. congestive heart failure
    D. angina pectoris

94. Most heart attacks are caused by the narrowing or occlusion of a _____ artery.
    A. cephalic   C. coronary
    B. brachial   D. carotid

95. Which of the following is the condition in which a portion of the myocardium dies because of oxygen starvation?
    A. angina pectoris
    B. mechanical pump failure
    C. cardiogenic shock
    D. acute myocardial infarction

96. An irregular heart rhythm is called
    A. mechanical pump failure.
    B. arrhythmia.
    C. cardiogenic shock.
    D. congestive heart failure.

97. Which term applies to a pulse slower than 60 beats per minute?
    A. bradycardia
    B. ventricular fibrillation
    C. tachycardia
    D. atrial fibrillation

98. An at-rest heart beating faster than 100 beats per minute is referred to as
    A. bradycardia.
    B. ventricular fibrillation.
    C. tachycardia.
    D. atrial fibrillation.

99. Which of the following is the condition caused by excessive fluid buildup in the lungs because of the inadequate pumping of the heart?
    A. congestive heart failure
    B. acute heart failure
    C. acute myocardial infarction
    D. chronic myocardial infarction

100. The conscious patient with a possible heart attack is best transported in the
   A. recovery position.
   B. medical coma position.
   C. traumatic coma position.
   D. position of comfort.

101. A diabetic found with a weak, rapid pulse and cold, clammy skin who complains of hunger pangs suffers from
   A. hypoglycemia.
   B. cardiogenic shock.
   C. hyperglycemia.
   D. ulcers.

102. Which of the following conditions frequently results in an acetone smell on the patient's breath?
   A. stroke
   C. ulcers
   B. hyperglycemia
   D. hypoglycemia

103. A conscious hypoglycemic patient who is able to swallow is frequently administered
   A. oral glucose.
   C. nitroglycerin.
   B. insulin.
   D. epinephrine.

104. If you cannot administer glucose to the diabetic patient because she is not alert enough to swallow, you should
   A. wait until her mental status improves.
   B. contact medical direction immediately.
   C. treat her like any other patient with altered mental status.
   D. place her in a position of comfort.

105. The first time a person is exposed to an allergen, the immune system
   A. reacts violently.
   B. shuts down.
   C. forms antibodies.
   D. ignores the allergen.

106. To be considered a severe allergic reaction, a patient must have signs and symptoms of shock and/or
   A. a history of allergies.
   B. massive swelling.
   C. respiratory distress.
   D. increased blood pressure.

107. A patient has no history of allergies and is having his first allergic reaction. What action should you take?
   A. Consult with medical direction.
   B. Treat for shock and transport immediately.
   C. Administer epinephrine via auto-injector.
   D. Attempt to determine the cause immediately.

108. Carbon monoxide, chlorine, and ammonia are examples of _____ poisons.
   A. ingested
   C. inhaled
   B. injected
   D. absorbed

109. It is important for the EMT-B to determine when the ingestion of a poison occurred because
   A. different poisons act on the body at different rates.
   B. those who ingest poison in the evening tend to vomit frequently.
   C. dilution of the poison is never effective after ten minutes.
   D. the antidote is more effective once the poison reaches the stomach.

110. The principal prehospital treatment of a patient who has inhaled poisonous gas is
   A. administering activated charcoal.
   B. administering high-concentration oxygen.
   C. rapidly administering an antidote.
   D. irrigating the respiratory tract with water.

111. Drinking alcohol along with taking other drugs frequently results in
   A. uncontrolled shivering.
   B. depressed vital signs.
   C. extreme agitation.
   D. all of the above.

112. Activated charcoal is contraindicated for patients who have ingested
   A. alkalis.
   C. acids.
   B. gasoline.
   D. all of the above.

113. Most cases of poisoning
   A. are intentional in nature.
   B. involve elderly patients.
   C. involve young children.
   D. lead to disability or death.

114. Poisons that are swallowed are _____ poisons.
   A. absorbed
   C. ingested
   B. inhaled
   D. injected

115. For a heat emergency, the patient with _____, dry skin requires rapid cooling and immediate transport.
   A. pale
   C. cool
   B. hot
   D. warm

116. As frostbite progresses and exposure continues, the skin will turn from white and waxy to
   A. blotchy and grayish yellow.
   B. pale and pinkish red.
   C. deep blue at the nose and cheeks.
   D. cherry red, except for the extremities.

117. To treat a patient with deep frostbite,
A. immerse the limb in 105°F water and transport the patient.
B. rub snow on the frozen area or apply cold packs if available.
C. cover the frostbitten area, handle it as gently as possible, and transport patient.
D. protect the frostbitten area by keeping it cold and transport the patient.

118. With frostbite, the
A. underlying tissues feel frozen to the touch.
B. skin is commonly mottled and grayish blue.
C. skin blisters and swells.
D. affected area feels frozen, but only on the surface.

119. The initial sign of hypothermia is
A. shivering.
B. numbness.
C. drowsiness and slow breathing.
D. white, waxy skin.

120. Extreme hypothermia is characterized by
A. unconsciousness, absence of discernible vital signs.
B. shivering, numbness, drowsiness.
C. flaccid muscles.
D. rapid breathing.

121. The emergency care steps for a hypothermic patient who is alert and responding include all of the following except
A. keep the patient still.
B. keep the patient dry.
C. apply heat to the patient's body.
D. encourage the patient to walk.

122. After calming a snakebite victim and treating for shock, you locate the fang marks. Next, you should
A. immobilize the affected extremity.
B. conserve patient body heat.
C. cleanse the wound site.
D. apply a full tourniquet.

123. A patient who was working in a hot environment complains of severe muscle cramps in the legs and feels faint. You should move the patient to a cool place and begin care by
A. administering oxygen by nonrebreather.
B. transporting the patient immediately.
C. administering oxygen by nasal cannula.
D. giving the patient water.

124. The first step in caring for a rescued near-drowning victim is to
A. expel water from the victim's lungs.
B. provide ventilations with oxygen.
C. establish an airway.
D. initiate chest compressions.

125. Your first step when called to care for any attempted suicide victim is to
A. gain access to the patient.
B. wait for police assistance.
C. survey for behavioral changes.
D. ensure your own safety.

126. You are unable to perform normal assessment and care procedures because the patient is aggressive and hostile. What action should you take?
A. Restrain the patient immediately.
B. Ask a family member to assist you.
C. Seek advice from medical direction.
D. Call the patient's physician.

127. When is the EMT-B allowed to use reasonable force?
A. only when the police are on the scene
B. to defend against attack by an emotionally disturbed patient
C. whenever a patient refuses treatment
D. whenever alcohol abuse is suspected

128. The developing unborn baby is called a
A. crowning.
B. fetus.
C. placenta previa.
D. stillborn.

129. The muscular organ in which the fetus develops is the
A. umbilical cord.
B. placenta.
C. uterus.
D. cervix.

130. The organ of pregnancy in which exchange of oxygen, nutrients, and wastes occurs between mother and fetus is the
A. placenta.
B. cervix.
C. vagina.
D. amniotic.

131. While developing, the fetus is protected by a thin, membranous "bag of waters" called the _____ sac.
A. uterine
B. placental
C. amniotic
D. peritoneal

132. When the presenting part of the baby first bulges from the vaginal opening, this is called
A. crowning.
B. dilating.
C. labor.
D. prolapsing.

133. The first stage of labor begins with
A. cervical dilation.
B. perineum.
C. uterine contractions.
D. afterbirth.

134. The second stage of labor ends with
A. cervical dilation.
B. infant delivery.
C. placental delivery.
D. uterine contractions.

135. The third stage of labor ends with
A. full cervical dilation.
B. perineum tearing.
C. delivery of the placenta.
D. delivery of infant.

136. If a woman is having her first baby, the first stage of labor will usually last _____ hours on the average.
A. 4   C. 12
B. 8   D. 16

137. During the most active stage of labor, the uterus usually contracts every _____ minutes.
A. 1 to 2   C. 5 to 9
B. 2 to 3   D. 10 to 15

138. If the amniotic sac does not break during delivery, the EMT-B should
A. do nothing; it will break after birth.
B. quickly remove with sterile scissors.
C. puncture it with a finger.
D. transport the patient immediately.

139. To assist the mother in delivering the baby, gently
A. pull at the baby's shoulders.
B. support the baby's head.
C. rotate the baby to the left or right.
D. push your gloved hand into the vagina.

140. After the delivery, which of the following should be done first?
A. Clamp and cut the cord.
B. Suction the baby's mouth and nose.
C. Lay the baby on his back.
D. Lift the baby by the feet and slap the buttocks.

141. Following the delivery, if spontaneous respiration does not begin after suctioning the baby's mouth and nose, the EMT-B should first
A. begin mouth-to-mouth-and-nose resuscitation.
B. apply mechanical resuscitation with 100% oxygen.
C. vigorously rub the baby's back.
D. transport immediately, administering 100% oxygen.

142. The first clamp placed on the umbilical cord should be about _____ inches from the baby.
A. 2   C. 10
B. 5   D. 12

143. If bleeding continues from the umbilical cord after clamping and cutting, the EMT-B should
A. clamp the cord again.
B. unclamp the cord and tie.
C. apply a sterile dressing.
D. transport the baby immediately.

144. Which of the following is the maximum amount of time the EMT-B should wait for the placenta to be delivered before transporting the mother and infant?
A. 20 minutes   C. 1 hour
B. 45 minutes   D. 2 hours

145. Delivery of the placenta is usually accompanied by the loss of no more than _____ of blood.
A. 500 cc   C. 800 cc
B. 600 cc   D. 1,000 cc

146. The first step to control vaginal bleeding after birth is to
A. apply a pressure dressing.
B. position a sanitary napkin.
C. massage the uterus.
D. pack the vagina with sterile gauze.

147. The presenting part of the baby in a breech birth is the
A. arms.   C. face.
B. buttocks or legs. D. head.

148. If during birth, the umbilical cord presents first, you should
A. gently push the cord back into the vagina.
B. gently push up on the baby's head or buttocks to keep pressure off the cord.
C. gently push on the cervix.
D. clamp and cut the cord.

149. If an arm presentation without a prolapsed cord is noted, the EMT-B should
A. reach up the vagina and turn the baby.
B. do nothing; the delivery will be normal.
C. transport immediately, providing O_2.
D. insert gloved hand and push back the vaginal wall.

150. A baby is considered premature if it weighs less than 5 pounds or is born before the _____ week of pregnancy.
A. 35th   C. 37th
B. 36th   D. 38th

Interim Exam Two Answer Sheet

Fill in the correct answer for each item. When scoring, note there are 150
questions valued at 0.666 points each.

1. [ ] A   [ ] B   [ ] C   [ ] D   37. [ ] A   [ ] B   [ ] C   [ ] D
2. [ ] A   [ ] B   [ ] C   [ ] D   38. [ ] A   [ ] B   [ ] C   [ ] D
3. [ ] A   [ ] B   [ ] C   [ ] D   39. [ ] A   [ ] B   [ ] C   [ ] D
4. [ ] A   [ ] B   [ ] C   [ ] D   40. [ ] A   [ ] B   [ ] C   [ ] D
5. [ ] A   [ ] B   [ ] C   [ ] D   41. [ ] A   [ ] B   [ ] C   [ ] D
6. [ ] A   [ ] B   [ ] C   [ ] D   42. [ ] A   [ ] B   [ ] C   [ ] D
7. [ ] A   [ ] B   [ ] C   [ ] D   43. [ ] A   [ ] B   [ ] C   [ ] D
8. [ ] A   [ ] B   [ ] C   [ ] D   44. [ ] A   [ ] B   [ ] C   [ ] D
9. [ ] A   [ ] B   [ ] C   [ ] D   45. [ ] A   [ ] B   [ ] C   [ ] D
10. [ ] A   [ ] B   [ ] C   [ ] D   46. [ ] A   [ ] B   [ ] C   [ ] D
11. [ ] A   [ ] B   [ ] C   [ ] D   47. [ ] A   [ ] B   [ ] C   [ ] D
12. [ ] A   [ ] B   [ ] C   [ ] D   48. [ ] A   [ ] B   [ ] C   [ ] D
13. [ ] A   [ ] B   [ ] C   [ ] D   49. [ ] A   [ ] B   [ ] C   [ ] D
14. [ ] A   [ ] B   [ ] C   [ ] D   50. [ ] A   [ ] B   [ ] C   [ ] D
15. [ ] A   [ ] B   [ ] C   [ ] D   51. [ ] A   [ ] B   [ ] C   [ ] D
16. [ ] A   [ ] B   [ ] C   [ ] D   52. [ ] A   [ ] B   [ ] C   [ ] D
17. [ ] A   [ ] B   [ ] C   [ ] D   53. [ ] A   [ ] B   [ ] C   [ ] D
18. [ ] A   [ ] B   [ ] C   [ ] D   54. [ ] A   [ ] B   [ ] C   [ ] D
19. [ ] A   [ ] B   [ ] C   [ ] D   55. [ ] A   [ ] B   [ ] C   [ ] D
20. [ ] A   [ ] B   [ ] C   [ ] D   56. [ ] A   [ ] B   [ ] C   [ ] D
21. [ ] A   [ ] B   [ ] C   [ ] D   57. [ ] A   [ ] B   [ ] C   [ ] D
22. [ ] A   [ ] B   [ ] C   [ ] D   58. [ ] A   [ ] B   [ ] C   [ ] D
23. [ ] A   [ ] B   [ ] C   [ ] D   59. [ ] A   [ ] B   [ ] C   [ ] D
24. [ ] A   [ ] B   [ ] C   [ ] D   60. [ ] A   [ ] B   [ ] C   [ ] D
25. [ ] A   [ ] B   [ ] C   [ ] D   61. [ ] A   [ ] B   [ ] C   [ ] D
26. [ ] A   [ ] B   [ ] C   [ ] D   62. [ ] A   [ ] B   [ ] C   [ ] D
27. [ ] A   [ ] B   [ ] C   [ ] D   63. [ ] A   [ ] B   [ ] C   [ ] D
28. [ ] A   [ ] B   [ ] C   [ ] D   64. [ ] A   [ ] B   [ ] C   [ ] D
29. [ ] A   [ ] B   [ ] C   [ ] D   65. [ ] A   [ ] B   [ ] C   [ ] D
30. [ ] A   [ ] B   [ ] C   [ ] D   66. [ ] A   [ ] B   [ ] C   [ ] D
31. [ ] A   [ ] B   [ ] C   [ ] D   67. [ ] A   [ ] B   [ ] C   [ ] D
32. [ ] A   [ ] B   [ ] C   [ ] D   68. [ ] A   [ ] B   [ ] C   [ ] D
33. [ ] A   [ ] B   [ ] C   [ ] D   69. [ ] A   [ ] B   [ ] C   [ ] D
34. [ ] A   [ ] B   [ ] C   [ ] D   70. [ ] A   [ ] B   [ ] C   [ ] D
35. [ ] A   [ ] B   [ ] C   [ ] D   71. [ ] A   [ ] B   [ ] C   [ ] D
36. [ ] A   [ ] B   [ ] C   [ ] D   72. [ ] A   [ ] B   [ ] C   [ ] D

73. [ ] A	[ ] B	[ ] C	[ ] D	112. [ ] A	[ ] B	[ ] C	[ ] D
74. [ ] A	[ ] B	[ ] C	[ ] D	113. [ ] A	[ ] B	[ ] C	[ ] D
75. [ ] A	[ ] B	[ ] C	[ ] D	114. [ ] A	[ ] B	[ ] C	[ ] D
76. [ ] A	[ ] B	[ ] C	[ ] D	115. [ ] A	[ ] B	[ ] C	[ ] D
77. [ ] A	[ ] B	[ ] C	[ ] D	116. [ ] A	[ ] B	[ ] C	[ ] D
78. [ ] A	[ ] B	[ ] C	[ ] D	117. [ ] A	[ ] B	[ ] C	[ ] D
79. [ ] A	[ ] B	[ ] C	[ ] D	118. [ ] A	[ ] B	[ ] C	[ ] D
80. [ ] A	[ ] B	[ ] C	[ ] D	119. [ ] A	[ ] B	[ ] C	[ ] D
81. [ ] A	[ ] B	[ ] C	[ ] D	120. [ ] A	[ ] B	[ ] C	[ ] D
82. [ ] A	[ ] B	[ ] C	[ ] D	121. [ ] A	[ ] B	[ ] C	[ ] D
83. [ ] A	[ ] B	[ ] C	[ ] D	122. [ ] A	[ ] B	[ ] C	[ ] D
84. [ ] A	[ ] B	[ ] C	[ ] D	123. [ ] A	[ ] B	[ ] C	[ ] D
85. [ ] A	[ ] B	[ ] C	[ ] D	124. [ ] A	[ ] B	[ ] C	[ ] D
86. [ ] A	[ ] B	[ ] C	[ ] D	125. [ ] A	[ ] B	[ ] C	[ ] D
87. [ ] A	[ ] B	[ ] C	[ ] D	126. [ ] A	[ ] B	[ ] C	[ ] D
88. [ ] A	[ ] B	[ ] C	[ ] D	127. [ ] A	[ ] B	[ ] C	[ ] D
89. [ ] A	[ ] B	[ ] C	[ ] D	128. [ ] A	[ ] B	[ ] C	[ ] D
90. [ ] A	[ ] B	[ ] C	[ ] D	129. [ ] A	[ ] B	[ ] C	[ ] D
91. [ ] A	[ ] B	[ ] C	[ ] D	130. [ ] A	[ ] B	[ ] C	[ ] D
92. [ ] A	[ ] B	[ ] C	[ ] D	131. [ ] A	[ ] B	[ ] C	[ ] D
93. [ ] A	[ ] B	[ ] C	[ ] D	132. [ ] A	[ ] B	[ ] C	[ ] D
94. [ ] A	[ ] B	[ ] C	[ ] D	133. [ ] A	[ ] B	[ ] C	[ ] D
95. [ ] A	[ ] B	[ ] C	[ ] D	134. [ ] A	[ ] B	[ ] C	[ ] D
96. [ ] A	[ ] B	[ ] C	[ ] D	135. [ ] A	[ ] B	[ ] C	[ ] D
97. [ ] A	[ ] B	[ ] C	[ ] D	136. [ ] A	[ ] B	[ ] C	[ ] D
98. [ ] A	[ ] B	[ ] C	[ ] D	137. [ ] A	[ ] B	[ ] C	[ ] D
99. [ ] A	[ ] B	[ ] C	[ ] D	138. [ ] A	[ ] B	[ ] C	[ ] D
100. [ ] A	[ ] B	[ ] C	[ ] D	139. [ ] A	[ ] B	[ ] C	[ ] D
101. [ ] A	[ ] B	[ ] C	[ ] D	140. [ ] A	[ ] B	[ ] C	[ ] D
102. [ ] A	[ ] B	[ ] C	[ ] D	141. [ ] A	[ ] B	[ ] C	[ ] D
103. [ ] A	[ ] B	[ ] C	[ ] D	142. [ ] A	[ ] B	[ ] C	[ ] D
104. [ ] A	[ ] B	[ ] C	[ ] D	143. [ ] A	[ ] B	[ ] C	[ ] D
105. [ ] A	[ ] B	[ ] C	[ ] D	144. [ ] A	[ ] B	[ ] C	[ ] D
106. [ ] A	[ ] B	[ ] C	[ ] D	145. [ ] A	[ ] B	[ ] C	[ ] D
107. [ ] A	[ ] B	[ ] C	[ ] D	146. [ ] A	[ ] B	[ ] C	[ ] D
108. [ ] A	[ ] B	[ ] C	[ ] D	147. [ ] A	[ ] B	[ ] C	[ ] D
109. [ ] A	[ ] B	[ ] C	[ ] D	148. [ ] A	[ ] B	[ ] C	[ ] D
110. [ ] A	[ ] B	[ ] C	[ ] D	149. [ ] A	[ ] B	[ ] C	[ ] D
111. [ ] A	[ ] B	[ ] C	[ ] D	150. [ ] A	[ ] B	[ ] C	[ ] D

Chapter Twenty-Six

BLEEDING AND SHOCK

MATCH TERMINOLOGY/DEFINITIONS

▶ PART A

A. Major artery of the upper arm

B. When the patient is developing shock, but the body is still able to maintain perfusion

C. Bleeding that is characterized by a slow, oozing flow of blood

D. Shock resulting from blood loss

E. Condition that occurs when the body can no longer compensate for low blood volume or lack of perfusion; late signs, such as falling blood pressure, develop.

F. Major artery supplying the thigh

G. Severe bleeding; a major cause of shock

H. Lack of perfusion brought on by inadequate pumping action of the heart

I. Optimum time limit between time of injury and surgery at the hospital; survival rates are best if surgery takes place within this time period.

J. Blood vessel with thick, muscular walls that carries blood away from the heart

_____ 1. Artery

_____ 2. Brachial artery

_____ 3. Capillary bleeding

_____ 4. Cardiogenic shock

_____ 5. Compensated shock

_____ 6. Decompensated shock

_____ 7. Femoral artery

_____ 8. Golden hour

_____ 9. Hemorrhage

_____ 10. Hemorrhagic shock

A. Device that closes off all blood flow to and from an extremity

B. Blood vessel that has one-way valves and carries blood back to the heart

C. Adequate circulation of blood throughout the body, filling the capillaries and supplying the cells and tissues with oxygen and nutrients

D. Site where a large artery lies near the surface of the body and directly over a bone; pressure on such a location can control profuse bleeding in the extremities.

E. When the body has lost the battle to maintain perfusion to the organ systems; cell damage occurs, especially to the liver and kidneys.

F. Another name for hypoperfusion

G. Bulky dressing held in position with a tightly wrapped bandage to help control bleeding

H. Shock resulting from uncontrolled bleeding or plasma loss

I. Shock resulting from uncontrolled dilation of blood vessels due to nerve paralysis (sometimes caused by spinal-cord injuries)

J. Inadequate circulation of the blood in which the body's cells and organs do not receive adequate supplies of oxygen and dangerous waste products build up

_____ 1. Hypoperfusion

_____ 2. Hypovolemic shock

_____ 3. Irreversible shock

_____ 4. Neurogenic shock

_____ 5. Perfusion

_____ 6. Pressure dressing

_____ 7. Pressure point

_____ 8. Shock

_____ 9. Tourniquet

_____ 10. Vein

MULTIPLE-CHOICE REVIEW

_____ 1. Blood that has been depleted of oxygen and loaded with carbon dioxide empties into the _____ , which carry it back to the heart.
A. arteries
B. veins
C. capillaries
D. tissues

_____ 2. Cells and tissues of the brain, spinal cord, and _____ are the most sensitive to inadequate perfusion.
A. kidneys
B. lungs
C. stomach
D. heart

_____ 3. The use of _____ is essential whenever bleeding is discovered or anticipated.
A. full protective gear
B. BSI precautions
C. universal isolation precautions
D. Tyvek overalls

_____ 4. Bleeding is classified as all of the following except
A. arterial.
B. venous.
C. cellular.
D. capillary.

_____ 5. Which statement about arterial bleeding is correct?
A. Clot formation takes place rapidly.
B. It is often rapid and profuse.
C. It is the least difficult to control.
D. It causes the blood pressure to rise.

_____ 6. A steady flow of dark red or maroon blood is a result of _____ bleeding.
A. arterial
B. venous
C. capillary
D. pulmonary

_____ 7. Bleeding described as oozing usually is a result of _____ bleeding.
   A. arterial
   B. venous
   C. capillary
   D. bronchiole

_____ 8. When a large bleeding vein in the neck sucks in debris or an air bubble, this can cause
   A. an evisceration.
   B. heart stoppage.
   C. infection.
   D. severe bleeding.

_____ 9. Sudden blood loss of _____ in an adult is considered serious.
   A. 250 cc
   B. 500 cc
   C. 600 cc
   D. 1,000 cc

_____ 10. Sudden blood loss of _____ in a child is considered serious.
   A. 200 cc
   B. 300 cc
   C. 400 cc
   D. 500 cc

_____ 11. Sudden blood loss of _____ in a 1-year-old infant is considered serious.
   A. 25 cc
   B. 50 cc
   C. 100 cc
   D. 150 cc

_____ 12. The body's natural responses to bleeding is constriction of the injured blood vessel and _____ .
   A. perfusion.
   B. hypoperfusion.
   C. compensation.
   D. clotting.

_____ 13. The EMT-B's assessment of external bleeding includes all of the following items except
   A. estimating the amount of blood lost in order to predict potential shock.
   B. waiting for signs and symptoms of shock to appear before beginning treatment.
   C. triaging, or prioritizing, bleeding patients properly.
   D. identifying bleeding that must be treated during the initial assessment.

_____ 14. The major methods used to control external bleeding include all of the following except
   A. direct pressure.
   B. elevation.
   C. pressure points.
   D. vessel clamps.

_____ 15. Why is administration of supplemental oxygen an important treatment for any trauma patient?
   A. It enhances blood clotting.
   B. It improves oxygenation of the tissues.
   C. It constricts the blood vessels.
   D. All of the above.

_____ 16. The most common and effective way to control external bleeding is by
   A. cold application.
   B. elevation.
   C. pressure points.
   D. direct pressure.

_____ 17. The initial dressing should not be removed from a bleeding wound because it
   A. can become a biohazard.
   B. takes too long to remove.
   C. is a necessary part of clot formation.
   D. may increase the chance of infection.

_____ 18. After controlling bleeding from an extremity using a pressure dressing, be sure to
   A. loosen the tourniquet.
   B. check the distal pulse.
   C. apply a PASG.
   D. administer oxygen by nasal cannula.

_____ **19.** Elevation is used to assist in bleeding control for all of the following
reasons <u>except</u>
  A. Bleeding slows.
  B. The limb is raised above the heart.
  C. Blood pressure in the limb is reduced.
  D. Pulse rate is speeded up.

_____ **20.** When is it inappropriate to use elevation to assist in bleeding control?
  A. as you apply direct pressure
  B. while trying to bandage an extremity
  C. if you suspect musculoskeletal injuries
  D. when a patient is found lying down

_____ **21.** A pressure point is a site where
  A. a main artery lies near the surface of the body directly over the bone.
  B. the blood pressure can be taken by auscultation.
  C. a large vein lies within the outer layer of the skin.
  D. excessive pressure causes the pulse rate to increase rapidly.

_____ **22.** Use of a pressure point may <u>not</u> be effective if the wound
  A. was caused by an impaled object.
  B. was accompanied by spinal injury.
  C. is at the distal end of a limb.
  D. is bleeding profusely.

_____ **23.** Which of the following is <u>true</u> about the use of an air splint?
  A. It is effective for controlling venous and capillary bleeding.
  B. It should be used only if there is no suspected bone injury.
  C. It is most effective for controlling arterial bleeding.
  D. It should be used before other manual methods of bleeding control.

_____ **24.** Which of the following is <u>not</u> a guideline for supplementing bleeding
control with cold application?
  A. Wrap the ice pack in a cloth or towel.
  B. Do not apply directly onto the skin.
  C. Do not leave the cold pack in place for more than 20 minutes.
  D. Insert the ice directly into the wound.

_____ **25.** Many experts agree that the pneumatic anti-shock garment is useful for
  A. controlling bleeding from head trauma.
  B. controlling bleeding from the areas the garment covers.
  C. penetrating chest trauma.
  D. the patient in cardiogenic shock.

_____ **26.** Bleeding from a clean-edged amputation is usually initially cared for with
  A. a pressure dressing.   **C.** a tourniquet.
  B. cold application.   **D.** a pneumatic anti-shock garment.

_____ **27.** Rough-edged amputations, usually produced by crushing or tearing injuries,
  A. are easily controlled by a pressure bandage.
  B. tend to stop bleeding on their own.
  C. often will bleed very heavily.
  D. will constrict quickly to control bleeding.

_____ **28.** Once a tourniquet is in place, it must
  A. not be removed or loosened unless ordered by medical direction.
  B. be covered immediately to prevent accidental removal.
  C. be loosened every 15 minutes to dislodge clots.
  D. be used under the pneumatic anti-shock garment.

_____ **29.** A blood pressure cuff
   A. can be used as a tourniquet if inflated to 70 mmHg.
   B. should never be used for bleeding control.
   C. can be used as a temporary tourniquet if inflated to 150 mmHg.
   D. should always be used to control arterial bleeding.

_____ **30.** If a patient has a head injury and you note bleeding or loss of cerebrospinal fluid from the patient's ears or nose, you should
   A. apply direct pressure to the skull.
   B. apply direct pressure to the ears and nose.
   C. apply cold packs to the ears and nose.
   D. allow the drainage to flow freely.

_____ **31.** The medical term for a nosebleed is
   A. hemorrhage.   **C.** epihemorrhage.
   B. epistaxis.   **D.** nostrium.

_____ **32.** To stop a nosebleed, try each of the following except
   A. place the patient in a sitting position, leaning forward.
   B. apply direct pressure by pinching the nostrils.
   C. keep the patient calm.
   D. apply cold packs to the bridge of the nose.

_____ **33.** The leading cause of internal injuries and bleeding is
   A. blunt trauma.   **C.** auto collisions.
   B. penetrating trauma.   **D.** large lacerations.

_____ **34.** Which is not an example of a penetrating trauma?
   A. blast injury   **C.** knife wound
   B. gunshot wound   **D.** ice-pick wound

_____ **35.** Signs of internal bleeding include all of the following except
   A. vomiting a coffee ground-like substance.
   B. bradycardia and a flushed face.
   C. dark, tarry stools.
   D. tender, rigid, or distended abdomen.

_____ **36.** A patient who has internal bleeding may have all of the following except
   A. painful, swollen, or deformed extremities.
   B. signs and symptoms of shock.
   C. bright red blood in the stool.
   D. laceration to the forearm.

_____ **37.** Inadequate tissue perfusion is referred to as
   A. hyperperfusion.   **C.** hypoperfusion.
   B. hypoxia.   **D.** hypotension.

_____ **38.** Shock may develop as a result of all of the following except
   A. pump failure.   **C.** dilated blood vessels.
   B. lost blood volume.   **D.** injury to the head.

_____ **39.** The type of shock most commonly seen by EMT-Bs is _____ shock.
   A. cardiogenic   **C.** neurogenic
   B. irreversible   **D.** hypovolemic

_____ **40.** The most common mechanism of shock for a heart attack patient is
   A. vasoconstriction.   **C.** pump failure.
   B. fluid loss.   **D.** vasodilation.

_____ **41.** Shock caused by the failure of the nervous system to control the diameter of blood vessels is called _____ shock.
   A. hypovolemic   **C.** neurogenic
   B. cardiogenic   **D.** reversible

_____ 42. When a patient is in shock but the body is still able to maintain perfusion to the vital organs, this is called _____ shock.
 A. compensated
 B. decompensated
 C. delayed
 D. irreversible

_____ 43. Early signs of shock that are actually the body's compensating mechanisms include all of the following except
 A. increased heart rate.
 B. increased respirations.
 C. pale, cool skin.
 D. decreased capillary refill time.

_____ 44. When the body has lost the battle to maintain perfusion to the organ systems, this is called _____ shock.
 A. delayed
 B. compensated
 C. decompensated
 D. irreversible

_____ 45. Why does a patient in shock feel nauseated?
 A. Blood is diverted from the digestive system.
 B. Blood rushes rapidly to the digestive system.
 C. Shock increases the production of digestive juices.
 D. The patient has swallowed a great amount of blood.

_____ 46. The pulse of a patient in shock will
 A. decrease.
 B. be absent.
 C. increase.
 D. be irregular.

_____ 47. A drop in blood pressure is
 A. an early sign of shock.
 B. an early sign of shock in a child.
 C. always present in shock.
 D. a late sign of shock.

_____ 48. Additional signs of shock may include any of the following except
 A. thirst.
 B. dilated pupils.
 C. cyanosis around the lips and nailbeds.
 D. flushed, warm skin.

_____ 49. The EMT-B should be especially careful when evaluating pediatric patients for shock because they
 A. cannot be administered oxygen at low flow rates.
 B. may display few signs/symptoms until a large percentage of blood volume is lost.
 C. will decompensate for blood loss in a short period of time.
 D. may exhibit erratic capillary refill times.

_____ 50. Which of the following is the best description of the "platinum ten minutes?"
 A. maximum on-scene time when caring for a trauma or shock patient
 B. optimum time limit from the time of injury until surgery
 C. maximum time limit for controlling arterial bleeding before shock occurs
 D. optimum time limit for applying PASG to the shock patient

COMPLETE THE FOLLOWING

1. List the three major types of shock.

 A. _____

 B. _____

 C. _____

2. List six of the signs and symptoms of shock.

A. _____

B. _____

C. _____

D. _____

E. _____

F. _____

VIRTUAL STREET SCENES

(First review the Street Scenes on pp. 520–521 of the textbook. Then answer the questions below.)

1. This patient may have broken a rib or two. What abdominal organs are protected by the rib cage?

2. Would an ALS unit be appropriate for this patient?

3. You observed that the patient's mental status was changing. What might this indicate to you?

WEB SIMULATION

For interactive case studies that will help you review and practice basic skills, visit the *Emergency Care 9e Companion Website* at www.bradybooks.com/emergencycare.

EMT-BASIC SKILL PERFORMANCE CHECKLISTS

▶ BLEEDING CONTROL/SHOCK MANAGEMENT

❑ Take BSI precautions.

❑ Apply direct pressure to the wound.

❑ Elevate the extremity.

❑ Apply a dressing to the wound.

❑ If wound continues to bleed, apply an additional dressing to the wound.

❑ If wound continues to bleed, locate and apply pressure to appropriate arterial pressure point.

❑ Administer high-concentration oxygen by nonrebreather mask.

(continued next page)

❑ Properly position the patient.

❑ Initiate steps to prevent heat loss from the patient.

❑ Determine need for immediate transportation.

▶ APPLICATION OF PASG

❑ Take BSI precautions.

❑ Assure patient meets local protocol for PASG.

❑ Check for contraindications (e.g., pulmonary edema or penetrating chest injury).

❑ Remove clothing and check for sharp objects.

❑ Quickly assess areas that will be under the PASG.

❑ Position PASG with top of abdominal section at or below the last set of ribs.

❑ Secure PASG around patient.

❑ Attach hoses.

❑ Check blood pressure.

❑ Begin inflation sequence.

❑ Stop inflation sequence (106 mm Hg or pop-off valves release).

❑ Operate PASG to maintain air pressure in device.

❑ Reassess patient's vital signs.

WARNING: Do not actually inflate a PASG on a mock victim in class.

CASE STUDY

▶ CONVENIENCE STORE SHOOTING

You respond to a local convenience store where there has been an armed robbery. The call was dispatched as a shooting in which the police have secured the scene. A bystander who pulled up at the store just as the shooter was running out the front door states that she found the injured clerk sitting on the floor.

1. What is the importance of a secure scene?

2. As you enter the store, what other scene size-up procedures are important?

You find the 17-year-old male clerk holding the right upper quadrant of his abdomen with a piece of cloth soaked in blood. He is conscious and alert, knows his name, where he is, and the day of the week. His name is Tom. He complains of pain and says he is very thirsty. You reach down and feel for his radial pulse. You can barely feel it because it is so fast and weak.

3. What important information have you just found out about this patient?

4. What phase and what type of shock is your patient in based upon the information you know?

5. What is the relevance of his being thirsty?

When you check Tom's carotid pulse, it is about 120 per minute and thready. His respirations are 24/shallow and regular. You quickly assess his chest and find no entry into the chest and equal breath sounds on both lungs. You immediately search for other injuries, ask him about other complaints, and find he has none. You do a very quick search from head to toe for additional external hemorrhage and an exit bullet wound. Your partner begins to control the bleeding and administer oxygen to the patient. Together, you and your partner carefully lay Tom down on a long spine board.

6. Since Tom was shot in the abdomen, what is the importance of listening to his lungs?

7. What device should be used and at what liter flow rate should the regulator be set for this patient?

8. Should an ALS unit be called for if one was not dispatched with you? If so, should you wait on the scene for ALS or arrange an intercept?

The patient is very pale and sweating profusely. He is beginning to get anxious about dying. You and your partner rapidly move him to the ambulance.

9. On a call like this, what is the maximum time you should spend on the scene? What is this time frame commonly called?

10. To give the surgeons a fighting chance to save Tom's life, what is the maximum time you should spend in assessment and transportation of the patient to the trauma center? What is this time frame commonly called?

The patient is loaded in the ambulance. His level of responsiveness is reassessed, and he is responding to painful stimuli only. ALS will intercept you en route.

11. Aside from reassessing the vitals, what airway care should be considered at this time?

12. Would the PASG be indicated in this case?

13. Is this patient critical?

You meet up with the ALS unit. They jump aboard your ambulance with their portable equipment. The driver quickly continues to the hospital.

14. What procedures would you expect an ALS unit to do en route to the hospital?

15. Briefly write down the radio report that you would give to the hospital en route. The patient initially told you he has no allergies, takes no medications, and has been healthy; his last meal was lunch a few hours ago. The paramedics establish two large bore IVs and prepare to endotracheally intubate the patient. His pulse oximeter reading is 85 and his ECG is sinus tachycardia at a rate of 136.

Radio Report:

Chapter Twenty-Seven

SOFT-TISSUE INJURIES

MATCH TERMINOLOGY/DEFINITIONS

▶ PART A

A. Swelling caused by the collection of blood under the skin or in damaged tissues as a result of an injured or broken blood vessel

B. Outer layer of the skin

C. Any material used to hold a dressing in place

D. Cut that can be smooth or jagged

E. Intestine or other internal organ protruding through a wound in the abdomen

F. Internal injury in which there is no open pathway from the outside to the injured site

G. Burn in which all the layers of the skin are damaged; also called a third-degree burn

H. Flap of skin or other tissue torn loose or pulled off completely

I. Any material used to cover a wound in an effort to control bleeding and help prevent additional contamination

J. Injury caused when force is transmitted from the body's exterior to its internal structures

K. Air bubble in the bloodstream

L. Layer of the skin found below the epidermis; it is rich in blood vessels, nerves, and specialized structures such as sweat glands, sebaceous (oil) glands, and hair follicles.

M. Bruise

N. Scrape or scratch in which the outer layer of the skin is damaged but all the layers are not penetrated

O. Surgical removal or traumatic severing of a body part, usually an extremity

_____ 1. Abrasion

_____ 2. Air embolus

_____ 3. Amputation

_____ 4. Avulsion

_____ 5. Bandage

_____ 6. Closed wound

_____ 7. Contusion

_____ 8. Crush injury

_____ 9. Dermis

_____ 10. Dressing

_____ 11. Epidermis

_____ 12. Evisceration

_____ 13. Full-thickness burn

_____ 14. Hematoma

_____ 15. Laceration

PART B

A. Large bulky dressing

B. Method for estimating the extent of a burn area in which areas on the body are assigned certain percentages of the body's total surface area

C. Open chest wound in which air is "drawn" into the chest cavity

D. Burn in which the epidermis is burned through and the dermis is damaged; also called a second-degree burn

E. Burn that involves only the epidermis, the outer layer of the skin; also called a first-degree burn

F. Injury in which the skin is interrupted, or broken, exposing the tissue underneath

G. Layers of fat and soft tissues below the dermis

H. Any dressing that forms an airtight seal

I. Method for estimating the extent of a burn area; the palm of the patient's hand, which equals about 1% of the body's surface area, is compared with the patient's burn to estimate its size.

J. Open wound caused by a sharp, pointed object that tears through the skin and destroys underlying tissues

_____ 1. Occlusive dressing

_____ 2. Open wound

_____ 3. Partial-thickness burn

_____ 4. Puncture wound

_____ 5. Rule of nines

_____ 6. Rule of palm

_____ 7. Subcutaneous layers

_____ 8. Sucking chest wound

_____ 9. Superficial burn

_____ 10. Universal dressing

MULTIPLE-CHOICE REVIEW

_____ 1. The soft tissues of the body include all of the following except
   A. skin, fatty tissue, muscles.   C. teeth, bones, cartilage.
   B. blood vessels and fibrous tissues.   D. nerves, membranes, glands.

_____ 2. Which of the following is not a function of the skin?
   A. protection   C. temperature regulation
   B. shock absorption   D. blood insulation

_____ 3. The layers of the skin include all of the following except
   A. epidermis.   C. subcutaneous.
   B. dermis.   D. epithelial.

_____ 4. The layer of the skin called the _____ is composed of dead cells, which are rubbed off or sloughed off and are replaced continuously.
   A. epidermis   C. subcutaneous
   B. dermis   D. epithelial

_____ 5. Specialized nerve endings in the skin layer called the _____ are involved with the senses of touch, cold, heat, and pain.
   A. epidermis   C. subcutaneous layers
   B. dermis   D. epithelial cells

_____ 6. Shock absorption and insulation are major functions of which layer of the skin?
   A. epidermis   C. subcutaneous
   B. dermis   D. epithelial

_____ 7. Wounds that usually result from the impact of a blunt object are called
   A. stabbings.   C. closed.
   B. lacerations.   D. perforations.

_____ 8. A closed wound that involves a large amount of tissue damage and a collection of blood at the injury site is called a
   A. crush injury.   C. contusion.
   B. hematoma.   D. penetration.

_____ 9. A soft-tissue injury caused by a force that can cause rupture or bleeding of internal organs is called a
   A. contusion.   C. crush injury.
   B. hematoma.   D. force injury.

_____ 10. A(n) _____ is an injury in which the skin is interrupted, exposing the tissues underneath.
   A. hematoma   C. open wound
   B. closed wound   D. crush injury

_____ 11. A minor ooze of blood from capillary beds is from an injury called a(n)
   A. amputation.   C. laceration.
   B. abrasion.   D. puncture.

_____ 12. A wound caused by a sharp-edged object such as a razor blade or broken glass is called a(n)
   A. abrasion.   C. laceration.
   B. puncture.   D. avulsion.

_____ 13. When a sharp, pointed object passes through the skin or other tissue, a(n) _____ wound has occurred.
   A. abrasion   C. amputation
   B. puncture   D. crush injury

_____ 14. When the tip of the nose is cut or torn off, this is a(n)
   A. avulsion.   C. crush injury.
   B. penetration.   D. amputation.

_____ 15. The priority when treating severe open wounds is to
   A. control bleeding.   C. prevent contamination.
   B. clean the wound.   D. bandage the wound.

_____ 16. Care for a laceration includes
   A. applying a tourniquet
   B. applying a butterfly bandage; then releasing the patient.
   C. pulling apart the edges to inspect the wound.
   D. checking the pulse distal to the injury.

_____ 17. Various types of guns fired at close range can cause all of the following except
   A. burns around the entry wound.   C. large contusion to the tissue.
   B. injection of air into the tissues. D. damage to underlying tissue.

_____ 18. Care in the field for a patient with an impaled object in the leg involves all of the following except
   A. stabilize the object.   C. leave the object in place.
   B. use direct pressure.   D. carefully remove the object.

_____ 19. Which of the following is not true about an injury caused by an impaled object?
   A. The object may plug bleeding from a major artery.
   B. Removal may cause further injury to the nerves, muscles, and soft tissue.
   C. Pressure should be applied to the object to stabilize it.
   D. All of the above.

_____ 20. To control profuse bleeding resulting from an injury caused by an impaled object,
  A. position your gloved hands on either side of the object and exert downward pressure.
  B. use a pressure point distal to the injury to control the bleeding.
  C. let the blood flow freely from the wound left by removal of the object.
  D. stabilize the object with gloved hands and then immediately apply a tourniquet.

_____ 21. Which of the following is <u>untrue</u> of an impaled object in the cheek?
  A. It should never be removed.
  B. It can create an airway obstruction.
  C. It can cause nausea and vomiting.
  D. It is pulled out in the direction it entered.

_____ 22. If a patient has an impaled object in the eye, your care should include use of a
  A. pressure bandage placed over the eye.
  B. loose bandage placed over the eye.
  C. combination of 4 × 4s and a paper cup.
  D. combination of 3-inch gauze and a Styrofoam cup.

_____ 23. When an avulsed flap of tissue has been torn loose but not off, the EMT-B should do all of the following <u>except</u>
  A. fold the skin back to its normal position.
  B. control bleeding and dress the wound.
  C. clean the wound surface.
  D. tear off the remainder of the flap and put it on ice.

_____ 24. Avulsed parts torn from the body should be wrapped and placed in a
  A. cup of dry ice placed in an airtight container.
  B. plastic bag filled with ice.
  C. plastic bag on top of a sealed bag of ice.
  D. saline and ice solution.

_____ 25. The most effective treatment for an amputation is to
  A. apply a tourniquet.
  B. place the amputated part in ice.
  C. place a snug pressure dressing over the stump.
  D. apply ice over the stump.

_____ 26. When treating an amputation, whenever possible
  A. place the amputated body part in ice and transport before the patient.
  B. transport the patient and the amputated body part in the same ambulance.
  C. apply a tourniquet after completing a partial amputation.
  D. immerse the amputated part in saline and transport before the patient.

_____ 27. An air bubble sucked into a large vein in the neck is called a(n)
  A. air embolus.   C. occlusion.
  B. blood clot.   D. case of the "bends."

_____ 28. The treatment of neck vein injury is aimed at all of the following <u>except</u> to
  A. compress the region of injury.   C. prevent cardiac arrest.
  B. prevent an embolus.   D. stop bleeding.

_____ 29. To treat a neck laceration, the EMT-B should use a(n)
  A. pressure bandage.   C. ACE bandage.
  B. thin dressing.   D. occlusive dressing.

_____ **30.** When applying pressure to a neck wound, be sure you do <u>not</u>
   A. apply pressure over the laceration.
   B. compress both carotids at the same time.
   C. administer oxygen to the patient.
   D. treat the patient for shock.

_____ **31.** The chest can be injured in a number of ways, including
   A. blunt trauma.   **C.** compression.
   B. penetrating objects.   **D.** all of the above.

_____ **32.** When the driver of a motor vehicle pitches forward after a head-on collision
   and strikes the chest on the steering column, this is called
   A. closed lung injury.   **C.** compression injury.
   B. penetrating trauma.   **D.** puncture trauma.

_____ **33.** All open wounds to the chest should be considered
   A. potentially infectious.   **C.** a low priority.
   B. life-threatening.   **D.** an indication for PASG.

_____ **34.** An injury that has both an entrance and an exit is called a _____ wound.
   A. puncture   **C.** perforating puncture
   B. penetrating   **D.** compression injury

_____ **35.** When the delicate pressure balance within the chest cavity is compromised,
   initially the
   A. diaphragm stops working.
   B. lung on the injured side will collapse.
   C. lung on the uninjured side will collapse.
   D. patient will stop breathing.

_____ **36.** When the chest cavity is open to the atmosphere, this is referred to as a
   A. flail chest.   **C.** sucking chest wound.
   B. hemothorax.   **D.** rib fracture.

_____ **37.** The treatment for an open chest wound includes all of the following <u>except</u>
   A. maintaining an open airway.
   B. binding the chest tightly.
   C. administering high-concentration oxygen.
   D. sealing the open wound.

_____ **38.** When air becomes trapped in the chest cavity, it can affect the body in all
   of the following ways <u>except</u>
   A. put pressure on the unaffected lung and heart.
   B. reduce cardiac output.
   C. affect oxygenation of the blood.
   D. increase the ventilatory volume of the chest.

_____ **39.** The signs of pneumothorax or tension pneumothorax include all of the
   following <u>except</u>
   A. tracheal deviation to the uninjured side.
   B. distended neck veins.
   C. uneven chest wall movement.
   D. increased depth of respiration.

_____ **40.** Which of the following is <u>not</u> a sign of traumatic asphyxia?
   A. distended neck veins
   B. coughed-up frothy blood
   C. head, neck, and shoulders that appear dark blue.
   D. bloodshot and bulging eyes

_____ 41. When taping an occlusive dressing in place,
  A. have the patient inhale as you tape.
  B. have the patient forcefully exhale as you tape.
  C. tape between breaths.
  D. have the patient hold his/her breath.

_____ 42. When an open wound to the abdomen is so large and deep that organs protrude through the opening, this is called an
  A. impaled object.   C. avulsion.
  B. evisceration.   D. amputated intestine.

_____ 43. The signs of an abdominal injury include all of the following <u>except</u>
  A. lacerations and puncture wounds to the lower back.
  B. large bruised area on the abdomen.
  C. indications of developing shock.
  D. contusions over the upper ribs.

_____ 44. Partially digested blood that is vomited looks like
  A. black and tarry material.   C. stained mucus.
  B. coffee grounds.   D. meconium staining.

_____ 45. Which of the following is <u>not</u> a symptom of an abdominal injury?
  A. cramps   C. headache
  B. nausea   D. thirst

_____ 46. Consider positioning the patient with an abdominal injury
  A. prone, with arms outstretched.   C. left lateral recumbent.
  B. supine, with legs flexed at knees. D. supine, with legs straight.

_____ 47. The treatment of an evisceration should <u>never</u> include
  A. using an occlusive dressing.
  B. cutting away the clothing.
  C. replacing or touching the exposed organ.
  D. applying a sterile, saline-soaked dressing.

_____ 48. When covering an exposed abdominal organ, you should apply a(n) _____ directly over the wound site.
  A. plastic wrap   C. saline-moistened dressing
  B. occlusive dressing   D. aluminum foil wrap

_____ 49. Burn injuries often involve structures below the skin, including muscles and
  A. nerves.   C. blood vessels.
  B. bones.   D. all of the above.

_____ 50. In addition to the physical damage caused by burns, patients often suffer
  A. heart attacks.
  B. emotional and psychological problems.
  C. diabetic emergencies.
  D. delayed reactions such as cancer.

_____ 51. When caring for a burn patient,
  A. think beyond the burn to possible medical causes and results.
  B. always begin transport before treatment.
  C. obtain the name of the product that caused the burn.
  D. determine the duration of the exposure.

_____ 52. When caring for a burn patient,
  A. do not neglect assessment to begin burn care.
  B. transport immediately.
  C. take the patient to the closest hospital.
  D. run cold water on the patient for at least 20 minutes.

_____ **53.** Examples of agents causing burns include all of the following <u>except</u>
    A. AC current.   **C.** dry lime.
    B. hydrochloric acid.   **D.** distilled water.

_____ **54.** A burn that involves only the epidermis is called a _____ burn.
    A. superficial   **C.** full-thickness
    B. partial-thickness   **D.** epi-thickness

_____ **55.** Which of the following burns will result in deep intense pain, blisters, and mottled skin?
    A. superficial   **C.** full-thickness
    B. partial-thickness   **D.** medium layer

_____ **56.** To distinguish between a partial-thickness burn and a full-thickness burn, look for _____ , which indicate a full-thickness burn.
    A. blisters   **C.** dry and white areas
    B. mottled skin   **D.** swelling

_____ **57.** Electrical burns are of special concern since they
    A. cause respiratory burns if superheated gas is inhaled.
    B. pose a great risk of severe internal injuries.
    C. may remain on the skin and continue to burn for hours.
    D. cause the patient to lose hair over time.

_____ **58.** Chemical burns are of special concern since they
    A. cause respiratory burns if superheated gas is inhaled.
    B. pose a great risk of internal injury.
    C. may remain on the skin and continue to burn for hours.
    D. jump from one extremity to another.

_____ **59.** Burns to the face are of special concern because they
    A. continue to burn for hours.   **C.** increase the potential for shock.
    B. can cause heart irregularities.   **D.** may involve airway injury.

_____ **60.** Burns that can interrupt circulation to distal tissues are called _____ burns.
    A. circulation   **C.** circumferential
    B. radiation   **D.** distal

_____ **61.** You are treating an adult patient who has partial-thickness burns to the entire left arm, chest, face, and neck. Using the rule of nines, approximate the size of the burn area.
    A. 18%   **C.** 27%
    B. 22%   **D.** 32%

_____ **62.** You are treating an adult patient who has partial-thickness burns totally covering the legs, chest, and abdomen. Using the rule of nines, approximate the size of the burn area.
    A. 18%   **C.** 45%
    B. 36%   **D.** 54%

_____ **63.** A burn the size of five palms would cover approximately _____ % of the body surface area.
    A. 5   **C.** 15
    B. 10   **D.** 20

_____ **64.** The age of the patient is an important factor in burns. Patients under _____ and over _____ years of age have the most severe body responses to burns.
    A. 3 : 50   **C.** 10 : 65
    B. 5 : 55   **D.** 15 : 70

_____ **65.** A partial-thickness burn that involves less than 15% of the body surface is classified as
    A. minor.   **C.** critical.
    B. moderate.   **D.** unnecessary to treat.

_____ 66. A partial-thickness burn that involves between 15% and 30% of the body surface area is classified as a _____ burn.
   A. minor
   B. moderate
   C. critical
   D. life-threatening

_____ 67. A partial-thickness burn that involves more than 30% of the body surface area is classified as a _____ burn.
   A. minor
   B. moderate
   C. critical
   D. fatal

_____ 68. Critical burns include all of the following except
   A. circumferential burns.
   B. moderate burns in a infant or elderly patient.
   C. burns complicated by musculoskeletal injuries.
   D. partial-thickness burns on the wrist.

_____ 69. A partial-thickness burn that involves between 10% and 20% of the body surface area of a child under 5 years of age is considered a _____ burn.
   A. minor
   B. moderate
   C. critical
   D. fatal

_____ 70. Which of the following is not considered a critical burn?
   A. entire genitalia area
   B. full-thickness burn to the entire chest and abdomen
   C. full-thickness burn to the front of the right forearm
   D. partial-thickness burn to both the lower extremities

_____ 71. If a patient has a partial-thickness burn to the entire back, the patient should be
   A. wrapped in a dry, sterile burn sheet.
   B. cooled down with ice for 15 minutes.
   C. wrapped in moist sterile dressings.
   D. dried and wrapped in an airtight dressing.

_____ 72. The primary care for a patient with a chemical burn is to
   A. wrap the patient in a dry sterile burn sheet.
   B. wash away the chemical with flowing water.
   C. dry the patient and wrap in an airtight dressing.
   D. wrap the patient with moist sterile dressings.

_____ 73. You are treating a patient who was burned. The patient is having visual difficulties, is restless and irritable, has an irregular pulse rate, and muscle tenderness. This patient probably has a(n) _____ burn.
   A. chemical
   B. thermal
   C. electrical
   D. radiation

_____ 74. If _____ is the burn agent, brush it from the patient's skin and then flush with water.
   A. dry lime
   B. electricity
   C. radiation
   D. acid

_____ 75. An occlusive dressing is used to
   A. form an airtight seal.
   B. stabilize an impaled object.
   C. control severe bleeding.
   D. secure sprain injuries.

COMPLETE THE FOLLOWING

1. List eight signs of abdominal injury.

   A. _____

   B. _____

   C. _____

   D. _____

   E. _____

   F. _____

   G. _____

   H. _____

2. List the parts of the adult body that account for 9% each in the rule of nines.

   A. _____

   B. _____

   C. _____

   D. _____

   E. _____

   F. _____

   G. _____

   H. _____

3. List five signs and symptoms of an electrical injury.

   A. _____

   B. _____

   C. _____

   D. _____

   E. _____

LABEL THE DIAGRAM

Fill in the name of each type of burn and how the skin is damaged.

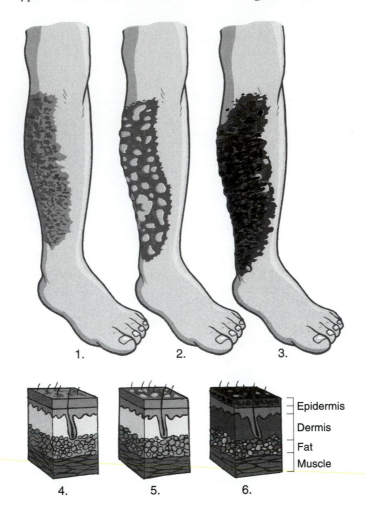

1.
2.
3.

Epidermis
Dermis
Fat
Muscle

4.
5.
6.

1. _____

2. _____

3. _____

4. _____

5. _____

6. _____

VIRTUAL STREET SCENES

(First review the Street Scenes on pp. 560–561 of the textbook. Then answer the questions below.)

1. Your patient had a serious laceration, but the bleeding had stopped by the time you arrived. Suppose it was a different situation, and when you uncovered the wound, blood spurted across the room. How should the bleeding be controlled?

2. Suppose that the patient's wound when uncovered was only bleeding slowly but there was a large piece of glass impaled in her arm. How would you manage this?

3. If upon assessment of the patient's vital signs, it is apparent that she already has low blood pressure, how should the patient be managed?

WEB SIMULATION

For interactive case studies that will help you review and practice basic skills, visit the *Emergency Care 9e Companion Website* at www.bradybooks.com/emergencycare.

Chapter Twenty-Eight

MUSCULOSKELETAL INJURIES

MATCH TERMINOLOGY/DEFINITIONS

A. Hard but flexible living structures that provide support for the body and protection for vital organs

B. Disruption or "coming apart" of a joint

C. Extremity injury in which the skin has been broken or torn through from the inside by an injured bone or from the outside by something that has caused a penetrating wound with associated injury to the bone

D. Special splint that applies constant pull along the length of the leg to help stabilize the fractured femur and reduce muscle spasms

E. Grating sensation or sound made when broken bone ends rub together

F. Bands of connective tissue that bind muscles to bones

G. Any break in a bone

H. Portion of the skeleton that includes the clavicles, scapulae, arms, wrists, hands, pelvis, thighs, legs, ankles, and feet

I. Connective tissue that covers the outside of the bone ends and acts as a surface for articulation allowing for smooth movement at joints

J. Muscle injury caused by overstretching or overexertion of the muscle

K. Process of applying tension to straighten and realign a fractured limb before splinting

L. Places where bones articulate, or meet

M. Stretching and tearing of ligaments

N. Injury to an extremity in which the skin is not broken

O. Connective tissue that supports joints by attaching the bone ends and allowing for a stable range of motion

_____ **1.** Bones

_____ **2.** Cartilage

_____ **3.** Closed extremity injury

_____ **4.** Crepitus

_____ **5.** Dislocation

_____ **6.** Extremities

_____ **7.** Fracture

_____ **8.** Joints

_____ **9.** Ligaments

_____ **10.** Manual traction

_____ **11.** Open extremity injury

_____ **12.** Sprain

_____ **13.** Strain

_____ **14.** Tendons

_____ **15.** Traction splint

_____ 1. As we age, our bones become
   A. deficient in magnesium.   C. high in iron.
   B. deficient in calcium.   D. high in potassium.

_____ 2. The strong white fibrous material covering the bones is called the
   A. perineum.   C. periosteum.
   B. marrow.   D. shell.

_____ 3. In children, the majority of the long bone growth occurs in the
   A. bone marrow.   C. periosteum.
   B. growth plate.   D. growth shaft.

_____ 4. Musculoskeletal injuries are caused by direct, indirect, and _____ forces.
   A. positive   C. negative
   B. penetrating   D. twisting

_____ 5. Fractures of the femur typically cause a _____ pint blood loss over the first two hours.
   A. 1   C. 3
   B. 2   D. 4

_____ 6. The death rate from closed fracture of the femur dropped from 80% to 20% in the post WWI period due to the invention of the
   A. PASG.   C. traction splint.
   B. IV bag.   D. tourniquet.

_____ 7. The coming apart of a joint is referred to as a
   A. dislocation.   C. sprain.
   B. fracture.   D. strain.

_____ 8. The stretching or tearing of ligaments is called a
   A. dislocation.   C. sprain.
   B. fracture.   D. strain.

_____ 9. A break in the continuity of the skin of a painful, swollen, deformed extremity is considered a(n) _____ bone or joint injury.
   A. simple   C. closed
   B. open   D. grating

_____ 10. Proper splinting of a possible closed fracture is
   A. done with an air splint and gentle traction.
   B. done with the pneumatic anti-shock garment.
   C. designed to prevent closed injuries from becoming open ones.
   D. completed in the hospital by a surgeon.

_____ 11. The signs and symptoms of a bone or joint injury include all of the following except
   A. grating.   C. vomiting.
   B. swelling.   D. bruising.

_____ 12. When a joint is locked into position, the EMT-B should
   A. splint the joint in the position found.
   B. pull traction and straighten the joint.
   C. use a long backboard as a full body splint.
   D. disregard splinting and transport immediately.

_____ 13. Which procedure is done at least twice whenever a splint is applied?
   A. elevation of the injured extremity.
   B. manual stabilization of the injured extremity.
   C. assessment for pulses, sensation, and movement distal to the injury.
   D. application of gentle manual traction.

_____ **14.** The treatment of a painful, swollen, deformed extremity includes the steps below.
   1. Take BSI precautions.
   2. Elevate the extremity.
   3. Splint the injury.
   4. Apply a cold pack.

   What is the correct order of the steps?
   A. 2, 3, 4, 1   **C.** 3, 2, 4, 1
   B. 1, 3, 2, 4   **D.** 1, 4, 2, 3

_____ **15.** Multiple fractures, especially of the _____ , can cause life-threatening external and internal bleeding.
   A. radius   **C.** femur
   B. ulna   **D.** tibia

_____ **16.** Applying a cold pack to a possible fracture will
   A. help to reduce the swelling.
   B. stop bleeding from the bone.
   C. eliminate the need for a pressure bandage.
   D. stop all the pain and discomfort.

_____ **17.** If the initial assessment of a patient with a musculoskeletal injury reveals the patient is unstable, care should include all of the following except
   A. manage the ABCs.
   B. immobilize on a long spine board.
   C. transport immediately.
   D. splint each injury individually.

_____ **18.** A splint properly applied to a closed bone injury should help prevent all of the following except
   A. damage to muscles, nerves, or blood vessels.
   B. an open bone injury.
   C. motion of bone fragments.
   D. circulation to the extremity.

_____ **19.** Complications of bone injuries include all of the following except
   A. excessive bleeding.   **C.** paralysis of the extremity.
   B. increased pain from movement.   **D.** increased distal circulation.

_____ **20.** The objective of realignment is to
   A. minimize blood loss and reduce pain.
   B. immobilize the bone ends and adjacent joints.
   C. assist in restoring circulation and to fit the extremity into a splint.
   D. prevent incorrect healing and avoid surgery.

_____ **21.** If there is a severe deformity of the distal extremity or it is cyanotic or pulseless, the EMT-B should
   A. align with gentle traction before splinting.
   B. apply PASG to align the extremity.
   C. delay splinting until en route to the hospital.
   D. contact medical direction immediately.

_____ **22.** The types of splints generally carried by EMT-Bs include
   A. rigid, formable, and traction.   **C.** padded, soft, and anatomical.
   B. PASG, board, and ladder.   **D.** air, cardboard, and vacuum.

_____ **23.** Which of the following is a false statement about rigid splints?
   A. They require the limb be moved into anatomical position.
   B. They tend to provide the greatest support.
   C. They are ideally used to splint long bones.
   D. They can immobilize joint injuries in the position found.

_____ 24. Traction splints are used specifically for fractures of the _____ .
  A. pelvis
  B. humerus
  C. femur
  D. clavicle

_____ 25. When splinting, the EMT-B should
  A. first move the patient to a stretcher.
  B. leave any open wounds exposed.
  C. replace protruding bones.
  D. immobilize the injury site and the joints above and below.

_____ 26. To ensure proper immobilization and increase patient comfort when using a rigid splint,
  A. place the patient on a stretcher before splinting.
  B. place the patient on a long spine board before splinting.
  C. pad the spaces between the body part and the splint.
  D. ensure that the splint conforms to the body curves.

_____ 27. The method of splinting is always dictated by
  A. the location of the injury and whether it is open or closed.
  B. the severity of the patient's condition and the priority decision.
  C. the number of available rescuers and the type of splints.
  D. all of the above.

_____ 28. If the patient with a musculoskeletal injury is unstable, the EMT-B should do all of the following except
  A. care for life-threatening problems first.
  B. align the injuries in an anatomical position.
  C. immobilize the entire body to a long spine board.
  D. apply a fixation splint before immobilizing on a long spine board.

_____ 29. Hazards of improper splinting include
  A. aggravation of a bone or joint injury.
  B. reduced distal circulation.
  C. delay in transport of patient with life-threatening injury.
  D. all of the above.

_____ 30. If the lower leg is cyanotic or lacks a pulse when a knee joint injury is assessed, the EMT-B should
  A. splint it in the position it was found.
  B. transport the patient to the hospital immediately.
  C. realign with gentle traction if no resistance is met.
  D. call for assistance from the paramedics.

_____ 31. Examples of a bipolar traction splint include all of the following except
  A. Hare
  B. Sagar
  C. Fernotrac
  D. half-ring

_____ 32. The amount of traction the EMT-B should pull when applying a Sager traction splint is
  A. enough until the patient verbalizes relief.
  B. about 10% of the patient's body weight up to 15 pounds.
  C. minimal since it doesn't require traction.
  D. about 15% of the patient's body weight up to 30 pounds.

_____ 33. The indications for a traction splint are a painful, swollen, deformed mid-thigh with
  A. either knee or ankle involvement.
  B. no joint or lower leg injury.
  C. extensive blood loss.
  D. an open fracture.

_____ **34.** Whenever possible, _____ rescuers should be used to apply a traction splint.
  A. two   **C.** four
  B. three   **D.** five

_____ **35.** If the patient has multiple leg fractures and exhibits signs of shock (hypoperfusion), the EMT-B should
  A. apply two traction splints and pull tension to 30 pounds.
  B. align in a normal position and transport on a backboard.
  C. apply PASG as a splint and treat for shock.
  D. apply a vacuum splint to each leg and transport quickly.

_____ **36.** Signs and symptoms of a knee injury include
  A. pain and tenderness.   **C.** deformity.
  B. swelling.   **D.** all of the above.

_____ **37.** Elderly patients are more susceptible to _____ fractures because of brittle bones or bones weakened by disease.
  A. hip   **C.** heel
  B. tibia   **D.** spine

_____ **38.** When a patient has a fractured hip, the injured limb
  A. will rarely be swollen.   **C.** often is lengthened.
  B. may appear shorter.   **D.** will have all of the above.

_____ **39.** When a patient, who was involved in a serious fall, has an unexplained sensation of having to empty her bladder, the patient may have a _____ fracture.
  A. femur.   **C.** pelvic
  B. hip   **D.** None of the above.

_____ **40.** When immobilizing a patient who has a pelvic injury, you should do all of the following except
  A. assure there is a spinal injury.   **C.** apply PASG if the patient is hypotensive.
  B. determine distal function.   **D.** raise the lower legs.

COMPLETE THE FOLLOWING

1. List eight signs and symptoms of musculoskeletal injury.

   A. _____

   B. _____

   C. _____

   D. _____

   E. _____

   F. _____

   G. _____

   H. _____

2. List eight signs and symptoms of a hip fracture.

   A. _____

   B. _____

   C. _____

   D. _____

   E. _____

   F. _____

   G. _____

   H. _____

LABEL THE DIAGRAM

Fill in the name of each bone on the line provided.

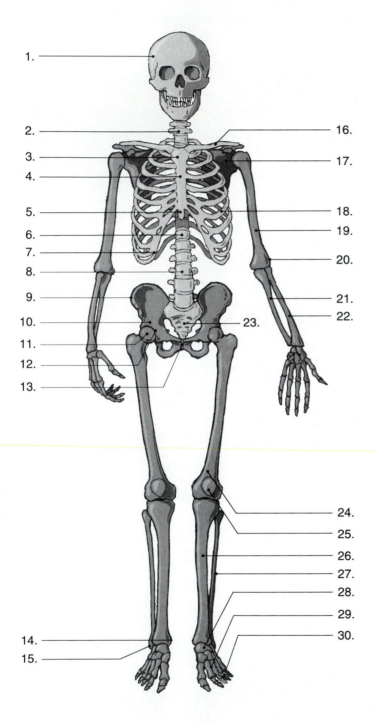

1. _____

2. _____

3. _____

4. _____

5. _____

6. _____

7. _____

8. _____

9. _____

10. _____

11. _____

12. _____

13. _____

14. _____

15. _____

16. _____

17. _____

18. _____

19. _____

20. _____

21. _____

22. _____

23. _____

24. _____

25. _____

26. _____

27. _____

28. _____

29. _____

30. _____

VIRTUAL STREET SCENES

(First review the Street Scenes on pp. 608–609 of the textbook. Then answer the questions below.)

1. When the injured leg was examined, it was found to be swollen. If it had been an open fracture, what would you have observed?

2. Imagine that the patient is found lying on the ground with the injured leg grossly deformed in the mid-shaft area. Should you attempt to straighten it? Explain.

3. Suppose the patient does not have a distal pulse in the injured leg. What can you do?

4. Should you have called for ALS in this case?

WEB SIMULATION

For interactive case studies that will help you review and practice basic skills, visit the *Emergency Care 9e Companion Website* at www.bradybooks.com/emergencycare.

EMT-BASIC SKILLS PERFORMANCE CHECKLISTS

▶ REALIGNING AN EXTREMITY

❏ Take BSI precautions.

❏ Assess distal pulse, motor function, and sensation in the injured extremity.

❏ One EMT-B grasps the distal extremity while a partner places one hand above and below the injury site.

❏ The partner supports the injury site while the first EMT-B pulls gentle manual traction in the direction of the long axis of the body. If resistance is felt or if it appears that bone ends will come through the skin, stop realignment and splint the extremity in the position found.

(continued next page)

❑ If no resistance is felt, maintain gentle traction until the extremity is properly splinted.

❑ Reassess distal pulse, motor function, and sensation.

▶ **IMMOBILIZATION: LONG BONE**

❑ Take BSI precautions.

❑ Apply manual stabilization.

❑ Assess distal pulse, motor function, and sensation in the injured extremity.

❑ Measure splint.

❑ Apply splint.

❑ Immobilize joints above and below the injury site.

❑ Secure the entire injured extremity in a distal to proximal direction.

❑ Immobilize hand/foot in the position of function.

❑ Reassess distal pulse, motor function, and sensation.

▶ **IMMOBILIZATION: JOINT INJURY**

❑ Take BSI precautions.

❑ Apply manual stabilization.

❑ Assess distal pulse, motor function, and sensation.

❑ Select proper splinting material.

❑ Immobilize the site of the injury and bones above and below.

❑ Reassess distal pulse, motor function, and sensation.

▶ **IMMOBILIZATION: TRACTION SPLINTING**

❑ Take BSI precautions.

❑ Manually stabilize the injured leg.

❑ Apply manual traction.

❑ Assess distal pulse, motor function, and sensation.

❑ Adjust and position splint at the injured leg.

❑ Apply proximal securing device (e.g., ischial strap).

❑ Apply distal securing device (e.g., ankle hitch).

❑ Apply mechanical traction.

❑ Position and secure support straps.

❑ Reassess distal pulse, motor function, and sensation.

❑ Secure patient's torso and traction splint to long backboard for transport.

Chapter Twenty-Nine

INJURIES TO THE HEAD AND SPINE

MATCH TERMINOLOGY/DEFINITIONS

A. Pairs of nerves that enter and exit the spinal cord between the vertebrae, twelve pairs of cranial nerves that travel between the brain and organs without passing through the spinal cord, and all of the body's other motor and sensory nerves

B. Mild closed head injury without detectable damage to the brain

C. Body system that is divided into two subsystems and that provides overall control of thought, sensation, and the voluntary and involuntary motor functions of the body

D. Cheek bone; also called the zygomatic bone

E. Bony bump on a vertebra that you can feel on a person's back

F. Bones of the spinal column

G. Movable joint formed between the mandible and the temporal bones; also called the TM joint

H. Bony structure making up the forehead, top, back, and upper sides of the skull

I. Fluid that surrounds the brain and spinal cord

J. Bruised brain caused when the force of a blow to the head is great enough to rupture blood vessels

K. Brain and the spinal cord

L. Bones that form part of the sides of the skull and floor of the cranial cavity

M. Bones that form the upper third, or bridge, of the nose

N. Bony structures, or sockets, around the eyes

O. Nervous system that consists of nerves that control involuntary functions such as the heartbeat and breathing

_____ **1.** Autonomic nervous system

_____ **2.** Central nervous system

_____ **3.** Cerebrospinal fluid (CSF)

_____ **4.** Concussion

_____ **5.** Contusion

_____ **6.** Cranium

_____ **7.** Malar

_____ **8.** Nasal bones

_____ **9.** Nervous system

_____ **10.** Orbits

_____ **11.** Peripheral nervous system

_____ **12.** Spinous process

_____ **13.** Temporal bones

_____ **14.** Temporomandibular joint

_____ **15.** Vertebrae

_____ 1. The function of the spinal column is to
   A. produce cerebrospinal fluid.
   B. protect the spinal cord.
   C. allow for back movement in all directions.
   D. manufacture platelets.

_____ 2. The spine is made up of _____ vertebrae.
   A. 35   C. 33
   B. 23   D. 38

_____ 3. When a patient has a scalp injury,
   A. expect minimal bleeding.   C. expect profuse bleeding.
   B. determine the wound depth.   D. palpate the site with fingertips.

_____ 4. A bruise behind the ear is called
   A. Cushing's syndrome.   C. Battle's sign.
   B. raccoon's eyes.   D. posturing syndrome.

_____ 5. Discoloration of the soft tissues under both eyes is called
   A. Cushing syndrome.   C. Battle's sign.
   B. raccoon's eyes.   D. posturing syndrome.

_____ 6. The signs and symptoms of a skull or brain injury include
   A. blood or fluid flowing from the ears and/or nose.
   B. yellow discoloration in the eyes.
   C. bruising around the base of the nose.
   D. pain at the base of the neck.

_____ 7. Skull or brain injury may result in
   A. airway swelling and dizziness.
   B. altered mental status and unequal pupils.
   C. difficulty moving below the waist.
   D. headache and hypoperfusion.

_____ 8. Which of the following is a late sign of brain or skull injury?
   A. temperature increase   C. irregular breathing patterns
   B. raccoon's eyes   D. Battle's sign

_____ 9. Which of the following is generally not a sign of head injury except in infants?
   A. bleeding from the nose and ears   C. hypoperfusion
   B. unequal pupils   D. seizures

_____ 10. What is the significance of an increase in carbon dioxide in the injured brain?
   A. It decreases the blood pressure.   C. It raises the heart rate.
   B. It causes brain tissue swelling.   D. It causes brain tissue shrinking.

_____ 11. In most EMS systems, a patient with a Glasgow Coma Scale (GCS) of less than _____ is taken to a trauma center.
   A. 8   C. 12
   B. 10   D. 15

_____ 12. If an object has penetrated, a patient's skull, the EMT-B should
   A. shorten lengthy objects, using any available tools.
   B. elevate the patient's legs immediately.
   C. remove the object and quickly control the bleeding.
   D. stabilize the object with bulky dressings.

_____ 13. The primary concern for emergency care of facial fractures or jaw injuries is
   A. the external bleeding.   C. the loss of teeth.
   B. the patient's airway.   D. a basilar skull fracture.

_____ 14. The vertebrae that are most frequently injured are the
  A. lumbar and sacral.
  B. thoracic and cervical.
  C. coccygeal and thoracic.
  D. cervical and lumbar.

_____ 15. When the spine is excessively pulled, which commonly occurs during a hanging, this is called a(n) _____ injury.
  A. excessive rotation
  B. lateral bending
  C. distraction
  D. compression

_____ 16. On your size-up of an automobile collision, you notice that both sides of the windshield have a spider-web crack. It is wise to call for a backup ambulance because
  A. every collision should have a two-ambulance response.
  B. patients hitting their heads on the windshield will be critical.
  C. both the driver and the passenger require spinal injury treatment.
  D. It takes four EMS personnel to properly immobilize one patient.

_____ 17. Which of the following would not create a high index of suspicion of a spine injury?
  A. motor vehicle or motorcycle collisions
  B. falls that cause open fractures to the ankles
  C. trauma patients who are found unconscious
  D. a fall from two times the patient's height

_____ 18. All of the following are examples of cervical-spine injuries that can result from a diving accident except
  A. excessive extension.
  B. compression.
  C. excessive flexion.
  D. lateral bending.

_____ 19. The unconscious trauma patient should be
  A. treated as if he has a potential spine injury.
  B. rolled immediately to check for back injuries.
  C. placed in the recovery position.
  D. placed in a prone position for fluid to drain.

_____ 20. The most reliable sign of spinal-cord injury in the conscious patient is
  A. pain with movement.
  B. impaired breathing.
  C. tenderness on the spine.
  D. paralysis of the extremities.

_____ 21. A lack of spinal pain does not rule out the possibility of spinal-cord injury because
  A. spinal injuries seldom cause pain.
  B. other painful injuries may mask it.
  C. spinal injuries are not painful until shock sets in.
  D. a patient may feel the pain but cannot verbalize it.

_____ 22. When assessing a suspected spine-injured patient, you note a reversal of the normal breathing pattern. This is likely a result of damage to the nerves that control the
  A. rib cage.
  B. diaphragm.
  C. abdomen.
  D. lungs.

_____ 23. If a patient is found on her back with arms extended above the head, this may indicate a _____ spine injury.
  A. thoracic
  B. lumbar
  C. sacral
  D. cervical

_____ 24. If a patient is up and walking around at the scene of a high-speed collision, the EMT-B should
  A. assess for a potential spinal injury.
  B. check with medical direction for orders.
  C. check with bystanders about the patient's mental status.
  D. assume that the patient is uninjured.

_____ 25. If a responsive patient has the mechanism of injury for a spinal injury, the EMT-B should do all of the following except
A. assess for spinal pain by asking the patient to move.
B. keep the patient still while asking him/her questions.
C. assess for equality of strength in the extremities.
D. assess for tingling in the extremities.

_____ 26. After performing the initial assessment and rapid trauma exam on a spine-injured patient, your next step is to
A. determine the patient's priority.
B. administer high-concentration oxygen.
C. immobilize the patient on a long spine board.
D. determine the mechanism of injury.

_____ 27. If a suspected spine-injured patient complains of pain when you attempt to place the head in a neutral in-line position,
A. pad the neck before immobilizing.
B. steady the head in the position found.
C. continue with the stabilization procedure.
D. contact medical direction immediately.

_____ 28. When treating a patient with a spine injury, one EMT-B should
A. strap the patient's head, then the torso, to the long spine board.
B. maintain constant manual in-line immobilization until the patient is secured to a backboard.
C. assess for range of cervical spine motion.
D. pad the neck before stabilizing.

_____ 29. Which of the following statements about the rigid cervical collar is false?
A. A wrong-sized collar can hyperextend the neck.
B. Maintain manual stabilization when applying.
C. The collar completely eliminates neck movement.
D. The collar should never obstruct the airway.

_____ 30. If a stable patient is found in a sitting position on the ground and is complaining about back pain, the EMT-B should
A. apply a cervical collar and rapidly transport the patient.
B. ask the patient to lie down, then immobilize.
C. immobilize with a short spine board or extrication vest.
D. perform a rapid take-down procedure with a long spine board.

_____ 31. The rapid extrication procedure is used in all of the following situations except
A. to rapidly move a patient from an unsafe scene.
B. when a stable, low-priority patient must be immobilized.
C. when more seriously injured patients must be accessed.
D. to move a high-priority patient.

_____ 32. When immobilizing a 6-year-old or younger child on a long backboard,
A. provide padding beneath the shoulder blades.
B. it is unnecessary to apply a cervical collar.
C. place a chin cup or chin strap on the patient.
D. secure the head first, then secure the torso.

_____ 33. Do not remove an injured patient's helmet
A. if it interferes with breathing management.
B. if it has a snug fit that allows no head movement.
C. by using a two-rescuer procedure.
D. if it hinders immobilization.

_____ **34.** Which is the correct order of steps for applying a short spine immobilization device?
1) Secure the device to the patient's torso.
2) Secure the patient's head to the device.
3) Position device behind the patient.
4) Evaluate torso fixation and pad behind neck as necessary.

A. 3, 2, 1, 4   **C.** 4, 3, 1, 2

B. 3, 1, 4, 2   **D.** 3, 4, 1, 2

_____ **35.** Prior to and after immobilization, the EMT-B should assess

A. pulses in all extremities.   **C.** sensation in all extremities.

B. motor function in all extremities.   **D.** all of the above.

COMPLETE THE FOLLOWING

1. List six signs of a skull fracture and brain injury.

A. _____

B. _____

C. _____

D. _____

E. _____

F. _____

2. List three types of brain injuries.

A. _____

B. _____

C. _____

LABEL THE DIAGRAM

Fill in the name of each division of the spine on the line provided.

1. _____

2. _____

3. _____

4. _____

5. _____

VIRTUAL STREET SCENES

(First review the Street Scenes on pp. 648–649 of the textbook. Then answer the questions below.)

1. Suppose that this patient had a lucid interval followed by decreasing mental status. What would be your highest priority in the treatment of this patient?

2. If the patient tells you he has no neck pain, why is it necessary to continue to immobilize him?

3. If the patient has a serious head injury, what would you expect to happen with his vital signs (provided he had no other injury)?

WEB SIMULATION

For interactive case studies that will help you review and practice basic skills, visit the *Emergency Care 9e Companion Website* at www.bradybooks.com/emergencycare.

EMT-BASIC SKILLS PERFORMANCE CHECKLISTS

▶ SPINAL IMMOBILIZATION: SUPINE PATIENT

❑ Take BSI precautions.

❑ Direct assistant to place/maintain head in neutral, in-line position and maintain manual stabilization until the patient is completely immobilized.

❑ Assess distal pulses, motor function, and sensation.

❑ Apply a properly sized rigid extrication collar.

❑ Position the immobilization device appropriately.

❑ Move patient onto device without compromising the integrity of the spine. Apply padding to voids between torso and board as necessary.

❑ Immobilize patient's torso to the device.

❑ Evaluate and pad behind the patient's head as necessary.

❑ Pad and immobilize patient's head.

❑ Secure patient's arms and legs to board.

❑ Reassesses distal pulses, motor function, and sensation.

▶ SPINAL IMMOBILIZATION: SEATED PATIENT

- ❑ Take BSI precautions.
- ❑ Direct assistant to manually stabilize head in neutral, in-line position.
- ❑ Assess distal pulses, motor function, and sensation.
- ❑ Apply a properly sized rigid extrication collar.
- ❑ Position immobilization device behind the patient.
- ❑ Secure device to the patient's torso.
- ❑ Evaluate and pad behind the patient's head as necessary.
- ❑ Secure patient's head to the device.
- ❑ Evaluate and adjust straps.
- ❑ Secure patient's wrists and legs and transfer to a long spine board.
- ❑ Reassess distal pulses, motor function, and sensation.

▶ RAPID TAKEDOWN TECHNIQUE: STANDING PATIENT

- ❑ Take BSI precautions.
- ❑ EMT-B #1 should be positioned behind the patient and hold manual in-line stabilization of the head and neck. Make sure the EMT-B in front of the patient explains the procedure to the patient so he does not move.
- ❑ EMT-B #1 behind the patient should not let go of the patient's head throughout the procedure.
- ❑ EMT-B #2 in front of the patient should quickly assess pulses, motor function, and sensation in all four extremities.
- ❑ EMT-B #2 applies a properly sized rigid extrication collar.
- ❑ EMT-B #2 and another rescuer position long spine board behind the patient, being careful not to disturb the manual stabilization in any way.
- ❑ EMT-B #2 and other rescuer, standing to each side of the patient, reach under the patient's armpit and grasp the spine-board handholds at the level of the armpit or higher. They both must hold the same level handhold.
- ❑ To keep patient's arms secure, EMT-B #2 and other rescuer use their other hand to grasp patient's arm just above the elbow and hold it against patient's body.
- ❑ They slowly lower the patient back, communicating with the EMT-B behind the board so it is clear when the scapulae are beginning to rest on the spine board. They lift with their legs, bending at the knees and not bending at the waist.
- ❑ EMT-B #1, who is holding the head, gently allows the head to come back to the spine board as the shoulders come back.
- ❑ Once the head is on the board, it never is lifted off the board again as EMT-B #1 kneels down at the patient's head.
- ❑ EMT-Bs reassess distal pulses, motor function, and sensation.

► **RAPID EXTRICATION PROCEDURE**

Step One: Assessment
❑ Take BSI precautions.

❑ EMT-B #1: Manually stabilize the patient's head/neck.

❑ EMT-B #2: Conduct initial assessment of patient and determine the need for rapid extrication based on patient status.

❑ EMT-B #2: Assess distal pulses, motor function, and sensation in all four extremities.

Step Two: Apply Collar
❑ EMT-B #2: Apply a properly sized rigid collar.

❑ EMT-B #1: Continue manual stabilization.

Step Three: Lift and Position Board
❑ EMT-B #2: Hold patient's armpit and join hands with EMT-B #3 under the patient's thighs.

❑ EMT-B #3: Hold patient by armpit and join hands with EMT-B #2 under patient's thighs.

❑ EMT-B #1: Call for a lift while maintaining manual stabilization.

❑ EMT-B #2: Lift patient approximately 2 inches off seat with EMT-B #3.

❑ EMT-B #3: Lift patient approximately 2 inches off seat with EMT-B #2.

❑ Bystander (or 4th EMT-B): Insert long backboard under patient on seat.

Step Four: Begin to Position for Extrication
❑ EMT B #2: Reach across patient's chest and support by both armpits.

❑ EMT-B #1: While maintaining manual stabilization, call for a 1/4 turn so patient is moved perpendicular to the steering wheel and ready to exit the car head first.

❑ EMT-B #3: Free the patient's lower legs from any obstructions.

❑ EMT-B #2: Begin to turn patient's back toward the door until EMT-B #1 says "stop turn."

❑ EMT-B #1: Turn patient. Call for "stop turn" just before being unable to hold patient's head anymore.

❑ EMT-B #3: Begin to turn patient's back toward door, freeing legs, then sliding up to the thighs until EMT-B #1 says "stop."

Step Five: Complete Another One-Fourth Turn
❑ EMT-B #2: Stop move and wait for EMT-B #3. Then take over manual stabilization of the head/neck from EMT-B #1.

❑ EMT-B #1: Maintain head/neck stabilization until EMT-B #2 takes over, allowing him to either exit car and work from outside or reach over the seat from inside if there is room or the roof has been removed.

❑ EMT-B #3: Move hands from thighs to patient's armpits, then replace EMT-B #2.

❑ Complete the patient turn another 1/4 turn.

Step Six: Lower Patient on Long Backboard
❑ EMT-B #2: Lower patient onto long backboard.

(continued next page)

❑ EMT-B #1: Call for move to lower patient's torso into a supine position on long backboard.

❑ EMT-B #3: Lower patient onto long backboard.

❑ Bystander (or 4th EMT-B): stabilize the board.

Step Seven: Position Patient on Backboard
❑ EMT-B #2: Slide patient as a unit.

❑ EMT-B #1: Call for move to slide patient toward head end of backboard. Once in position, tell partners to "stop." Slide the chest as a unit.

❑ EMT-B #3: Slide pelvis as a unit until EMT-B #1 says to "stop."

❑ Bystander (or 4th EMT-B): Stabilize the head end of long backboard.

Step Eight: Secure Patient to Backboard
❑ Crew carefully straps patient's torso first and head last, and then moves backboard to the stretcher.

❑ Reassess distal pulses, motor function, and sensation.

▶ **CHILD SAFETY SEAT IMMOBILIZATION: ASSESSMENT**

❑ Take BSI precautions.

❑ EMT-B #1 positions behind patient and holds manual in-line stabilization of the head/neck. This remains his job throughout the procedure.

❑ Based on the initial assessment and the patient's status, determine if the infant/toddler should be immobilized in the child safety seat or rapidly extricated from the seat.

❑ EMT-B #2 assesses distal pulses, motor function, and sensation in all four extremities before and after the immobilization.

▶ **IMMOBILIZING PATIENT IN A CHILD SAFETY SEAT**

❑ Take BSI precautions.

❑ EMT-B #1: Stabilize child safety seat in an upright position. Maintain manual head/neck stabilization of head and neck throughout procedure until patient is completely immobile.

❑ EMT-B #2: Prepare equipment. Apply rigid extrication collar or improvise with rolled hand towel for the newborn/infant.

❑ EMT-B #2: Place a small blanket or bath towel on the child's lap. Either strap or use wide tape to secure the pelvis and chest area to the seat.

❑ EMT-B #2: Place a towel roll on both sides of the head to fill the voids. Tape the forehead in place. Then place tape across collar or maxilla. Avoid taping chin, which would place pressure on the child's neck.

❑ EMT-B #1: Carry child and seat to ambulance and strap onto the stretcher with the stretcher head raised.

❑ Reassess distal pulses, motor function, and sensation.

▶ **RAPID EXTRICATION FROM A CHILD SAFETY SEAT**

❑ Take BSI precautions.

(continued next page)

❏ EMT-B #1: Stabilize the child safety seat in upright position. Maintain manual stabilization of head and neck throughout procedure until patient is completely immobilized.

❏ EMT-B #2: Prepare the equipment. Loosen or cut the seat straps and raise the front guard.

❏ Apply the rigid extrication collar or improvise with a rolled hand towel in the newborn/infant.

❏ EMT-B #2: Place the child safety seat on the center of the long backboard and slowly tilt it back into a supine position, being careful not to allow the child to slide out of the chair. If the child has a large head, it is helpful to place a towel under the area where his shoulders will end up on the board.

❏ EMT-B #1: Call for a coordinated long axis move onto the board.

❏ EMT-B #2: Grasp the chest and axilla with each hand and do a coordinated long axis move onto the board. Make sure the child is positioned at the end of the board and not in the middle.

❏ EMT-B #2: Place a rolled blanket on each side of the patient.

❏ EMT-B #2: Strap the pelvis and upper chest to the board. Do not strap abdomen down. Tape the lower legs to the board with wide tape.

❏ EMT-B #2: Place a towel roll on both sides of the head to fill the voids. Tape the forehead in place. Then place tape across the collar or the maxilla. Do not tape across the chin to avoid pressure on the child's neck.

CASE STUDY

▶ DEEP DIVE IN A SHALLOW POOL

You respond to a call for an injury in a pool at a private residence in your district. The EMS dispatcher tells you they have received numerous 9-1-1 calls on this incident and they are trying to calm someone down to obtain better information. Fortunately, your EMS station is about a mile from the location. As you pull up in front, you see there are lots of cars parked outside. A bystander runs up to the ambulance and says, "Please come quickly. He is still in the swimming pool. Can I help you carry anything?" Hearing this, you notify the dispatcher to continue the ALS unit and have the police respond also.

Both you and your partner are experienced swimmers. As you enter the backyard with your equipment, you ask her quickly, "Wet or dry?" She says, "Go. I'll take care of coordinating the poolside activities."

When you first see the patient, he is face up and being assisted in floating on his back by one other person in the pool, who states his name is Bill. He says he was a lifeguard 20 years ago. The patient is an adult male about 40 years old, and in about $5\frac{1}{2}$ feet of water. There is some blood in the pool from a large laceration to the patient's forehead.

You quickly empty your pockets, remove your shoes, hand the radio to your partner, and carefully enter the shallow end of the pool without making any waves. You also happen to notice that everyone has a soccer team shirt on.

1. What would you want to know about the patient from Bill right away?

2. How would you move the patient from the deep water to the shallow end of the pool?

Seeing that most of the adults are a bit intoxicated and most of the children at poolside are a bit small, you ask your partner to get an ETA on the backup unit. Just then they come walking into the backyard. There are two paramedics and an EMT-B who is a student in the paramedic course. You ask them to assist with the patient removal (if they are good swimmers).

3. What equipment will be needed?

In talking with Bill, you find that the party is a celebration for the children winning the soccer tournament. The patient, whose name is Tom, is the coach and apparently is not a drinker, so after two beers he did something he never would have done normally. Apparently, they were horsing around near the edge of the pool and he flipped head first into the shallow end. The laceration was from striking his head. He was initially unconscious. Bill had entered the pool and carefully turned him over, as he was trained years ago to do, and Tom regained consciousness after a moment or two. Bill said that he did not believe Tom swallowed any water.

4. What other information should you obtain?

As one of the medics and the student enter the water with a long backboard and a rigid collar, you instruct Bill to continue to stabilize the patient's head and neck in a neutral position. You assist the patient in floating. The patient is very scared because he is unable to feel his arms or legs.

5. When the patient asks you what are you going to do, what should you tell him?

You carefully float the patient to the shallow end of the pool and do the immobilization there. The voids are padded, and the patient is strapped to the board. By this time, the police have arrived and have asked the soccer team and their parents to move up to the deck area and watch from there. Your partner has found two more helpers who are not intoxicated to assist in the lifting at poolside. Your in-water team lifts the immobilized patient onto the edge of the pool, and the out-of-water team carefully lifts the patient and backboard onto a stretcher.

6. What are some of the initial management steps your partner should take while you get out of the pool?

Once it was clear that your patient does not have any movement of his arms and legs, your partner and the paramedic call for a helicopter and ask the police to set up a landing zone. Fortunately, there is an elementary school with a large field about two blocks away. The patient will be going directly to the Regional Trauma Center and a paramedic will be going along.

When the patient is loaded into your ambulance, the paramedic inserts an IV, the patient's clothing is cut off and he is covered with a blanket, the pulse oximeter is attached, and ECG electrodes are placed on him. His vital signs are still within normal range at this time.

After the patient and paramedic fly off in the helicopter, you look at your partner and say, "Can you imagine? Forty years old. Life can change so fast!" You talk about the call as you clean up back at the station. Although the situation is very sad, and life will change dramatically for the patient and his family, you are satisfied that the response, assessment, management, and teamwork went well. You and your partner agree that you will both stop at the hospital tomorrow to visit the patient. The report that was relayed back to you from the helicopter team was that the patient sustained a fracture of C-4, which severed his spinal cord.

7. Before handing in your PCR, is there anything that you should make sure is clearly documented? If so, what?

Chapter Thirty

PUTTING IT ALL TOGETHER FOR THE TRAUMA PATIENT

MATCH TERMINOLOGY/DEFINITIONS

A. Optimum limit of time between the moment of injury and surgery at the hospital

B. Quick assessment of the head, neck, chest, abdomen, pelvis, extremities, and posterior of the body to detect signs and symptoms of injury

C. Cooperation of crew members, each knowing their role and working together to manage the serious patient

D. Patient with more than one serious injury

E. Action or forces that may have caused or contributed to the injury

F. Swelling caused by a collection of blood under the skin or in damaged tissues as a result of an injured or broken blood vessel

G. Inability of the body to adequately circulate blood to the body's cells to supply them with oxygen and nutrients

H. A procedure designed to move a patient in a hurry when the situation of safety warrants it

_____ 1. Multiple-trauma patient

_____ 2. Teamwork

_____ 3. Rapid trauma assessment

_____ 4. Hypoperfusion

_____ 5. Golden hour

_____ 6. Emergency move

_____ 7. Hematoma

_____ 8. Mechanism of injury

_____ 1. The patient with a fractured right leg and a crushed pelvis is called
a _____ patient.
- **A.** lower extremity
- **B.** multiple trauma
- **C.** shock
- **D.** stable

_____ 2. When a patient has an obvious angulated forearm and is unresponsive, what
is the priority?
- **A.** splinting
- **B.** immobilization
- **C.** the airway
- **D.** distal pulses

_____ 3. At what point is the multiple-trauma patient most likely stabilized?
- **A.** at the emergency department
- **B.** once splints have been provided
- **C.** in the surgical suite
- **D.** once the PASG is applied

_____ 4. The three "Ts" involved in the management of a multiple-trauma patient
are timing, transport, and:
- **A.** teamwork.
- **B.** trauma.
- **C.** treatment.
- **D.** thorax.

_____ 5. A reasonable goal for scene time when dealing with a critical trauma patient
is _____ minutes.
- **A.** 60
- **B.** 45
- **C.** 10
- **D.** 2

_____ 6. When a trauma patient is making gurgling sounds as he breathes, what should
you do?
- **A.** Ventilate him.
- **B.** Suction the airway.
- **C.** Hyperextend the neck.
- **D.** Apply high-concentration oxygen.

_____ 7. Sometimes a _____ can act as a full-body splint when the critical patient
must be immobilized quickly.
- **A.** wheeled stretcher
- **B.** short KED
- **C.** warm blanket
- **D.** long backboard

_____ 8. When a patient has two fractured femurs, a crushed pelvis, and a possible
abdominal injury, you should
- **A.** not apply a traction splint.
- **B.** consider the PASG.
- **C.** set up an ALS intercept en route to the hospital.
- **D.** do all of the above.

_____ 9. When you must minimize the scene care of a multiple-trauma patient, you
can perform any of the following except
- **A.** suction the airway.
- **B.** ventilate with a BVM.
- **C.** bandage all the lacerations.
- **D.** immobilize the cervical spine.

_____ 10. Even when you are trying to cut scene time for a multiple-trauma patient,
the one thing you do not cut out is
- **A.** applying a traction splint if needed.
- **B.** the detailed physical exam.
- **C.** scene safety.
- **D.** immobilization.

COMPLETE THE FOLLOWING

1. List the five treatments that would be appropriate on the scene of a critical trauma patient.

A. _____

B. _____

C. _____

D. _____

E. _____

VIRTUAL STREET SCENES

(First review the Street Scenes on pp. 656–657 of the textbook. Then answer the questions below.)

1. In this case, the use of rapid extrication seems appropriate, considering the mechanism of injury and the patient findings. But suppose the patient was alert, obviously pregnant, lying supine on the seat, and complaining of dizziness. Would rapid extrication still be appropriate? Explain.

2. Imagine that after immobilizing the patient on a long backboard, she developed breathing difficulty due to blood in the airway. What might you consider doing to help her ?

3. If the patient has a fractured femur, would a traction splint be appropriate?

4. What should be your concern for the other patients on the scene?

WEB SIMULATION

For interactive case studies that will help you review and practice basic skills, visit the ***Emergency Care 9e Companion Website*** at www.bradybooks.com/emergencycare.

Chapter Thirty-One

INFANTS AND CHILDREN

MATCH TERMINOLOGY/DEFINITIONS

A. Child from 12 to 18 years of age

B. "Soft spot" at the front of an infant's skull where bones have not yet fused together

C. Flowing oxygen over the face of a small child so it will be inhaled

D. Child from 6 to 12 years of age

E. Child from 1 to 3 years of age

F. Feeding tube placed through the abdominal wall directly into the stomach

G. Child between birth and 1 year of age

H. Child from 3 to 6 years of age

I. Bacterial infection that produces swelling of the epiglottis and partial airway obstruction

J. Sudden unexplained death during sleep of an apparently healthy baby in its first year of life

K. Complication of a rapidly rising temperature

L. Group of viral illnesses that cause inflammation of the larynx, trachea, and bronchi

M. Tube placed through the neck into the trachea to create an open airway

N. Intravenous line that is placed close to the heart

O. Drainage device that runs from the brain to the abdomen to relieve excess cerebrospinal fluid

_____ 1. Adolescent

_____ 2. Blow-by oxygen

_____ 3. Central line

_____ 4. Croup

_____ 5. Epiglottitis

_____ 6. Febrile seizure

_____ 7. Fontanelle

_____ 8. Gastrostomy tube

_____ 9. Newborn or infant

_____ 10. Preschooler

_____ 11. School-aged child

_____ 12. Shunt

_____ 13. SIDS

_____ 14. Toddler

_____ 15. Tracheostomy tube

_____ 1. When a child is considered a toddler, his/her age group is between
_____ year(s).
    A. birth and 1   **C.** 3 and 6
    B. 1 and 3   **D.** 6 and 12

_____ 2. When a child is considered school age, his/her age group is between
_____ years.
    A. 1 and 3   **C.** 6 and 12
    B. 3 and 6   **D.** 12 and 18

_____ 3. Which of the following is <u>not</u> appropriate when assessing the toddler?
    A. Have the child sit on the parent's lap.
    B. Avoid lying to the patient.
    C. Explain what you are doing.
    D. Perform the head exam first.

_____ 4. Until about age 4, a child's head is proportionately _____ than the adult's.
    A. smaller and lighter   **C.** larger and heavier
    B. smaller and heavier   **D.** larger and lighter

_____ 5. The soft spot on an infant's skull is called a
    A. croup.   **C.** depression.
    B. fontanelle.   **D.** shunt.

_____ 6. A sunken fontanelle may indicate
    A. dehydration.   **C.** external hemorrhage.
    B. rising intracranial pressure.   **D.** hypertension.

_____ 7. A bulging fontanelle may indicate
    A. dehydration.   **C.** external hemorrhage.
    B. elevated intracranial pressure.   **D.** hypertension.

_____ 8. Newborns usually breathe
    A. over sixty times a minute.   **C.** through their mouths.
    B. less than eight times a minute.   **D.** through their noses.

_____ 9. In an infant, hyperextension of the neck
    A. is necessary to open the airway.
    B. may result in airway obstruction.
    C. is necessary if trauma is suspected.
    D. is a procedure reserved for respiratory distress.

_____ 10. If the EMT-B suctions a child's airway for longer than a few seconds at a
time, this could lead to
    A. gag reflex activation.   **C.** airway blockage.
    B. vagus nerve stimulation.   **D.** cardiac arrest.

_____ 11. The tongues of infants and children are more likely than an adult's to fall
back into and block the airway because their tongues are
    A. proportionately larger than an adult's.
    B. larger than an adult's.
    C. proportionately smaller than an adult's.
    D. smaller than an adult's.

_____ 12. The insertion procedure for an oropharyngeal airway in an infant or a child
is performed
    A. much more quickly than in an adult.
    B. with the tip pointing toward the tongue and throat.
    C. the same way it is done for adults.
    D. without inserting a tongue depressor.

_____ **13.** When assessing the capillary refill of a child 5 years old or younger, peripheral perfusion is considered satisfactory if the color returns in less than _____ seconds.
   A. 2
   B. 3
   C. 4
   D. 5

_____ **14.** Which of the following is <u>not</u> a sign of a partial airway obstruction in an infant or a child?
   A. pink skin
   B. adequate peripheral perfusion
   C. stridor and crowing
   D. loss of consciousness

_____ **15.** Signs of a severe partial airway obstruction or complete airway obstruction in an infant or a child include all of the following <u>except</u>
   A. cyanosis.
   B. altered mental status.
   C. crying or coughing.
   D. inability to speak.

_____ **16.** The effects of hypoxia on an infant and a child are
   A. slowed heart rate and improved mental status.
   B. increased heart rate and decreased mental status.
   C. slowed heart rate and altered mental status.
   D. increased heart rate and coma.

_____ **17.** All of the following are appropriate guidelines to follow when ventilating the infant or child <u>except</u>
   A. avoid breathing too hard through the pocket face mask.
   B. avoid using excessive bag pressure and volume.
   C. use a properly sized mask to assure a good mask seal.
   D. omit the use of infection control barriers.

_____ **18.** The flow-restricted, oxygen-powered ventilation device is
   A. used with caution in an infant.
   B. contraindicated in infants and children.
   C. preferred during the resuscitation of a child.
   D. is only used with the pop-off valve engaged in children.

_____ **19.** Common causes of shock in children include infection, trauma, blood loss, and
   A. meningitis.
   B. heart failure.
   C. dehydration.
   D. lack of insulin.

_____ **20.** Less common causes of shock in a child include all of the following <u>except</u>
   A. allergic reactions.
   B. cardiac events.
   C. poisoning.
   D. croup.

_____ **21.** The blood volume of infants and children is approximately _____ of the total body weight.
   A. 6%
   B. 8%
   C. 10%
   D. 12%

_____ **22.** When children are in shock, they do all of the following <u>except</u>
   A. compensate for a long time.
   B. appear better than they actually are.
   C. decompensate very rapidly.
   D. decompensate very slowly.

_____ **23.** When a child is bleeding internally, the EMT-B should avoid
   A. administering too much oxygen.
   B. transporting too quickly.
   C. waiting for signs of decompensated shock before treating for shock.
   D. placing the child in the Trendelenburg position if respiratory distress is not evident.

_____ **24.** Decreased urine output and absence of tears are signs of _____ in infants and children.
  A. epiglottitis
  B. shock
  C. hypothermia
  D. croup

_____ **25.** When treating a child in shock, unless there are injuries that would contraindicate it, the EMT-B should
  A. lower the patient's legs.
  B. elevate the patient's legs.
  C. have the patient sit up.
  D. have the patient lie supine.

_____ **26.** Because children have a large skin surface area in proportion to their body mass, they can easily become victims of
  A. hypothermia.
  B. high fever.
  C. airway obstruction.
  D. hypovolemia.

_____ **27.** If a child has an airway respiratory disease, it is very important that the EMT-B avoid
  A. opening the airway.
  B. inserting a tongue blade into the mouth.
  C. positioning the child in the parent's lap.
  D. administering blow-by oxygen.

_____ **28.** A child with signs of an airway disease should be transported as quickly as possible. The signs include all of the following except
  A. stridor on inspiration.
  B. breathing effort on exhalation.
  C. rapid breathing.
  D. wheezing.

_____ **29.** A viral illness that causes inflammation of the upper airway and bronchi, which is often accompanied by a "seal bark" cough is called
  A. bronchitis.
  B. asthma.
  C. croup.
  D. epiglottitis.

_____ **30.** About _____ of all pediatric trauma deaths are related to airway mismanagement.
  A. one-fifth
  B. one-fourth
  C. one-third
  D. one-half

_____ **31.** Causes of fever in children include all of the following except
  A. upper respiratory infection.
  B. hypothermia.
  C. pneumonia.
  D. infection.

_____ **32.** In the prehospital setting, which of the following is used to determine an infant's skin temperature?
  A. ungloved hand
  B. rectal thermometer
  C. oral thermometer
  D. pulse oximeter

_____ **33.** When treating an infant or a child with a high fever,
  A. submerge the patient in cold water.
  B. use rubbing alcohol to cool the patient.
  C. monitor for shivering while cooling with tepid water.
  D. cover the patient with a towel soaked in ice water.

_____ **34.** Infants are more susceptible to _____ because, compared to adults, a greater percentage of their body is water.
  A. shock
  B. dehydration
  C. high fever
  D. all of the above.

_____ **35.** Which of the following is not true of seizures in the pediatric patient?
  A. Seizures require medical evaluation.
  B. Seizures should be considered life-threatening.
  C. Seizures are rarely caused by fever.
  D. Seizures may be a sign of an underlying condition.

_____ **36.** Severe aspirin poisoning in children can cause all of the following <u>except</u>
  A. seizures.   **C.** coma.
  B. dehydration.   **D.** shock.

_____ **37.** A common cause of lead poisoning in children is
  A. ingesting chips of lead-based paint.
  B. chewing on pencils.
  C. drinking water from a well.
  D. eating fish from fresh water lakes.

_____ **38.** You are treating a child who accidentally ingested a handful of her mother's vitamin tablets. Should you be concerned?
  A. No! The body eliminates excess vitamins.
  B. No! The child will just have diarrhea for a few days.
  C. Yes! Many vitamin pills contain iron, which can be fatal to a child.
  D. Yes! Adult vitamins are too concentrated for children.

_____ **39.** The majority of meningitis cases occur between the ages of one month and
  A. 6 months.   **C.** 3 years.
  B. 1 year.   **D.** 5 years.

_____ **40.** In cases of sudden infant death syndrome, the EMT-B should
  A. not deliver care and transport immediately.
  B. pronounce the infant's death.
  C. look for evidence of child neglect.
  D. provide resuscitation and transport.

_____ **41.** The number one cause of death in infants and children is
  A. respiratory arrest.   **C.** cardiac arrest.
  B. trauma.   **D.** child abuse.

_____ **42.** The child who has been struck by a vehicle may present with a triad of injuries that include head injury, lower extremity injury, and _____ injury.
  A. chest   **C.** abdominal
  B. neck   **D.** upper extremity

_____ **43.** Which of the following is <u>true</u> of a head-injury child?
  A. The most frequent sign is altered mental status.
  B. Respiratory arrest is a common secondary effect.
  C. Suspect internal injuries whenever the patient presents with shock.
  D. All of the above.

_____ **44.** Because the musculoskeletal structures of the chest are less developed in infants and children,
  A. they are able to maintain rapid respiratory rates for a long time.
  B. they are more likely than adults to fracture their ribs.
  C. the chest is less easily deformed.
  D. they are more likely to incur injury to structures beneath the ribs.

_____ **45.** Because the abdominal muscles of infants and small children are immature,
  A. they have less visible signs of breathing difficulty.
  B. they use their chest muscles for breathing.
  C. there is less protection for underlying organs.
  D. they rarely have distention of the abdomen.

_____ **46.** When using a PASG on a pediatric patient, the EMT-B should remember
  A. to place the infant in the leg of an adult garment.
  B. the abdominal section is not generally used on children.
  C. it is contraindicated with pelvic instability.
  D. it is contraindicated in children younger than 12 years old.

_____ **47.** Guidelines for managing pediatric burn patients include all of the following
<u>except</u>
   A. use the rule of nines to estimate the extent of burns.
   B. identify candidates for transportation to burn centers.
   C. cover the burn with sterile dressing.
   D. keep the patient cool to reduce pain.

_____ **48.** Indications that child abuse may be occurring include all of the following
<u>except</u>
   A. repeated responses to provide care for the same child or family.
   B. poorly healing wounds or improperly healed fractures.
   C. indications of past injuries.
   D. a parent who seems concerned about the child's injuries.

_____ **49.** When you respond to the home of a person that you think may be a child
abuser, observe for all of the following <u>except</u>
   A. a family member who has trouble controlling anger.
   B. indications of alcohol and drug abuse.
   C. torn clothing on the child.
   D. any adult who appears in a state of depression.

_____ **50.** Which of the following is <u>not</u> a role of the EMT-B when child abuse is
suspected?
   A. Control your emotions and hold back accusations.
   B. Gather information from parents/caregiver away from the child.
   C. Talk to the child separately and ask her if she has been abused.
   D. Report your suspicions of abuse to the emergency department.

COMPLETE THE FOLLOWING

1. List ten signs of respiratory distress in a child.

   A. _____   **F.** _____

   B. _____   **G.** _____

   C. _____   **H.** _____

   D. _____   **I.** _____

   E. _____   **J.** _____

2. List five potential problems that can occur when caring for a special needs
child with a tracheostomy tube.

   A. _____

   B. _____

   C. _____

   D. _____

   E. _____

3. List four possible complications of central venous lines.

A. _____

B. _____

C. _____

D. _____

COMPLETE THE CHART

Fill in each numbered box to complete the chart.

Artificial Ventilation

	Child over 8 years	Child 1 to 8 years	Infant birth to 1 year
Ventilation duration	1.	2.	3.
Ventilation rate	4.	5.	6.

VIRTUAL STREET SCENES

(First review the Street Scenes on pages 682–683 in the textbook. Then answer the questions beow.)

1. The mother reported seeing her child "shake." What do you suppose happened to this child?

2. This child's mental status improved. Suppose it had not improved and the child was warm to the touch and had a rash. What BSI precautions would be appropriate?

3. Why would it be important for you to follow up on the hospital admission of this child?

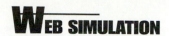
WEB SIMULATION

For interactive case studies that will help you review and practice basic skills, visit the *Emergency Care 9e Companion Website* at www.bradybooks.com/emergencycare.

CASE STUDY

▶ **THE CASE OF THE POISONED JUICE**

You are dispatched to a community day care center that called 9-1-1 because a number of the children suddenly became ill after lunch. Upon arrival, you determine the scene is safe to enter and size up the situation. There are at least six children of different ages, ranging from infant to six years old, who have become nauseated after drinking apple juice that was left over from a few days ago. They are vomiting and complaining of stomach cramps. You have decided to call for an ALS unit and another BLS unit for backup at this time.

1. What BSI precautions should you take?

2. How could you prepare for additional patients with the assistance of the day care workers?

As your crew begins to evaluate each of the children, the day care supervisor notifies you that all the parents of the sick children have been called. It appears that all of the children are in various stages of vomiting and most also have diarrhea. Initial assessment doesn't reveal any patients who are high priority except one infant who normally requires special care.

3. What can be a complication of children vomiting and having diarrhea?

4. The infant who receives special care is normally healthy except she is closely watched because she has had a shunt installed since birth. What is a shunt and why are they used frequently in infants?

The other ambulances arrive and the decision is made to immediately transport the infant with the shunt as a high priority and call for an additional ambulance to respond to the scene. Each of the EMT-Bs begins obtaining complete sets of vital signs on the remaining children. Most of the sixty children in the day care center are being evaluated for complaints and a full set of vitals; a prehospital care report has been completed on each child. Most of the children are not sick; however, you are noticing a trend of "sympathy" pains from children who could not possibly have had a drink from the contaminated can of juice.

5. What would be the normal vital signs to expect from the infants?

6. What would be the normal vital signs to expect from the toddlers?

7. What would be the normal vital signs to expect from the preschoolers?

8. As you examine the infants, are there any assessment strategies that would be helpful?

9. As you examine the toddlers, are there any assessment strategies that would be helpful?

10. As you examine the preschoolers, are there any assessment strategies that would be helpful?

When the parents arrive, some of them decide to sign the appropriate documentation and to take their children to their pediatricians. Eight other parents have agreed to be transported with their children to the local hospital so the children can be examined further in the emergency department.

11. For the infants and toddlers who are being transported by ambulance, what is the safest way to transport them provided they are not unstable and their parents are nearby to assist?

12. For the infants being transported by ambulance, what is the best way to determine their level of responsiveness with the assistance of their parents?

13. One of the paramedics suggests taking a sample of the juice that all the children drank. Why might this be helpful?

CHAPTER Thirty-Two

AMBULANCE OPERATIONS

MATCH TERMINOLOGY/DEFINITIONS

A. Legal term, which appears in most states' driving laws, referring to the responsibility of the emergency vehicle operator to drive safely and keep the safety of all others in mind at all times

B. Emergency Medical Dispatcher

C. Call in which the driver of the emergency vehicle responds with lights and siren because he/she is of the understanding that loss or life or limb is possible

D. Large, flat area without aerial obstruction in which a helicopter can land to pick up a patient

E. Special thermometer that is designed to go down to 82°F

F. Traction splint for the immobilization of a painful, swollen, deformed thigh

G. Automated external defibrillator

H. Cervical immobilization device

I. Automatic transport ventilator

J. Mechanical compressor for performing CPR that is especially helpful to services with transport time to the hospital over 15 minutes

_____ **1.** AED

_____ **2.** ATV

_____ **3.** CID

_____ **4.** Due regard

_____ **5.** EMD

_____ **6.** Hypothermia thermometer

_____ **7.** Landing zone (LZ)

_____ **8.** Sager

_____ **9.** Thumper

_____ **10.** True emergency

_____ 1. The federal agency that develops specifications for ambulance vehicle designs is the
   A. U.S. Department of Motor Vehicles.
   B. Food and Drug Administration.
   C. U.S. Department of Transportation.
   D. U.S. Department of Health, Education, and Welfare.

_____ 2. The purpose(s) for carrying an EPA-registered, intermediate-level disinfectant on the ambulance is to
   A. clean up blood spills.
   B. destroy mycobacterium tuberculosis.
   C. disinfect patient wounds.
   D. do all of the above.

_____ 3. Which of the following is not a piece of equipment that should be in the portable first-in kit, which is taken directly to a patient's side?
   A. suction unit
   B. rigid cervical collar
   C. blood pressure cuff
   D. telemetry repeater

_____ 4. Supplies used for the "C" step of the initial assessment of a trauma victim includes all of the following except
   A. disposable gloves.
   B. occlusive dressings.
   C. the AED.
   D. a suction unit.

_____ 5. Each of the following is a piece of equipment used to obtain vital signs except
   A. rubber bulb syringe.
   B. adult and pediatric stethoscope.
   C. sphygmomanometer kit.
   D. pen light.

_____ 6. A device used to carry patients over long distances is called a
   A. Stokes basket.
   B. scoop stretcher.
   C. Reeves stretcher.
   D. wheeled ambulance stretcher.

_____ 7. Which one of the following pieces of patient transfer equipment is incorrectly matched with its function?
   A. wheeled ambulance stretcher : transporting patients in sitting, supine, or Trendelenburg position
   B. folding stair chair : moving patients down stairs in a sitting position
   C. Reeves stretcher : carrying patients from a high-angle rescue
   D. scoop stretcher : picking up patients found in tight spaces

_____ 8. Components of a typical fixed oxygen delivery system include
   A. 3,000-liter reservoir.
   B. a two-stage regulator.
   C. the necessary reducing valve and yokes.
   D. all of the above.

_____ 9. Of the following devices carried on the ambulance for prehospital respiratory care, which is an optional item?
   A. six adult and four pediatric nasal cannula
   B. flow-restricted, oxygen-powered ventilation device
   C. automatic transport ventilator
   D. plastic cup for blow-by oxygen

_____ 10. The fixed suction unit in the ambulance should
   A. provide an airflow of over 15 liters per minute.
   B. be usable by a person seated beside the patient.
   C. have a current hydrostat test date.
   D. reach a vacuum of at least 300 mmHg within 4 seconds.

_____ 11. Which of the following pieces of equipment carried on ambulances for defibrillation or assisting with cardiopulmonary resuscitation is optional?
   A. short or long spine board
   B. mechanical CPR compressor
   C. automated external defibrillator
   D. kit with oral and nasal airways

_____ 12. Equipment that is carried on an ambulance for immobilization include all of the following except
   A. a Hare traction splint.
   B. triangular bandages.
   C. padded aluminum splints.
   D. a burn sheet.

_____ 13. Chemical cold packs are carried on an ambulance primarily for use with _____ injuries.
   A. musculoskeletal
   B. abdominal
   C. respiratory
   D. cardiac

_____ 14. Supplies used for wound care should include all of the following except
   A. sterile burn sheets.
   B. 5 × 9 inch combine dressings.
   C. self-adhering roller bandages.
   D. Hare traction device.

_____ 15. What is the purpose of carrying sterilized aluminum foil on the ambulance?
   A. to wrap body parts in
   B. to maintain body heat
   C. to make a shield over an avulsed eye
   D. for warming minor abrasions

_____ 16. The supplies for childbirth include all of the following except
   A. a rubber bulb syringe.
   B. sanitary napkins.
   C. large safety pins.
   D. sterile surgical gloves.

_____ 17. Every shift, both you and your partner should
   A. wash and wax the ambulance.
   B. change the oil on the ambulance.
   C. complete the equipment checklist.
   D. do preventative maintenance on the ambulance.

_____ 18. Of the following items checked on the ambulance, which is checked with the engine off?
   A. dash mounted gauges
   B. battery
   C. windshield wiper operation
   D. vehicle's warning lights

_____ 19. The responsibilities of the Emergency Medical Dispatcher include all of the following except
   A. dispatching and coordinating EMS resources.
   B. interrogating the caller and prioritizing the call.
   C. coordinating with other public safety agencies.
   D. advising the caller that an ambulance is not needed.

_____ 20. When an Emergency Medical Dispatcher questions a patient or caller, which of the following is not routinely asked?
   A. What is the exact location of the patient?
   B. What's the problem?
   C. Has the patient been in the hospital recently?
   D. How old is the patient?

_____ 21. When speaking with a caller who is at the scene of a traffic collision, the Emergency Medical Dispatcher should ask all of the following except
   A. Is traffic moving?
   B. What brand vehicle was involved in the collision?
   C. How many lanes of traffic are open?
   D. Are any of the vehicles on fire?

_____ 22. To be a safe ambulance operator, the EMT-B should
   A. be tolerant of other drivers.
   B. always wear glasses or contact lenses if required.
   C. have a positive attitude about his/her ability as a driver.
   D. do all of the above.

_____ 23. Every state has statutes that regulate the operation of emergency vehicles. Under certain circumstances, vehicle operators can do all of the following except
   A. park the vehicle anywhere so long as it does not damage personal property.
   B. proceed past red stop signals, flashing red stop signals, and stop signs.
   C. exceed the posted speed limit as long as life and property are not endangered.
   D. pass a school bus that has its red lights blinking.

_____ 24. At the scene of a collision, you examine a patient and find that he is stable. This situation is no longer a
   A. true emergency.   C. cold response.
   B. due regard.   D. priority one response.

_____ 25. Which guideline for the use of the ambulance siren is inappropriate?
   A. Use the siren sparingly.
   B. Never assume that all motorists will hear your signal.
   C. Be prepared for erratic movements of motorists.
   D. Keep it on until the call is completed.

_____ 26. Which of the following is true about the use of lights and sirens?
   A. Motorists are more inclined to give way to ambulances when sirens are continually sounded.
   B. The decision about their use should be based on the patient's medical condition.
   C. The use of the siren has little effect on the ambulance operator.
   D. Four-way flashers should be used in addition to emergency lights.

_____ 27. Use of escorts or multi-vehicle responses are a
   A. very quick and successful means of response.
   B. very dangerous means of response.
   C. means of decreasing the chance of collision.
   D. standard operating procedure in most communities.

_____ 28. Factors that can affect ambulance response include all of the following except
   A. time of the day.
   B. weather.
   C. road maintenance and construction.
   D. type of emergency.

_____ 29. You are the first vehicle on the scene of an auto collision in which one of the automobiles is on fire. You should park your vehicle _____ the wreckage.
   A. 50 feet from   C. beyond
   B. in front of   D. downwind from

_____ 30. A sequence of operations to ready a patient for transfer is called
   A. stabilization.   C. transport.
   B. packaging.   D. removal.

_____ 31. An unconscious patient who has no potential spine injury should be positioned in the ambulance
   A. in the recovery position.   C. in the supine position.
   B. with legs raised 8 to 12 inches. D. a sitting-up position.

_____ **32.** Which of the following is an action you would <u>not</u> perform en route to the hospital?
  A. Recheck the patient's bandages and splints.
  B. Form a general impression of the patient.
  C. Perform ongoing assessment and continue to monitor vital signs.
  D. Notify the receiving facility of your estimated time of arrival.

_____ **33.** If a patient develops cardiac arrest en route to the hospital, the EMT-B's <u>first</u> action should be to
  A. apply and operate the AED.
  B. begin cardiopulmonary resuscitation.
  C. notify the emergency department.
  D. tell the operator to stop the ambulance.

_____ **34.** When delivering the patient to the hospital, the EMT-B should <u>never</u>
  A. complete the prehospital care report at the hospital.
  B. move a patient onto the hospital stretcher and leave.
  C. transfer the patient's personal effects.
  D. obtain your release from the hospital.

_____ **35.** When approaching a helicopter, first wait for the pilot or medic to wave you in. Then approach from the _____ of the craft.
  A. rear   **C.** front or side
  B. uphill slope side   **D.** downhill slope rear

COMPLETE THE FOLLOWING

1. List the seven questions an EMD should ask a caller who is reporting a medical emergency.

  A. _____

  B. _____

  C. _____

  D. _____

  E. _____

  F. _____

  G. _____

2. List seven factors that can affect an ambulance response.

  A. _____

  B. _____

  C. _____

  D. _____

  E. _____

  F. _____

  G. _____

3. List the four major ways the EMT-B on the scene of a collision should describe the landing zone to the air rescue service.

A. _____

B. _____

C. _____

D. _____

LABEL THE PHOTOGRAPHS

Fill in the name of each level of disinfecting shown in the photo on the line provided.

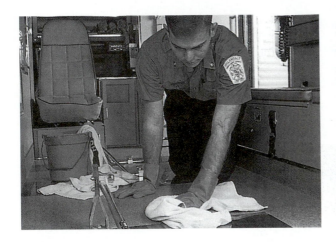

1. _____

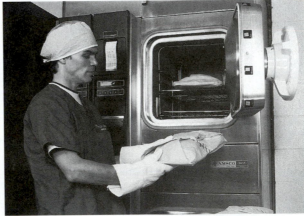

2. _____

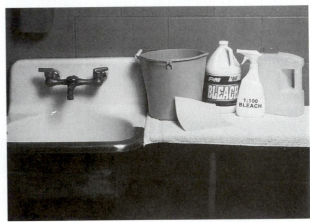

3. _____

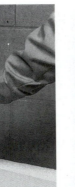

4. _____

Virtual Street Scenes

(First review the Street Scenes on pp. 714–715 of the textbook. Then answer the questions below.)

1. Imagine that the ambulance had gone through a red light and had a collision en route to the call. What should you do right away?

2. If the collision involved another motorist, whose fault would it be?

3. Why is it an unsafe practice to drive an ambulance through a red light?

Web Simulation

For interactive case studies that will help you review and practice basic skills, visit the **Emergency Care 9e Companion Website** at www.bradybooks.com/emergencycare.

EMT-Basic Skills Performance Checklists

▶ **Transferring the Patient**

❑ Take BSI precautions.

❑ Transfer the patient as soon as possible. In a routine admission or when an illness or injury is not life-threatening, first check to see what is to be done with the patient.

❑ An EMT-B should remain with the patient until transfer is complete.

❑ Assist the emergency department staff as required.

❑ Give a complete verbal report of the patient's condition and treatment administered.

❑ Complete your prehospital care report and turn a copy over to the hospital staff.

❑ Transfer the patient's personal effects.

❑ Obtain your release from the hospital if required in your region.

▶ **Actions To Be Taken at the Hospital**

❑ Take BSI precautions.

(continued next page)

❑ Clean the ambulance interior as required by your service exposure control plan.

❑ Replace respiratory equipment as required.

❑ Replace disposable items according to local policies.

❑ Exchange equipment according to local policies.

❑ Make up the ambulance stretcher.

▶ **CHECKING THE AED**

❑ Check the AED for the following:

- Unit, cables, and connectors for cleanliness.

- Supplies carried with the AED.

- Power supply and its operation.

- Indicators on the ECG display.

- ECG recorder operation.

- Charge display cycle with a simulator.

- Pacemaker feature if applicable.

❑ File a written report on the status of the AED.

NOTE: The specifics can be found on the FDA Automated Defibrillator: Operator's Shift Checklist.

CASE STUDY

▶ **THE AMBULANCE COLLISION**

You are notified by dispatch to respond to the neighboring district for a mutual aid call—an ambulance has collided with a passenger vehicle at an intersection. Responding with emergency lights and siren, the ambulance had approached the red light and had attempted to pass through it without stopping. The other vehicle's occupants are an elderly couple who were on their way to the store.

As you arrive on the scene, it is obvious that there are a number of very seriously injured patients due to the speed and size of the ambulance that broadsided the car. You are assigned to look after the ambulance operator who has minor cuts and scrapes. Fortunately for him, he was wearing his seat belt. His EMT-B partner was not as fortunate; another ambulance had already removed her from the scene with serious head and neck injuries from being ejected through the windshield of the ambulance. She had not been wearing her shoulder harness. Two other ambulance crews are in the process of removing the elderly man, who is in critical condition, and his wife, who has sustained leg fractures and is having a heart attack from the stress of the incident.

1. Was this a preventable collision?

2. Could the serious injuries to the female EMT-B have been prevented?

3. What happened to the patient to whom the ambulance was responding?

4. What is the first rule of medicine?

The next day, the headlines in the local newspaper are: "Ambulance Kills Two En Route to Third." The story goes on to say how the initial patient had basically minor medical problems and was taken by an ambulance to the local hospital for the flu and released within three hours. The newspaper concludes with "The driver was suspended. The District Attorney requests a grand jury."

5. Aside from the reputation of the EMT-B who was driving, what might this "negative publicity" cost the service and other EMT-Bs who work there?

6. Why can the district attorney request a grand jury for this incident?

7. Is the operator of an emergency vehicle held to a higher standard than other motorists?

8. Who pays for the court defense of the EMT-B who was driving?

9. Could the EMT-B be personally sued for the injuries (deaths) that occurred?

10. How can an ambulance service prevent a collision like this from happening in its community?

CHAPTER Thirty-Three

GAINING ACCESS AND RESCUE OPERATIONS

MATCH TERMINOLOGY/DEFINITIONS

A. When moving towards the rear of the vehicle, the second post you see, which supports the roof

B. Glass used in an automobile's side and rear windows designed to break into small rounded pieces rather than sharp fragments

C. Named after a well-known consumer advocate, this case-hardened pin is held by the cams of an automobile's door locking system

D. Decreasing circles of voltage on the ground surrounding a point where a charged wire is down

E. When a patient is pinned and requires assistance, sometimes mechanical, to free him

F. To crib or block a vehicle or structure to prevent further unintended, uncontrolled movement

G. Gear designed to prevent the rescuer from being injured while working in the inner circle

H. Post in front of the driver's compartment which supports the roof and windshield

I. Safety glass used in the windshields of automobiles made of two sheets of plate glass bonded to a sheet of tough plastic

J. Blocks of hardwood usually 4 × 4 × 18-inch or 2 × 4 × 18-inch used to stabilize a vehicle

K. Area immediately around and including the wrecked vehicle

L. Access that requires tools or special equipment to reach the patient

M. Three-part procedure used by rescue personnel to free a patient trapped in a vehicle

N. Process by which entrapped patients are rescued from vehicles, buildings, tunnels, or other places

O. Saw that is designed to cut laminated windshield glass

_____ **1.** A Post

_____ **2.** B Post

_____ **3.** Complex

_____ **4.** Cribbing

_____ **5.** Disentanglement

_____ **6.** Entrapment

_____ **7.** Extrication

_____ **8.** Glas-Master

_____ **9.** Ground gradient

_____ **10.** Inner circle

_____ **11.** Laminated glass

_____ **12.** Nader Pin

_____ **13.** Protective gear

_____ **14.** Stabilization

_____ **15.** Tempered glass

_____ 1. Trench, dive, ice, and high-angle rescue is frequently carried out by
    A. industrial rescue teams.   C. police rescue services.
    B. specialty rescue teams.   D. commercial rescue services.

_____ 2. The phases of extrication include all of the following except
    A. gaining access to the patient.   C. disentangling the patient.
    B. defining patient care.   D. sizing up the situation.

_____ 3. An important part of a rescue scene size-up is
    A. determining the extent of entrapment.
    B. starting IVs on the patient.
    C. removing shattered glass from around the patient.
    D. informing the patient about the extent of vehicle damage.

_____ 4. During size-up of a collision, you must be able to read a collision and develop an action plan based on your knowledge of rescue operations and your
    A. previous experience at collision scenes.
    B. judgment of the extent of vehicle damage.
    C. estimate of the patient's condition and priority.
    D. evaluation of the resources available.

_____ 5. When developing an action plan for patient extrication, always keep in mind the
    A. potential for observation by bystanders.
    B. "golden hour" concept of trauma management.
    C. cost of further damage to the vehicle.
    D. type of vehicle that is involved in the incident.

_____ 6. If a vehicle has an air bag which deployed, the manufacturer recommends
    A. airing out the car for 15 minutes prior to treating the patient.
    B. placing masks on patients before treating.
    C. lifting the bag and examining the steering wheel and dash.
    D. using HEPA masks before gaining access.

_____ 7. The unsafe act that contributes most to collision scene injuries is failure to
    A. eliminate or control hazards during operations.
    B. wear protective gear during rescue operations.
    C. recognize mechanisms of injury early on.
    D. select the proper tool for the task.

_____ 8. Factors that may contribute to injuries of rescuers at a collision include all of the following except
    A. careless attitude toward personal safety.
    B. a lack of skill in tool and equipment use.
    C. physical problems that impede strenuous effort.
    D. limiting the inner circle to rescuers who are in protective gear.

_____ 9. Good protective gear at the scene of a collision includes all of the following except
    A. firefighter or leather gloves.
    B. fire-resistant trousers or turnout pants.
    C. steel toe, high-top work shoes.
    D. plastic "bump caps."

_____ **10.** To ensure adequate eye protection at the collision scene, the EMT-B should wear
  A. safety goggles with a soft vinyl frame.
  B. a hinged plastic helmet shield.
  C. a thermal mask or shield.
  D. safety glasses with small lenses.

_____ **11.** During an extrication, an aluminized rescue blanket may be used to
  A. maintain the rescuer's body heat.
  B. smother fire in the engine compartment.
  C. protect the patient from poor weather and flying particles.
  D. None of the above.

_____ **12.** When using flares, the EMT-B should
  A. watch for spilled fuel or other combustibles prior to igniting.
  B. throw them out of the moving vehicle to save time.
  C. use them as a traffic wand to divert traffic.
  D. always walk with oncoming traffic while positioning them.

_____ **13.** When there is an electrical hazard, the safe zone
  A. should be established as soon as the power company arrives.
  B. does not exist due to the numerous dangers of an electrical hazard.
  C. should be far enough away to assure an arcing wire does not cause injury.
  D. is located at least ten feet from the ground gradient.

_____ **14.** A material or object that will carry electricity is
  A. dangerous to stand near.   **C.** always energized.
  B. not a hazard unless it is arcing.   **D.** called a conductor.

_____ **15.** If a vehicle collides with a broken utility pole with wires down, you should
  A. ignore it since the vehicle will not conduct electricity.
  B. tell the vehicle's occupants to stay in the vehicle.
  C. immediately shut off the vehicle's ignition switch.
  D. don full protective gear and remove downed wires.

_____ **16.** In wet weather, a phenomenon known as _____ may provide your first clue that a wire is down.
  A. an arc   **C.** lightning
  B. ground gradient   **D.** flash point

_____ **17.** As you approach a scene with an electrical hazard, you feel a tingling sensation in your legs and lower torso. Which action should you take?
  A. Turn 180 degrees and shuffle with both feet together to safety.
  B. Turn 90 degrees and walk as quickly as possible to safety.
  C. Ask your partner for his hand and have him pull you to safety.
  D. Turn 180 degrees and crawl to safety.

_____ **18.** If there is a fire in the car's engine compartment and people are trapped in the vehicle, you should do all of the following except
  A. quickly and carefully remove the patient.
  B. assure that the fire department has been called.
  C. don protective gear and use your fire extinguisher.
  D. apply a short spine board to the driver right away.

_____ **19.** When a vehicle's hood is closed and there is an engine fire, you should do all of the following except
  A. use emergency moves to remove occupants.
  B. let the fire department extinguish the fire.
  C. fully open the hood to extinguish the fire.
  D. let the fire burn under the closed hood.

_____ **20.** When a vehicle rolls off the roadway into a field of dried grass, it is possible that a fire may be caused by the
  A. catalytic converter.
  C. ground gradient.
  B. leaking radiator fluid.
  D. airbag deployment.

_____ **21.** "Try Before You Pry" is the foundation for the _____ procedure.
  A. disentanglement
  C. simple access
  B. stabilization
  D. entanglement

_____ **22.** Once a vehicle is stabilized and an entry point is gained, the EMT-B should immediately do all of the following except
  A. begin the initial assessment.
  B. crawl inside the vehicle.
  C. provide manual cervical stabilization.
  D. pull the patient out of the access hole.

_____ **23.** If an unconscious patient is in a sitting position behind the wheel with legs pinned by the vehicle, which is the best approach to disentanglement?
  A. Displace the doors, cut the roof, then displace the dash.
  B. Pull the dash, cut the doors, then push the seat.
  C. Cut the roof, displace the doors, and then displace the dash.
  D. Cut the roof, displace the dash, then displace the doors.

_____ **24.** Which of the following is not a reason for disposing of the roof to access a patient?
  A. It makes the entire interior of the vehicle accessible.
  B. It creates a large exitway through which to remove a patient.
  C. It provides fresh air and helps cool off the patient.
  D. It helps to quickly stabilize the vehicle.

_____ **25.** An extrication involves displacing the dash or steering wheel but the air bag has not yet deployed. What should you do?
  A. Apply heat to the steering wheel.
  C. Disconnect the battery cable.
  B. Drill a hole into the air bag module.
  D. Displace the steering column.

COMPLETE THE FOLLOWING

1. List the ten phases of the rescue process.

A. _____

B. _____

C. _____

D. _____

E. _____

F. _____

G. _____

H. _____

I. _____

J. _____

2. List six factors that can increase the potential for an injury at a collision site.

A. _____

B. _____

C. _____

D. _____

E. _____

F. _____

LABEL THE PHOTOGRAPHS

Label each procedure on the lines provided.

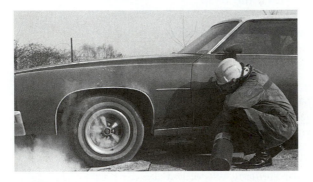

1. _____

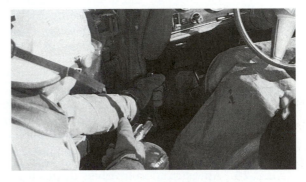

2. _____

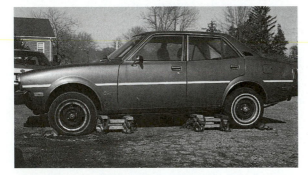

3. _____

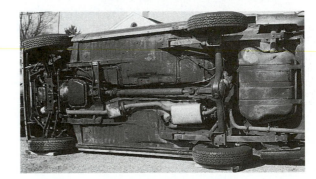

4. _____

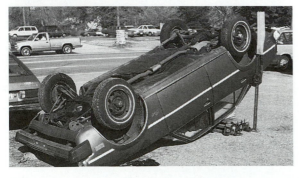

5. _____

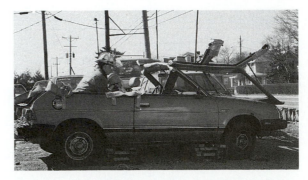

6. _____

VIRTUAL STREET SCENES

(First review the Street Scenes on pp. 736–737 of the textbook. Then answer the questions below.)

1. Suppose the patient had been trapped under the dashboard. Would it make more sense to pop open the doors and then take off the roof? Or should the roof come off first?

2. What is the significance of a vehicle with ten feet of intrusion?

3. Should ALS be requested for this patient?

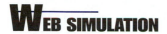

WEB SIMULATION

For interactive case studies that will help you review and practice basic skills, visit the *Emergency Care 9e Companion Website* at www.bradybooks.com/emergencycare.

CHAPTER Thirty-Four

SPECIAL OPERATIONS

MATCH TERMINOLOGY/DEFINITIONS

A. Color-coded tag indicating the priority group to which a patient has been assigned

B. Area in which secondary triage takes place at a multiple-casualty incident

C. Process of quickly assessing patients in a multiple-casualty incident and assigning each a priority for receiving emergency care or transportation to definitive care

D. Person responsible for overseeing triage at a multiple-casualty incident

E. Area in which patient care is delivered at a multiple-casualty incident

F. Person responsible for overseeing treatment of patients who have been triaged at a multiple-casualty incident

G. Person responsible for communicating with sector officers and hospitals to manage transportation of patients to hospitals from the scene of a multiple-casualty incident

H. Area in which ambulances are parked and other resources are held until needed

I. Person responsible for overseeing and keeping track of ambulances and ambulance personnel at a multiple-casualty incident and who directs ambulances to treatment areas at the request of the transportation officer

J. Any medical or trauma event involving three or more patients that places a great demand on EMS equipment and personnel

K. System used for the management of a large-scale multiple-casualty incident, involving assumption of responsibility for command and designation and coordination of such elements as triage, treatment, transport, and staging

L. Senior EMS person on the scene who establishes an EMS command post and oversees the medical aspects of a multiple-casualty incident

M. Any substance or material in a form which poses an unreasonable risk to health, safety, and property when transported in commerce

N. Area immediately surrounding a dangerous goods incident that extends far enough to prevent adverse effects from released dangerous goods to personnel outside the zone

O. Area in which the command post and support functions that are necessary to control the incident are located

_____ **1.** Cold zone

_____ **2.** EMS Command

_____ **3.** Hazardous material

_____ **4.** Hot zone

_____ **5.** Incident Management System (IMS)

_____ **6.** Multiple-casualty incident (MCI)

_____ **7.** Staging officer

_____ **8.** Staging sector

_____ **9.** Transportation officer

_____ **10.** Treatment officer

_____ **11.** Treatment sector

_____ **12.** Triage

_____ **13.** Triage officer

_____ **14.** Triage sector

_____ **15.** Triage tag

MULTIPLE-CHOICE REVIEW

_____ **1.** Using the *North American Emergency Response Guidebook,* the EMT-B would find that ethyl acetate is a chemical that
- **A.** irritates the eyes and respiratory tract.
- **B.** destroys the bone marrow.
- **C.** damages internal organs.
- **D.** is extremely explosive.

_____ **2.** Using the *North American Emergency Response Guidebook,* the EMT-B would find that Benzene (benzol) is a chemical that
- **A.** damages the eyes by eliminating moisture.
- **B.** has toxic vapors which can be absorbed through the skin.
- **C.** is used as an industrial blasting agent.
- **D.** is used in surgical techniques to control pain.

_____ **3.** The regulations that require training in hazardous materials for responders to hazmat incidents are
- **A.** Ryan White CARE Act.
- **B.** NFPA 1200.
- **C.** FEMA 1910.1030.
- **D.** OSHA 1910.120

_____ **4.** The level of training for those who initially respond to releases or potential releases of hazardous materials in order to protect people, property, and the environment is called
- **A.** First Responder Awareness.
- **B.** First Responder Operations.
- **C.** Hazardous Materials Technician.
- **D.** Hazardous Materials Specialist.

_____ **5.** The level of training for those who are likely to witness or discover a hazardous substance release is called
- **A.** First Responder Awareness.
- **B.** First Responder Operations.
- **C.** Hazardous Materials Technician.
- **D.** Hazardous Materials Specialist.

_____ **6.** The standard that deals with competencies for EMS personnel at a hazardous material incident is called
- **A.** OSHA 1910.1030.
- **B.** NFPA 472.
- **C.** NFPA 473.
- **D.** OSHA 1910.1200.

_____ **7.** Which of the following is not likely to be a potential hazardous material location?
- **A.** garden center
- **B.** chemical plant
- **C.** trucking terminal
- **D.** pet store

_____ **8.** Unless EMS personnel are trained to the level of _____ , they must remain in the cold zone.
- **A.** First Responder Awareness.
- **B.** First Responder Operations.
- **C.** Hazardous Materials Technician.
- **D.** Hazardous Materials Specialist.

_____ **9.** All victims leaving the _____ zone should be considered contaminated until proven otherwise.
- **A.** cold
- **B.** warm
- **C.** hot
- **D.** decontamination

_____ **10.** What is the primary concern at the scene of a hazardous material incident?
- **A.** the safety of the EMT-B and crew, patients, and the public
- **B.** stabilizing the incident as fast as possible
- **C.** quickly removing all exposed patients from the scene
- **D.** determining the extent and cost of the damage

_____ 11. Upon arrival at a tanker truck crash where the vehicle has overturned and is rapidly leaking its contents onto the street, the EMT-B should
   A. quickly apply a short spine board to the truck driver in the tanker.
   B. isolate the area and call for the appropriate backup assistance.
   C. try to stop or seal the leak as quickly as possible.
   D. send the least senior EMT-B in to assess the patient.

_____ 12. The "safe zone" of a hazardous materials incident should be established in a _____ location.
   A. downwind/downhill
   B. upwind/same level
   C. downwind/same level
   D. upwind/downhill

_____ 13. The role of the incident commander at a hazardous material incident is to delegate responsibility for all of the following except
   A. directing bystanders to a safe area.
   B. establishing a perimeter.
   C. immediately initiating rescue attempts.
   D. evacuating people if necessary.

_____ 14. When a contaminated victim of a hazardous material incident comes in contact with other people who are not contaminated, this is referred to as _____ contamination.
   A. secondary
   B. chemical
   C. contact
   D. clone

_____ 15. The designations on the sides of tanker trucks are called hazardous material
   A. license plates.
   B. waybills.
   C. placards.
   D. shipping papers.

_____ 16. The commonly used placard system for fixed facilities is called the
   A. MSDS.
   B. NFPA 704.
   C. CHEM 369.
   D. UN Classification System.

_____ 17. All employers are required to post in an obvious spot the information about all the chemicals in the workplace on a form called a
   A. NFPA 704.
   B. MSDS.
   C. OSHA Chemical listing.
   D. Fair trade posting.

_____ 18. Resources that the EMT-B should use at a hazardous materials incident include all of the following except
   A. copies of NFPA rules.
   B. the local hazmat team.
   C. the _North American Emergency Response Guidebook_.
   D. CHEM-TEL.

_____ 19. What is CHEMTREC?
   A. 24-hour service for identifying hazardous materials
   B. oil refinery and manufacturer
   C. national hazmat response team
   D. round-the-clock special rescue teams

_____ 20. EMS personnel at the scene of a hazardous material incident are responsible for taking care of the injured and
   A. identifying and controlling the substance involved.
   B. monitoring and rehabilitating hazmat team members.
   C. decontaminating patients exiting the hot zone.
   D. moving patients from the hot zone to the warm zone.

_____ **21.** Which of the following is <u>not</u> a characteristic of the rehab sector at a hazardous material incident?
  A. located in the warm zone
  B. protected from the weather
  C. easily accessible to EMS
  D. free from exhaust fumes

_____ **22.** As soon as possible after a hazmat team member exits the hot zone, the EMT-B should
  A. have him drink a pint of water.
  B. remove his protective clothing.
  C. begin the decontamination process.
  D. reassess his vital signs.

_____ **23.** You are confronted with a patient at risk for causing secondary contamination in which treatment calls for irrigation with water. The hazmat team has not yet arrived. Which of the following actions is <u>not</u> recommended?
  A. Cut the patient's clothes off.
  B. Irrigate the patient with tepid water.
  C. Flush runoff water down the nearest drain.
  D. Use disposable equipment for treatment.

_____ **24.** Which of the following is <u>not</u> a feature of a good local disaster plan?
  A. All emergency responders should be familiar with the plan.
  B. The plan must be based on the actual availability of resources.
  C. The plan must be rehearsed to ensure it works correctly.
  D. The plan should be generic and meet national standards.

_____ **25.** Upon arrival of the first EMS unit at the scene of an MCI, the crew leader should do all of the following <u>except</u>
  A. assume EMS command.   **C.** call for backup.
  B. conduct a scene walk through.   **D.** begin patient treatment.

_____ **26.** Which of the following is <u>not</u> a principle of good communication at an MCI?
  A. The person responsible for incident management should have unique Command name.
  B. Responding units should be informed that a disaster plan is in effect.
  C. The majority of communications should be done via radio transmission.
  D. Communications between Command and sector officers should be face-to-face.

_____ **27.** If an MCI involves hazardous materials, an additional _____ sector would be needed.
  A. hazmat   **C.** rehabilitation
  B. extrication   **D.** decontamination

_____ **28.** The individual at an MCI who is responsible for the sorting and prioritizing of the patients is the _____ officer.
  A. triage   **C.** transportation
  B. treatment   **D.** extrication

_____ **29.** Patients who are assessed to have decreased mental status at an MCI are considered Priority
  A. 1.   **C.** 3.
  B. 2.   **D.** 4.

_____ **30.** Patients who are assessed to have shock (hypoperfusion) at an MCI are considered Priority
  A. 1.   **C.** 3.
  B. 2.   **D.** 4.

_____ **31.** Patients who are assessed to have multiple-bone or joint injuries at an MCI are considered Priority
  A. 1.   **C.** 3.
  B. 2.   **D.** 4.

_____ **32.** Patients who are assessed to have died at the MCI scene are considered Priority
  A. 1.   **C.** 3.
  B. 2.   **D.** 4.

_____ **33.** The individual at an MCI who is responsible for maintaining a supply of vehicles and personnel at a location away from the incident site is the _____ officer.
  A. extrication   **C.** staging
  B. transportation   **D.** triage

_____ **34.** The individual at an MCI who is responsible for determining patient destinations and notifying the hospitals of the incoming patients is the _____ officer.
  A. triage   **C.** transportation
  B. treatment   **D.** extrication

_____ **35.** Patient transport decisions at an MCI are based upon all of the following except
  A. prioritization.   **C.** transportation resources.
  B. destination facilities. **D.** patient's family preferences.

COMPLETE THE FOLLOWING

1. List the information you should be prepared to give when you call for assistance from CHEMTREC.

_____

_____

_____

_____

_____

_____

_____

_____

2. List four characteristics of the rehab sector at a hazardous material incident.

  A. _____

  B. _____

  C. _____

  D. _____

COMPLETE THE CHART

Fill in the blanks to complete the chart.

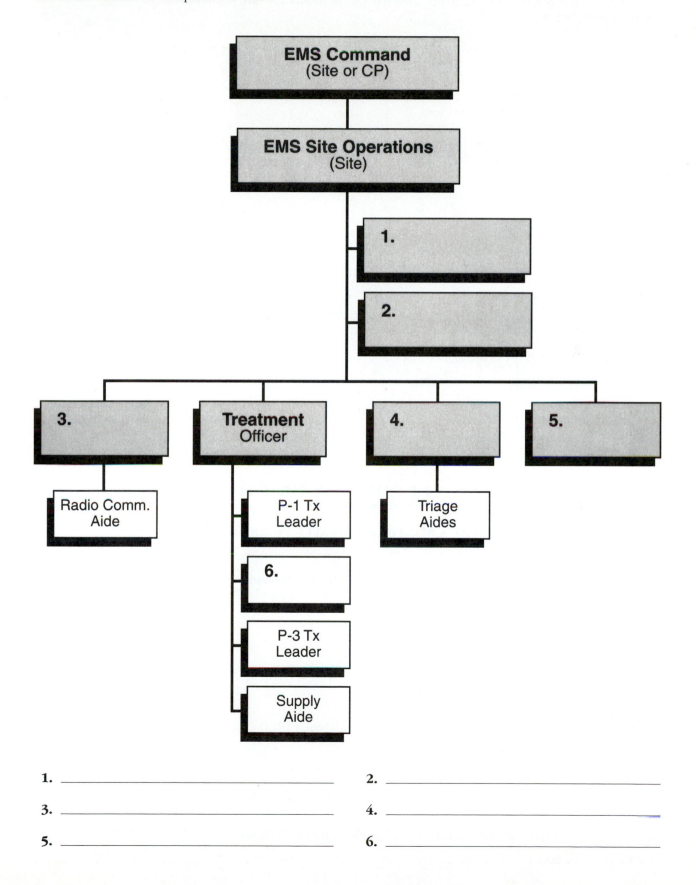

1. _____   2. _____

3. _____   4. _____

5. _____   6. _____

(First review the Street Scenes on pp. 760–761 of the textbook. Then answer the questions below.)

1. For this call, would it have been appropriate to request a helicopter if it was available?

2. How could you find enough additional ambulances?

3. Suppose there was a bus involved at this scene and there were 20 low priority patients. How could you transport them?

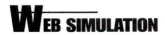
WEB SIMULATION

For interactive case studies that will help you review and practice basic skills, visit the *Emergency Care 9e Companion Website* at www.bradybooks.com/emergencycare.

EMT-BASIC SKILLS PERFORMANCE CHECKLIST

▶ **ESTABLISHING COMMAND AT A MULTIPLE-CASUALTY INCIDENT (MCI)**

❑ Perform a scene size-up.

❑ Locate the police and fire officers and establish a unified command post.

❑ Don the EMS command vest.

❑ Notify the EMS dispatcher:

- Declare an MCI.
- Describe extent of incident.
- Characterize it as ongoing or contained.
- Give approximate number of patients.
- Give the location of the command posts.
- Request number of BLS and ALS units.

❑ Designate a triage officer.

❑ Designate a staging officer and a location for staging, and notify dispatcher to have all additional ambulances respond to staging.

❑ Request the dispatcher roll call the local hospitals for bed availability.

(continued next page)

❑ Designate treatment officer and location for this sector (as needed).

❑ Designate transportation officer and location for this sector (as needed).

❑ Consider the need for aeromedical evacuation and appropriate landing zone nearby the scene.

❑ Consider the usefulness of a school bus to transport the "walking wounded" low-priority patients. Make sure everyone on the bus is medically examined and that medical personnel also ride the bus.

❑ Consider the need for extrication sector (if not already established).

❑ Consider the need for a safety officer (as needed).

❑ Consider the need for a follow-up CISD and rehab of personnel.

❑ Keep the dispatcher and other service chiefs in close contact throughout the incident.

❑ Along with the police and fire officers, consider the need for a public information officer to work with the arriving media representatives.

CASE STUDY

▶ THE SCHOOL BUS MCI

You are dispatched to a school-bus collision in a major intersection in town. En route the dispatcher notifies you that he has received numerous calls on the collision, and the police as well as the fire department are en route. Callers state that a large truck collided with the bus in an intersection at a high rate of speed, overturning the bus full of school children. As you near the center of town, the traffic is backed up in both directions for about five blocks. The police have arrived on the scene and are beginning to re-route the traffic after confirming that there are many injured children on and near the bus.

1. What would be your initial role as the crew leader of the first arriving ambulance at the scene?

2. A) Which vest from the MCI kit should you wear and, B) what are your responsibilities?

After declaring the MCI, confirming the incident with dispatch, and establishing contact with the police and fire officers, you begin to estimate the number of patients with the assistance of your two crew members.

3. What would be the most likely job to designate to one of your partners?

4. What are his/her specific functions?

Upon size-up of the situation, it is determined that there were 40 children on the bus, half of which have numerous contusions and cuts and who are walking around the scene crying. You decide to designate a nearby store as the location for the P-3 patients. You have one of your partners make a PA announcement that the walking wounded should go to that location. In addition, you call for 10 ambulances and another school bus to respond.

5. Where would be the best place to stage the ambulances?

6. What should be the role of the crew leader on the first ambulance arriving at the staging sector?

7. Should any ambulances report directly to the scene?

8. Are there any other sector officers needed at this time?

The fire department has cleared the bus for entry now that it is stabilized and no longer leaking any fuel. Inside there are 15 patients who need to be removed from the bus. Many of the patients have head injuries, fractures, contusions, and glass cuts.

9. How should these patients be removed from the bus if it is possible?

10. Once removed from the bus, where should the patients be taken?

Prioritize the patients described below into the following categories: P-1 (critical and unstable), P-2 (potentially unstable), P-3 (stable walking wounded), P-4 (dead).

11. A 7-year-old female who complains of a swollen deformed right lower arm and a contusion to the head with no loss of consciousness. She is alert and has vital signs that are normal for her age.

12. A 9-year-old male who has a seizure disorder who has been unconscious since the collision and has already had two observed grand-mal seizures without a lucid interval.

13. A 10-year-old male who was thrown through the front window of the bus because he was standing up talking to the bus driver. He was ejected from the vehicle, was found approximately 50 feet from the bus, and has a large contusion, depressed skull fracture, and no vital signs.

14. A 8-year-old female who has a bruise on the left upper quadrant and the forehead. She denies any loss of consciousness but is pale, clammy, and has a rapid heart rate for her age.

The treatment officer has set up a treatment sector across the street from the collision in the gas station parking lot. He has set out a large yellow and a large red tarp. There is also a smaller black tarp inside the gas station for the P-4 patients. As the incident proceeds, you are able to obtain additional assistance from the firefighters at the scene for lifting the patients being removed from the bus and carried on backboards to the treatment sector. Also, the area is becoming quite congested because a number of parents are arriving at the scene.

15. What is the best thing to do with the parents?

16. As a smooth flow of ambulances begins to arrive from the staging sector, who should coordinate the destinations of the patient transports and communicate with the hospitals?

17. What might this person want to know immediately from the local hospitals?

18. Other than the bus that was ordered for the P-3 patients, is there any other form of transportation that should be considered for this incident?

19. How should the decision be made as to who rides on the bus to a hospital?

20. As the incident is wrapped up, how could you, as the incident commander, deal with the media and the emotional and physical needs of your personnel?

Interim Exam Three

Use the answer sheet on pages 283–284 to complete this exam. It is perforated so it can be easily removed from this book.

1. The circulation of blood throughout the body, filling the capillaries and supplying the cells and tissues with oxygen and nutrients is called
   - **A.** physiology.
   - **B.** perfusion.
   - **C.** bleeding.
   - **D.** metabolism.

2. With one exception, arteries carry _____ blood _____ the heart.
   - **A.** deoxygenated : back to
   - **B.** deoxygenated : away from
   - **C.** oxygenated : back to
   - **D.** oxygenated : away from

3. With one exception, veins carry _____ blood _____ the heart.
   - **A.** deoxygenated : back to
   - **B.** deoxygenated : away from
   - **C.** oxygenated : back to
   - **D.** oxygenated : away from

4. Once an adult loses approximately a _____ of blood, his/her condition is considered serious.
   - **A.** pint
   - **B.** gallon
   - **C.** milliliter
   - **D.** liter

5. Once a child loses approximately _____ of blood, his/her condition is considered serious.
   - **A.** a milliliter
   - **B.** 250 cc
   - **C.** 500 ml
   - **D.** 1 liter

6. Once an infant loses approximately _____ of blood volume, his/her condition is considered serious.
   - **A.** 75 cc
   - **B.** 150 cc
   - **C.** 250 cc
   - **D.** 500 cc

7. Since internal bleeding is not visible, you must base severity of blood loss on
   - **A.** signs and symptoms exhibited.
   - **B.** what the patient tells you.
   - **C.** the size of the contusion.
   - **D.** advice from medical direction.

8. The factors on which severity of bleeding depends include all of the following <u>except</u>
   - **A.** rate of bleeding and the amount of blood loss.
   - **B.** patient's age and weight.
   - **C.** ability of the patient's body to respond and defend against blood loss.
   - **D.** the patient's history of diabetes.

9. Blood that oozes and is dark red is most likely from a
   - **A.** vein.
   - **B.** capillary.
   - **C.** artery.
   - **D.** lymphatic vessel.

10. You are treating a patient who has a slashed wrist, which is spurting bright red blood. After trying direct pressure and elevation to control the bleeding, the next step would be to
    - **A.** apply a tourniquet to the arm.
    - **B.** apply an air splint to the arm.
    - **C.** press on the brachial artery.
    - **D.** press on the femoral artery.

11. When all other methods have failed to control bleeding, the EMT-B should
    - **A.** apply the PASG.
    - **B.** apply an air splint.
    - **C.** press harder on the pressure point.
    - **D.** apply a tourniquet.

12. Signs of internal bleeding include all of the following <u>except</u>
    - **A.** painful, swollen, or deformed extremities.
    - **B.** a tender rigid abdomen.
    - **C.** vomiting bile.
    - **D.** bruising.

13. Examples of penetrating trauma include all of the following <u>except</u>
    - **A.** hand-gun bullet wound.
    - **B.** carving-knife wound.
    - **C.** fall from a height.
    - **D.** screwdriver stab wound.

14. Examples of blunt trauma include all of the following <u>except</u>
    - **A.** blast injuries.
    - **B.** auto-pedestrian collisions.
    - **C.** gunshot wounds.
    - **D.** falls.

15. The signs and symptoms of internal bleeding are
    - **A.** the same as those of shock.
    - **B.** identical to those of external bleeding.
    - **C.** usually not present in elderly patients.
    - **D.** easy to stabilize in the field.

16. Which is not considered a type of shock?
    - **A.** hypovolemic
    - **B.** hydrophobic
    - **C.** cardiogenic
    - **D.** neurogenic

17. At a point when the body can no longer compensate for the low blood volume, _____ shock begins.
   A. compensated
   B. anaphylactic
   C. decompensated
   D. terminal

18. What are the major components of the central nervous system?
   A. cranial nerves
   B. peripheral nerves
   C. brain and spinal cord
   D. vessels and support tissue

19. Which of the following is not a division of the nervous system?
   A. central
   B. peripheral
   C. autonomic
   D. voluntary

20. The skull is made up of the cranium and the facial bones. The cranium consists of the _____ areas of the skull.
   A. temporal, mandible, and maxilla
   B. frontal, parietal, and distal
   C. anterior, forehead, and lateral
   D. forehead, top, back, and upper sides

21. The bones forming the face include all of the following except
   A. vertebrae.
   B. zygomatic
   C. mandible
   D. maxillae.

22. The brain and spinal cord are bathed in
   A. cerebrospinal fluid.
   C. synovial fluid.
   B. lymphatic fluid.
   D. mucous secretion.

23. The spine is divided into sections called
   A. joints.
   B. vertebrae.
   C. coccygeal.
   D. compartments.

24. The lumbar area of the spine includes _____ vertebrae.
   A. 3
   B. 5
   C. 8
   D. 12

25. The cervical area of the spine includes _____ vertebrae.
   A. 3
   B. 5
   C. 7
   D. 9

26. When a patient strikes her head and states she feels groggy and has a headache, she most likely has a(n)
   A. abrasion.
   B. concussion.
   C. contrecoup.
   D. none of the above.

27. A 50-year-old male driver who was involved in an automobile collision states he did not loose consciousness. However, a bystander says he ran to the car after the collision and tried to talk to the driver, but said the driver "just sat there staring off into space for a few minutes." This patient may have any of the following except
   A. contusion.
   B. concussion.
   C. coup injury.
   D. attention deficit.

28. When a patient has some memory loss after a head injury, this is referred to as
   A. bruising.
   B. amnesia.
   C. verbally responsive.
   D. "seeing stars."

29. When a bruising of the brain occurs on the side of the injury, this is referred to as a _____ injury.
   A. contrecoup
   B. hematoma
   C. coup
   D. epidural

30. A collection of blood within the skull or the brain is called a _____ hematoma.
   A. subdural
   B. epidural
   C. intracerebral
   D. all of the above.

31. All of the following make a head injury worse except
   A. limited room for expansion inside the skull.
   B. increased pressure in the skull.
   C. increased carbon dioxide level in the brain.
   D. decreased respiration leading to increased cellular perfusion.

32. An assessment strategy used to check an extremity for injury or paralysis in a conscious patient is
   A. checking for a proximal pulse.
   B. assessing equality of strength.
   C. checking for foot wave.
   D. confirming sensitivity.

33. The type of immobilization device used for a patient depends on
   A. patient priority.
   B. availability.
   C. medical direction's advice.
   D. all of the above.

34. If a patient has a brain injury with skull fracture, the patient's pupils will tend to be
   A. equal.
   B. dilated.
   C. constricted.
   D. unequal.

35. Which of the following describes the blood pressure and pulse for a patient with a brain injury?
   A. decreased blood pressure, increased pulse
   B. decreased blood pressure, decreased pulse
   C. increased blood pressure, increased pulse
   D. increased blood pressure, decreased pulse

36. Consider the possibility of a cranial fracture whenever you note
   A. deep lacerations or severe bruises to the scalp or forehead.
   B. a deformed femur.
   C. facial deformity.
   D. blood or other fluids in the airway.

37. The spinal column is made up of _____ shaped bones.
   A. 33 regularly
   B. 33 irregularly
   C. 12 regularly
   D. 12 irregularly

38. Any blunt trauma above the clavicles may damage the _____ vertebrae.
   A. lumbar
   B. cervical
   C. sacral
   D. thoracic

39. Priapism is
   A. a persistent erection of the penis.
   B. spasms to the hands and feet.
   C. apparent only in unconscious patients.
   D. uncontrolled muscle twitches of the thighs.

40. Often with a cervical-spine injury, the patient in a supine position may have his arms
   A. straight out at his side.
   B. stretched out above his head.
   C. down at his side.
   D. across his chest.

41. The first step in the care of a scalp injury is to
   A. control bleeding.
   B. apply a sterile dressing.
   C. cut away hair around the site.
   D. apply a water-moistened dressing.

42. An unstable object impaled in the cheek wall should be
   A. stabilized from the outside.
   B. stabilized from the inside.
   C. pulled out if easily done.
   D. stabilized from the inside and the outside.

43. If possible, a patient with facial fractures should be transported on a long spine board in the _____ position.
   A. supine
   B. Trendelenburg
   C. head elevated
   D. prone

44. The pressure point for controlling bleeding from the leg is the
   A. carotid artery.
   B. brachial artery.
   C. subclavian vein.
   D. femoral artery.

45. Care for an open wound includes all of the following except
   A. pick embedded particles out of the cut.
   B. control bleeding.
   C. bandage the dressing in place.
   D. clean the wound surface.

46. The best method for control of nasal bleeding is
   A. packing the nose with cotton.
   B. pinching the nostrils together.
   C. packing the nose with gauze.
   D. applying pressure to the facial artery.

47. The first step in caring for possible internal bleeding after ensuring respiration and circulation and controlling life-threatening external bleeding is
   A. administering liquids by mouth to the patient.
   B. applying a bulky dressing.
   C. treating for shock.
   D. placing the patient in a sitting position.

48. A razor blade cut is an example of a(n)
   A. incision.
   B. abrasion.
   C. contusion.
   D. laceration.

49. The injury in which flaps of skin and tissues are torn loose or pulled off completely is called
   A. laceration.
   B. amputation.
   C. incision.
   D. avulsion.

50. If a patient has an object impaled in the forearm, after the control of profuse bleeding, you should
   A. remove the object.
   B. place a pressure dressing over the site.
   C. stabilize the object.
   D. apply firm pressure to a pressure point.

51. Which of the following is a sign of shock?
   A. high blood pressure
   B. constricted pupils
   C. slowed pulse rate
   D. pale, cool, clammy skin

52. An object impaled in the eye should be
   A. stabilized with gauze and protected with a disposable cup.
   B. removed carefully and a pressure dressing applied.
   C. shielded with a cup taped over the orbit.
   D. removed and a dressing applied with minimum pressure.

53. A lacerated eyelid or injury to the eyeball should be
    A. flushed with water.
    B. covered with a cold pack.
    C. covered with folded 4 × 4s.
    D. covered with dark patches.

54. All open wounds to the chest should be considered
    A. life-threatening.
    B. potentially infectious.
    C. a low priority.
    D. an indication for PASG.

55. Before moving a supine patient with possible spinal injuries onto a long spine board, you should always
    A. align the teeth and tape the jaw in place.
    B. apply a short spine board.
    C. apply a rigid collar.
    D. secure a KED to the patient.

56. The initial effort to control bleeding from a severed neck artery should be
    A. direct pressure or pinching.
    B. applying tape.
    C. pressure points.
    D. occlusive dressing.

57. The most reliable sign of spinal-cord injury in conscious patients is
    A. pain without movement.
    B. paralysis of extremities.
    C. pain with movement.
    D. tenderness along the spine.

58. When caring for an open abdominal wound with evisceration,
    A. replace the organ but cover with occlusive material.
    B. replace the organ but cover with a bulky dressing.
    C. do not replace the organ but cover with occlusive material.
    D. do not replace the organ but cover with a moistened dressing.

59. A patient in acute abdominal distress without vomiting should be transported
    A. in the Trendelenburg position with legs straight.
    B. in the coma position.
    C. face up with the knees bent.
    D. in the recumbent position with one knee bent.

60. When a joint is locked into position, the EMT-B should
    A. pull traction on the extremity.
    B. straighten it.
    C. splint it in the position found.
    D. skip splinting and transport immediately.

61. A splint properly applied to an extremity should prevent all of the following except
    A. circulation to the extremity.
    B. an open bone injury.
    C. motion of bone fragments.
    D. damage to muscles and blood vessels.

62. A fractured clavicle is best cared for with a
    A. padded splint.
    B. sling and swathe.
    C. wrist sling.
    D. bulky pressure dressing.

63. A fracture to the humerus shaft is best cared for by immobilizing with a(n)
    A. wrist sling.
    B. rigid splint or sling and swathe.
    C. air-inflated splint.
    D. sling and swathe.

64. A fracture to the proximal end of the humerus is best cared for by immobilizing with a(n)
    A. wrist sling and swathe.
    B. padded board, sling, and swathe.
    C. air-inflated splint.
    D. sling and swathe.

65. The best way to immobilize a fractured elbow when the arm is found in the bent position and there is a distal pulse is to
    A. straighten the arm and apply an air-inflated splint.
    B. keep the arm in its found position and apply a short padded board splint.
    C. keep the arm in its found position and apply an air-inflated splint.
    D. straighten the arm and apply a wire-ladder splint.

66. When splinting, if a severe deformity exists or distal circulation is compromised, you should
    A. push protruding bones back into place.
    B. align to anatomical position under gentle traction.
    C. immediately move the patient to a stretcher.
    D. immobilize in the position found.

67. The first step in immobilizing a fractured wrist with distal pulse is to
    A. correct angulation of the wrist.
    B. secure a padded board splint to the wrist.
    C. place the broken hand in its position of function.
    D. tape the wrist.

68. A patient with a fractured pelvis should be immobilized on an orthopedic stretcher or long spine board with
    A. legs bound together with wide cravats.
    B. long padded boards secured down each side of the body.
    C. stabilizing sandbags placed between the legs.
    D. straps securing the torso and pelvis.

69. A fractured femur is best immobilized with a(n) _____ splint.
    A. long padded
    B. air-inflated
    C. rigid vacuum
    D. traction

70. Before immobilizing a fractured knee,
    A. assess distal PMS function.
    B. straighten the angulation.
    C. apply firm traction.
    D. flex the leg at the knee.

71. The best method for immobilizing a suspected ankle fracture is a(n) _____ splint.
    A. traction
    B. pillow splint
    C. padded board
    D. air-inflated

72. A sprain is an injury in which
    A. tendons are torn.
    B. ligaments are torn.
    C. cartilage is crushed.
    D. muscles spasm.

73. Which of the following is not true of open extremity injuries?
    A. The skin has been broken or torn.
    B. There is increased likelihood of infection.
    C. Definitive care is provided in the prehospital setting.
    D. Such injuries require surgery at the hospital.

74. Muscle is attached to bone by
    A. cartilage.
    B. ligaments.
    C. smooth muscles.
    D. tendons.

75. A partial-thickness burn involves the
    A. epidermis.
    B. epidermis and dermis.
    C. epidermis, dermis, and subcutaneous layers.
    D. epidermis, dermis, subcutaneous layers, and muscles.

76. The entire back of an adult patient's right arm and her entire chest have been burned. What percentage of surface burn would you report?
    A. 13.5%
    B. 18%
    C. 27%
    D. 36%

77. A moderate burn involves
    A. partial- and full-thickness burns of the face and hands.
    B. full-thickness burns over less than 2% of the body surface.
    C. superficial burns covering more than 50% of the body surface .
    D. superficial burns covering less than 20% of the body surface.

78. Partial-thickness burns cause
    A. swelling and blistering.
    B. nerve damage.
    C. slight swelling.
    D. scarring.

79. A patient is suffering from chemical burns to the skin caused by dry lime. Your first step should be to
    A. wash the area with running water.
    B. remove the lime with phenol.
    C. remove the lime with alcohol.
    D. brush away the lime.

80. Acid burns to the eyes should be flooded with water for at least _____ minute(s).
    A. 1
    B. 5
    C. 10
    D. 20

81. A method for estimating the extent of a burn is the
    A. rule of nines.
    B. rule of percentages.
    C. rule of degree.
    D. burn assessment rule.

82. The number-one priority for all EMS personnel at a collision scene is
    A. wearing the appropriate protective clothing.
    B. keeping the bystanders clear of the scene.
    C. assuring the patient's safety first.
    D. contacting medical control for instructions.

83. When arriving at the scene of a collision, the first thing an EMT-B should do is
    A. evaluate hazards and calculate the need for additional support.
    B. determine whether patients are low or high priority.
    C. check to see if the vehicles involved have deployed air bags.
    D. determine the extent of patient entrapment and the means of extrication.

84. The EMT-B is responsible for protecting the patient from all of the following except
   A. broken glass from the wrecked car.
   B. sharp metal in the wrecked car.
   C. the environment.
   D. injuries sustained by not wearing a seatbelt.

85. At the scene of an auto collision, the EMT-B should try to do all of the following except
   A. keep the patient's safety in mind.
   B. inform the patient of the unique aspects of the extrication.
   C. keep his/her own personal safety in mind.
   D. describe the extrication procedures to bystanders.

86. A vehicle involved in a collision that is determined to be a simple access will
   A. not require towing.
   B. not require stopping traffic.
   C. not require equipment to get to the patient.
   D. require only basic air-powered tools.

87. Which of the following is untrue of applying a short spine board?
   A. Secure the torso first, and then the head.
   B. Pad between the patient's head and the spine board.
   C. Apply a single chin strap prior to moving the patient.
   D. Reassess the patient after the device is placed.

88. To assist with patient access, the EMT-B should initially do each of the following except
   A. try opening each car door.
   B. roll down windows.
   C. ask the patient to unlock the doors.
   D. pull the patient out the side windows.

89. What dictates the specific technique used for spinal immobilization of a patient at a collision extrication?
   A. requirements for speed of removal
   B. how many rescuers are available for removal
   C. whether an air bag has deployed
   D. none of the above.

90. Which step in the phases of the rescue process is out of order: 1) sizing up the situation, 2) gaining the access, 3) disentangling the patient, 4) stabilizing the vehicle?
   A. 1   C. 3
   B. 2   D. 4

91. Considerations for size-up of a collision include all of the following except
   A. potential hazards.
   B. need for additional EMS units.
   C. number of patients involved.
   D. number of ambulances in the region.

92. To minimize injuries at a collision, the EMT-B should
   A. use a limited number of tools.
   B. deactivate the safety guards on tools.
   C. wear highly visible clothing.
   D. wait until the police arrive on the scene.

93. The vehicle's catalytic converter can be a source of ignition at a collision because it
   A. often emits sparks.
   B. is often over 1200°F.
   C. may leak gasoline.
   D. pumps high pressure fumes.

94. The three-step process of disentanglement described in the text includes all of the following except
   A. open the trunk and cut the battery cable.
   B. create exitways by displacing doors and roof posts.
   C. disentangle occupants by displacing front end.
   D. gain access by disposing of the roof.

95. Which of the following is true about dealing with a collision vehicle's electrical system?
   A. It should be disabled by cutting a battery cable.
   B. If it must be disrupted, disconnect the ground cable from the battery.
   C. Cutting the battery cable can assist in rescue operations.
   D. Disconnecting the ground cable will produce a spark that can ignite battery gases.

96. When positioning flares, use a formula that includes the stopping distance for the posted speed plus the
   A. angle of the road.
   B. radius of the danger zone.
   C. reaction distance.
   D. margin of safety.

97. Once the vehicle has been stabilized, the second part of an extrication procedure for patient rescue is to
   A. dispose of the vehicle's roof.
   B. displace the front end of the vehicle.
   C. displace doors and roof posts.
   D. none of the above.

98. The Emergency Medical Dispatcher has told you the exact location of a collision, how many and what kinds of vehicles are involved, and any known hazards. What other information would you like the EMD to provide concerning this collision?
  A. how many persons are injured
  B. the direction designator
  C. how to contact the person who reported the collision
  D. the nature of the emergency

99. Which of the following is an <u>unnecessary</u> question for the Emergency Medical Dispatcher to ask when receiving a call for help?
  A. How old is the patient?
  B. What's the patient's sex?
  C. What's the patient's name?
  D. Is the patient conscious?

100. When operating a siren, be aware that
  A. the continuous sound of a siren could worsen a patient's condition.
  B. all motorists will hear and honor your signal.
  C. the siren must be used continuously when carrying injured patients.
  D. it's necessary to pull up close to vehicles and sound the siren.

101. All of the following are factors that affect an ambulance's response to a scene <u>except</u>
  A. day of the week.   **C.** detours.
  B. time of the day.   **D.** danger zones.

102. If a patient develops cardiac arrest during transport, have the operator of the ambulance
  A. adjust the ambulance's speed.
  B. stop the ambulance.
  C. contact the hospital emergency department.
  D. assist you with CPR.

103. When transferring a non-emergency patient to the emergency department personnel, you should
  A. wait for emergency staff to call for the patient.
  B. off-load, wheel to the designated area, and stay with the patient.
  C. check to see what is to be done with the patient.
  D. off-load, wheel to the designated area, and leave the patient.

104. The last step when transferring a patient is to
  A. wait to help the emergency department staff.
  B. transfer the patient's valuables.
  C. obtain your release.
  D. transfer patient information.

105. At the hospital, as soon as you are free from patient care activities, you should
  A. notify dispatch you are back in service.
  B. quickly clean the vehicle's patient compartment.
  C. prepare the prehospital care report.
  D. check on patient status with the emergency department.

106. Which of the following is <u>not</u> a biohazard?
  A. suction catheters
  B. contaminated dressings
  C. blood-soaked linen
  D. unopened gauze bandages

107. Which of the following is <u>not</u> a benefit of an EMS/hospital equipment exchange program?
  A. Patients are not subjected to injury-aggravating movement.
  B. Delay of the crew at the hospital is prevented.
  C. Ambulances can return to quarters fully equipped.
  D. Completeness and operability of equipment is ensured.

108. Vigorous cleaning of the ambulance while parked at the hospital is prevented or restricted by all of the following limitations <u>except</u>
  A. time.   **C.** space.
  B. equipment.   **D.** law.

109. While en route to your quarters,
  A. radio dispatch that you are returning.
  B. disinfect and decontaminate the ambulance.
  C. clean and sanitize the patient compartment.
  D. clean any equipment that touched the patient.

110. When you return to quarters, do all of the following <u>except</u>
  A. replenish oxygen cylinders.
  B. prepare for service.
  C. clean the interior of the ambulance.
  D. air the ambulance if necessary.

111. A poison-control kit should include all of the following except
    A. paper cups.
    B. activated charcoal.
    C. drinking water.
    D. antivenin solution.

112. Which of the following is not a piece of equipment in the first-in kit?
    A. stethoscope
    B. penlight
    C. fixed suction system
    D. rigid cervical collar

113. The first thing to inspect on the ambulance when the engine is off is the
    A. body of the vehicle.
    B. battery.
    C. siren.
    D. fuel level.

114. Rescue tools should always be examined for
    A. electrolyte levels.
    B. rust and dirt.
    C. water pressure.
    D. dead batteries.

115. Along with physical and mental fitness, ambulance operators should be able to
    A. move other vehicles off the roadway.
    B. perform under stress.
    C. always be up for a run.
    D. justify feelings of superiority.

116. When driving an ambulance, you should realize that there are no state laws that grant the
    A. use of controlled additional speed.
    B. passage through traffic signals.
    C. privilege of special parking at the scene.
    D. absolute right of way.

117. The headlights of an ambulance should be turned on
    A. only at night.
    B. whenever the vehicle is on the road.
    C. during the day, but only when raining.
    D. and off in a blinking fashion.

118. When a car collides with a utility pole, the EMT-B should assume all of the following except
    A. obviously dead wires could be energized at any moment.
    B. that severed conductors may be energizing every wire.
    C. wires may be charged at the highest voltage present.
    D. there is no electrical hazard.

119. The easiest way to break tempered window glass is with a
    A. blunt object.
    B. spring-loaded center punch.
    C. Glas Master window saw.
    D. sledge hammer.

120. Which of the following signs is not an indication that a child has an airway disease?
    A. wheezing
    B. breathing effort on exhalation
    C. rapid breathing
    D. lack of airway passage swelling

121. The soft spot on top of an infant's head is called a
    A. contusion.
    B. depression site.
    C. fontanelle.
    D. suture.

122. Small children are referred to as _____ breathers.
    A. neck
    B. abdominal
    C. head
    D. chest

123. A child's compensating mechanisms for shock fails at approximately _____ blood loss.
    A. 10%
    B. 20%
    C. 30%
    D. 40%

124. In cases of sudden infant death syndrome, the EMT-B should
    A. hunt for evidence of child abuse.
    B. hold off on care and simply transport the body.
    C. declare the patient dead.
    D. provide resuscitation and transport to the hospital.

125. Which injuries might lead you to consider child abuse?
    A. multiple skinned knees
    B. a burn from chewing an electric cord
    C. injuries to the center of the back and upper arms
    D. both ankles are sprained

126. A child who is hypoxic will
    A. have a slowed heart rate.
    B. have an increased heart rate.
    C. forget to breathe.
    D. complain of neck pain.

127. Artificial ventilations for an infant or child under 8 years of age should be provided at a rate of _____ per minute.
    A. 8
    B. 12
    C. 16
    D. 20

128. If you suspect respiratory distress in a conscious toddler, you should <u>not</u>
    A. administer high-concentration oxygen.
    B. insert anything into the patient's mouth.
    C. open the airway.
    D. allow the child to sit up.

129. How do children usually get lead poisoning?
    A. eating pencils
    B. eating fish
    C. eating paint chips
    D. breathing asbestos

130. Common causes of shock in children include infections, trauma, blood loss, and
    A. meningitis.   C. dehydration.
    B. heart failure   D. lack of insulin.

131. A sunken fontanelle may indicate
    A. elevated intracranial pressure.
    B. hypertension.
    C. dehydration.
    D. fever.

132. Flowing oxygen over the face of a small child so it will be inhaled is referred to as the _____ technique.
    A. blow-by   C. supplemental
    B. rebreather   D. flow-by

133. A complication of a rapidly rising temperature in a child is often
    A. hyperactivity.
    B. a seizure.
    C. vomiting.
    D. ringing in the ears.

134. A group of viral illnesses that results in inflammation of the larynx, trachea, and bronchi is called
    A. meningitis.   C. asthma.
    B. anaphylaxis.   D. croup.

135. A child ages three to six is referred to as
    A. trouble.   C. preschooler.
    B. preadolescent.   D. toddler.

136. The strong, white, fibrous material covering the bones is called the
    A. shell.   C. marrow.
    B. perineum.   D. periosteum.

137. The coming apart of a joint is referred to as a
    A. fracture.   C. dislocation.
    B. sprain.   D. strain.

138. Over-stretching or over-exertion of a muscle is called a
    A. strain.   C. dislocation.
    B. sprain.   D. fracture.

139. Proper splinting of a closed fracture is
    A. done with the PASG.
    B. designed to prevent closed injuries from becoming open ones.
    C. completed in the hospital by a surgeon.
    D. done with an air splint.

140. Any force strong enough to fracture the pelvis also can cause injury to the
    A. clavicle.   C. rib cage.
    B. spine.   D. tibia.

141. Examples of a bipolar traction splint include all of the following <u>except</u>
    A. Hare.   C. half-ring.
    B. Fernotrac.   D. Sager.

142. The indications for a traction splint are painful, swollen, deformed mid-thigh with
    A. an open fracture of the lower leg.
    B. extensive blood loss and shock.
    C. no joint or lower leg injury.
    D. either ankle or knee involvement.

143. The level of training established by OSHA for those who actually plug, patch, or stop the release of a hazardous material is called
    A. First Responder Awareness.
    B. First Responder Operations.
    C. Hazardous Materials Technician.
    D. Paramedic.

144. At a hazardous materials accident site, the "safe zone" should be located
    A. downwind/downhill.
    B. downwind/same level.
    C. upwind/same level.
    D. upwind/downhill.

145. A resource that must be maintained at the work site by the employer and that must be available to all employees working with hazardous materials is called
    A. NFPA 704.
    B. Material Safety Data Sheet
    C. *North American Emergency Response Guidebook.*
    D. shipping manifest.

146. The responsibilities of EMS personnel at a hazmat incident include caring for the injured and
    A. staging personnel and equipment in the warm zone.
    B. monitoring and rehabilitating the hazmat team members.
    C. decontaminating those exiting the hot zone.
    D. notifying medical direction about the incident.

147. When a patient is categorized as Priority 1 at a MCI, this means the patient
   A. is serious, but does not have life-threatening injuries or illness.
   B. has minor musculoskeletal or soft-tissue injuries.
   C. is dead or fatally injured.
   D. has treatable life-threatening illness or injuries.

148. The MCI officer responsible for communicating with each treatment sector to determine the number and priority of the patients in that sector is called the _____ officer.
   A. staging
   B. triage
   C. treatment
   D. transportation

149. When identifying a patients treatment priority at an MCI, a Priority 2 patient would be color-coded as
   A. black
   B. green
   C. yellow
   D. red

150. At an MCI, patients who are assessed to have minor injuries should be categorized as Priority
   A. 1
   B. 2
   C. 3
   D. 4

Chapter Exam Three Answer Sheet

Fill in the correct answer for each item. When scoring, note there are 150
questions valued at 0.666 points each.

1. [ ] A   [ ] B   [ ] C   [ ] D
2. [ ] A   [ ] B   [ ] C   [ ] D
3. [ ] A   [ ] B   [ ] C   [ ] D
4. [ ] A   [ ] B   [ ] C   [ ] D
5. [ ] A   [ ] B   [ ] C   [ ] D
6. [ ] A   [ ] B   [ ] C   [ ] D
7. [ ] A   [ ] B   [ ] C   [ ] D
8. [ ] A   [ ] B   [ ] C   [ ] D
9. [ ] A   [ ] B   [ ] C   [ ] D
10. [ ] A   [ ] B   [ ] C   [ ] D
11. [ ] A   [ ] B   [ ] C   [ ] D
12. [ ] A   [ ] B   [ ] C   [ ] D
13. [ ] A   [ ] B   [ ] C   [ ] D
14. [ ] A   [ ] B   [ ] C   [ ] D
15. [ ] A   [ ] B   [ ] C   [ ] D
16. [ ] A   [ ] B   [ ] C   [ ] D
17. [ ] A   [ ] B   [ ] C   [ ] D
18. [ ] A   [ ] B   [ ] C   [ ] D
19. [ ] A   [ ] B   [ ] C   [ ] D
20. [ ] A   [ ] B   [ ] C   [ ] D
21. [ ] A   [ ] B   [ ] C   [ ] D
22. [ ] A   [ ] B   [ ] C   [ ] D
23. [ ] A   [ ] B   [ ] C   [ ] D
24. [ ] A   [ ] B   [ ] C   [ ] D
25. [ ] A   [ ] B   [ ] C   [ ] D
26. [ ] A   [ ] B   [ ] C   [ ] D
27. [ ] A   [ ] B   [ ] C   [ ] D
28. [ ] A   [ ] B   [ ] C   [ ] D
29. [ ] A   [ ] B   [ ] C   [ ] D
30. [ ] A   [ ] B   [ ] C   [ ] D
31. [ ] A   [ ] B   [ ] C   [ ] D
32. [ ] A   [ ] B   [ ] C   [ ] D
33. [ ] A   [ ] B   [ ] C   [ ] D
34. [ ] A   [ ] B   [ ] C   [ ] D
35. [ ] A   [ ] B   [ ] C   [ ] D
36. [ ] A   [ ] B   [ ] C   [ ] D

37. [ ] A   [ ] B   [ ] C   [ ] D
38. [ ] A   [ ] B   [ ] C   [ ] D
39. [ ] A   [ ] B   [ ] C   [ ] D
40. [ ] A   [ ] B   [ ] C   [ ] D
41. [ ] A   [ ] B   [ ] C   [ ] D
42. [ ] A   [ ] B   [ ] C   [ ] D
43. [ ] A   [ ] B   [ ] C   [ ] D
44. [ ] A   [ ] B   [ ] C   [ ] D
45. [ ] A   [ ] B   [ ] C   [ ] D
46. [ ] A   [ ] B   [ ] C   [ ] D
47. [ ] A   [ ] B   [ ] C   [ ] D
48. [ ] A   [ ] B   [ ] C   [ ] D
49. [ ] A   [ ] B   [ ] C   [ ] D
50. [ ] A   [ ] B   [ ] C   [ ] D
51. [ ] A   [ ] B   [ ] C   [ ] D
52. [ ] A   [ ] B   [ ] C   [ ] D
53. [ ] A   [ ] B   [ ] C   [ ] D
54. [ ] A   [ ] B   [ ] C   [ ] D
55. [ ] A   [ ] B   [ ] C   [ ] D
56. [ ] A   [ ] B   [ ] C   [ ] D
57. [ ] A   [ ] B   [ ] C   [ ] D
58. [ ] A   [ ] B   [ ] C   [ ] D
59. [ ] A   [ ] B   [ ] C   [ ] D
60. [ ] A   [ ] B   [ ] C   [ ] D
61. [ ] A   [ ] B   [ ] C   [ ] D
62. [ ] A   [ ] B   [ ] C   [ ] D
63. [ ] A   [ ] B   [ ] C   [ ] D
64. [ ] A   [ ] B   [ ] C   [ ] D
65. [ ] A   [ ] B   [ ] C   [ ] D
66. [ ] A   [ ] B   [ ] C   [ ] D
67. [ ] A   [ ] B   [ ] C   [ ] D
68. [ ] A   [ ] B   [ ] C   [ ] D
69. [ ] A   [ ] B   [ ] C   [ ] D
70. [ ] A   [ ] B   [ ] C   [ ] D
71. [ ] A   [ ] B   [ ] C   [ ] D
72. [ ] A   [ ] B   [ ] C   [ ] D

73. [ ] A	[ ] B	[ ] C	[ ] D		112. [ ] A	[ ] B	[ ] C	[ ] D
74. [ ] A	[ ] B	[ ] C	[ ] D		113. [ ] A	[ ] B	[ ] C	[ ] D
75. [ ] A	[ ] B	[ ] C	[ ] D		114. [ ] A	[ ] B	[ ] C	[ ] D
76. [ ] A	[ ] B	[ ] C	[ ] D		115. [ ] A	[ ] B	[ ] C	[ ] D
77. [ ] A	[ ] B	[ ] C	[ ] D		116. [ ] A	[ ] B	[ ] C	[ ] D
78. [ ] A	[ ] B	[ ] C	[ ] D		117. [ ] A	[ ] B	[ ] C	[ ] D
79. [ ] A	[ ] B	[ ] C	[ ] D		118. [ ] A	[ ] B	[ ] C	[ ] D
80. [ ] A	[ ] B	[ ] C	[ ] D		119. [ ] A	[ ] B	[ ] C	[ ] D
81. [ ] A	[ ] B	[ ] C	[ ] D		120. [ ] A	[ ] B	[ ] C	[ ] D
82. [ ] A	[ ] B	[ ] C	[ ] D		121. [ ] A	[ ] B	[ ] C	[ ] D
83. [ ] A	[ ] B	[ ] C	[ ] D		122. [ ] A	[ ] B	[ ] C	[ ] D
84. [ ] A	[ ] B	[ ] C	[ ] D		123. [ ] A	[ ] B	[ ] C	[ ] D
85. [ ] A	[ ] B	[ ] C	[ ] D		124. [ ] A	[ ] B	[ ] C	[ ] D
86. [ ] A	[ ] B	[ ] C	[ ] D		125. [ ] A	[ ] B	[ ] C	[ ] D
87. [ ] A	[ ] B	[ ] C	[ ] D		126. [ ] A	[ ] B	[ ] C	[ ] D
88. [ ] A	[ ] B	[ ] C	[ ] D		127. [ ] A	[ ] B	[ ] C	[ ] D
89. [ ] A	[ ] B	[ ] C	[ ] D		128. [ ] A	[ ] B	[ ] C	[ ] D
90. [ ] A	[ ] B	[ ] C	[ ] D		129. [ ] A	[ ] B	[ ] C	[ ] D
91. [ ] A	[ ] B	[ ] C	[ ] D		130. [ ] A	[ ] B	[ ] C	[ ] D
92. [ ] A	[ ] B	[ ] C	[ ] D		131. [ ] A	[ ] B	[ ] C	[ ] D
93. [ ] A	[ ] B	[ ] C	[ ] D		132. [ ] A	[ ] B	[ ] C	[ ] D
94. [ ] A	[ ] B	[ ] C	[ ] D		133. [ ] A	[ ] B	[ ] C	[ ] D
95. [ ] A	[ ] B	[ ] C	[ ] D		134. [ ] A	[ ] B	[ ] C	[ ] D
96. [ ] A	[ ] B	[ ] C	[ ] D		135. [ ] A	[ ] B	[ ] C	[ ] D
97. [ ] A	[ ] B	[ ] C	[ ] D		136. [ ] A	[ ] B	[ ] C	[ ] D
98. [ ] A	[ ] B	[ ] C	[ ] D		137. [ ] A	[ ] B	[ ] C	[ ] D
99. [ ] A	[ ] B	[ ] C	[ ] D		138. [ ] A	[ ] B	[ ] C	[ ] D
100. [ ] A	[ ] B	[ ] C	[ ] D		139. [ ] A	[ ] B	[ ] C	[ ] D
101. [ ] A	[ ] B	[ ] C	[ ] D		140. [ ] A	[ ] B	[ ] C	[ ] D
102. [ ] A	[ ] B	[ ] C	[ ] D		141. [ ] A	[ ] B	[ ] C	[ ] D
103. [ ] A	[ ] B	[ ] C	[ ] D		142. [ ] A	[ ] B	[ ] C	[ ] D
104. [ ] A	[ ] B	[ ] C	[ ] D		143. [ ] A	[ ] B	[ ] C	[ ] D
105. [ ] A	[ ] B	[ ] C	[ ] D		144. [ ] A	[ ] B	[ ] C	[ ] D
106. [ ] A	[ ] B	[ ] C	[ ] D		145. [ ] A	[ ] B	[ ] C	[ ] D
107. [ ] A	[ ] B	[ ] C	[ ] D		146. [ ] A	[ ] B	[ ] C	[ ] D
108. [ ] A	[ ] B	[ ] C	[ ] D		147. [ ] A	[ ] B	[ ] C	[ ] D
109. [ ] A	[ ] B	[ ] C	[ ] D		148. [ ] A	[ ] B	[ ] C	[ ] D
110. [ ] A	[ ] B	[ ] C	[ ] D		149. [ ] A	[ ] B	[ ] C	[ ] D
111. [ ] A	[ ] B	[ ] C	[ ] D		150. [ ] A	[ ] B	[ ] C	[ ] D

CHAPTER Thirty-Five

ADVANCED AIRWAY MANAGEMENT

MATCH TERMINOLOGY/DEFINITIONS

▶ PART A

A. Fork at the lower end of the trachea where the two mainstem bronchi branch

B. Insertion of a tube

C. Tube designed to be inserted into the trachea; oxygen, medication, or a suction catheter can be directed into the trachea through an endotracheal tube.

D. Area directly above the openings of both the trachea and the esophagus

E. Inadequate oxygenation, or oxygen starvation

F. Opening to the trachea

G. Tube that leads from the pharynx to the stomach

H. To provide ventilations at a higher rate to compensate for oxygen not delivered during intubation or suctioning

I. Leaf-shaped structure that acts as covering to the opening of the trachea and that prevents food and foreign matter from entering it

J. Ring-shaped structure that circles the trachea at the lower portion of the larynx

K. Two large sets of branches that come off the trachea and enter the lungs

L. Voice box

M. Microscopic sacs of the lungs where exchange of oxygen and carbon dioxide takes place

N. Illuminating instrument that is inserted into the pharynx to permit visualization of the pharynx and larynx

O. Esophageal intubation detector device that may be used to detect incorrect placement (or to verify correct placement) of the endotracheal tube

_____ 1. Alveoli

_____ 2. Bronchi

_____ 3. Carina

_____ 4. Cricoid cartilage

_____ 5. EIDD

_____ 6. Endotracheal tube

_____ 7. Epiglottis

_____ 8. Esophagus

_____ 9. Glottic opening

_____ 10. Hyperventilate

_____ 11. Hypopharynx

_____ 12. Hypoxia

_____ 13. Intubation

_____ 14. Laryngoscope

_____ 15. Larynx

PART B

A. Placement of an endotracheal tube through the mouth and into the trachea

B. "Windpipe"; structure that connects the pharynx to the lungs

C. Two thin folds of tissue within the larynx that vibrate as air passes between them, producing sounds

D. Long, thin, flexible metal probe

E. Either of the two (right or left) large sets of branches that come off the trachea and enter the lungs

F. Groove-like structure anterior to the epiglottis

G. Tube designed to be passed through the nose, nasopharynx, and esophagus. It is used to relieve distention of the stomach in an infant or child patient.

H. Area directly posterior to the nose

I. Area directly posterior to the mouth

J. Pressure applied to the cricoid cartilage to suppress vomiting and bring the vocal cords into view; also called cricoid pressure

_____ **1.** Mainstem bronchi

_____ **2.** Nasogastric tube (NG tube)

_____ **3.** Nasopharynx

_____ **4.** Oropharynx

_____ **5.** Orotracheal intubation

_____ **6.** Sellick's maneuver

_____ **7.** Stylet

_____ **8.** Trachea

_____ **9.** Vallecula

_____ **10.** Vocal cords

MULTIPLE-CHOICE REVIEW

_____ **1.** The area directly above the openings of both the trachea and the esophagus is called the
   A. vallecula.
   B. larynx.
   C. hypopharynx.
   D. oropharynx.

_____ **2.** The groove-like structure anterior to the epiglottis is called the
   A. carina.
   B. vallecula.
   C. epiglottis.
   D. vocal cord.

_____ **3.** Why is food more apt to be aspirated into the right mainstem bronchus rather than the left mainstem bronchus?
   A. It splits off the carina at more of an angle than the left.
   B. It splits off the carina at less of an angle than the left.
   C. It is much larger in diameter than the left.
   D. It is much smaller in diameter than the left.

_____ **4.** The brain's center for respiratory control is located in the
   A. brainstem.
   B. cerebellum.
   C. pons.
   D. cerebrum.

_____ **5.** The endotracheal tube is primarily intended to
   A. be placed into the esophagus.
   B. provide a medication route.
   C. be inserted into the trachea.
   D. be used as a means of suctioning the hypopharynx.

_____ **6.** Orotracheal intubation allows direct ventilation of the lungs, bypassing the
   A. entire upper airway.
   B. entire lower airway.
   C. vocal cords.
   D. oropharynx.

7. When placing the endotracheal tube, EMT-Bs use
   A. a rapid-sequence technique.
   C. direct visualization.
   B. a blind technique.
   D. a surgical technique.

8. The advantage of orotracheal intubation is that it offers complete control of the airway and it
   A. minimizes the risk of aspiration.
   B. allows for better oxygen delivery.
   C. allows for deeper suctioning of the airway.
   D. all of the above.

9. All of the following are complications of orotracheal intubation except
   A. hypoxia from prolonged intubation attempts.
   B. soft tissue trauma to the lips, gums, or airway structures.
   C. increased heart rate from vagal stimulation.
   D. gagging and vomiting from airway stimulation.

10. When the endotracheal tube is advanced too deeply, this commonly results in
    A. vallecula injury.
    C. esophageal intubation.
    B. right-mainstem intubation.
    D. left-mainstem intubation.

11. The most serious complication of endotracheal intubation is
    A. left-mainstem intubation.
    B. bradycardia from airway stimulation.
    C. esophageal intubation.
    D. airway trauma.

12. The EMT-B should reassess endotracheal tube placement each time the patient is moved to prevent disastrous complications from
    A. accidental extubation.
    C. right mainstem intubation.
    B. vomiting.
    D. occlusion of the ET tube.

13. Most adult patients can be intubated using a size _____ straight blade or size _____ curved blade.
    A. 0 or 1 : 1
    C. 2 or 3 : 3
    B. 1 or 2 : 2
    D. 3 or 4 : 4

14. The straight blade is designed so that the tip of the blade is placed
    A. into the vallecula.
    C. under the epiglottis.
    B. into the carina.
    D. behind the epiglottis.

15. The curved blade is designed so the tip of the blade is inserted
    A. into the carina.
    C. into the glottis.
    B. under the epiglottis.
    D. into the vallecula.

16. The cuff at the distal end of the endotracheal tube
    A. usually seals with 8 to 10 cc of air.
    B. is called the pilot balloon.
    C. has a standard 15 millimeter adapter.
    D. holds 5 cc of air in an infant tube.

17. When using an endotracheal tube on an infant or child less than eight years of age, do not expect to see
    A. the child's vocal cords.
    C. a cuff on the tube.
    B. a Murphy eye.
    D. a variety of tube sizes.

18. No matter what the internal diameter of the endotracheal tube, it
    A. will always fit into a large adult.
    B. has a standard 15-millimeter adapter.
    C. will have an inflation valve.
    D. will have a pilot balloon.

_____ 19. It is generally accepted that the adult male should receive either a(n) _____ mm tube.
A. 6.0 or 6.5
B. 7.0 or 7.5
C. 8.0 or 8.5
D. 9.0 or 9.5

_____ 20. In an adult, the properly placed tube will have the _____ cm mark at the teeth.
A. 18
B. 20
C. 22
D. 24

_____ 21. Once the lubricated stylet is inserted, the endotracheal tube should be shaped like a
A. hairpin.
B. horseshoe.
C. "C".
D. hockey stick.

_____ 22. Prior to securing an endotracheal tube, do all of the following except
A. insert an oral airway as a bite block.
B. listen to both lungs.
C. listen over the epigastrium.
D. suction down the tube.

_____ 23. Items that should be checked prior to an intubation attempt include all of the following except the
A. laryngoscope light bulb.
B. cuff on the tube.
C. length of the tube.
D. shape of the tube and stylet.

_____ 24. The laryngoscope is designed to be
A. used as a fulcrum pivoting on the teeth.
B. placed in the left corner of the patient's mouth.
C. held in the left hand.
D. held in the right hand.

_____ 25. The Sellick's maneuver is designed to help
A. reduce the risk of vomiting.
B. move the vallecula into view.
C. move the carina into view.
D. compress the trachea.

_____ 26. The correct order for verifying tube placement by auscultation is
A. right, then left, then epigastrium.
B. epigastrium, then left, then right.
C. epigastrium, then right, then left.
D. left, then right, then epigastrium.

_____ 27. If the breath sounds are diminished or absent on the left but present on the right, it is likely the tube has advanced into the
A. esophagus.
B. left lung.
C. right mainstem bronchus.
D. carina.

_____ 28. It is recommended that the EMT-B make no more than _____ attempt(s) at orotracheal intubation.
A. one
B. two
C. three
D. four

_____ 29. The narrowest point of the infant's or small child's airway is the
A. glottic opening.
B. carina.
C. epiglottis.
D. cricoid ring.

_____ 30. The preferred laryngoscope blade size in infants and small children is
A. #2 straight.
B. #1 straight.
C. #5 curved.
D. #2 curved.

_____ 31. A nasogastric tube is commonly used in an infant or child patient to
A. suction out the esophagus.
B. perform deep and extensive suctioning.
C. decompress the stomach and proximal bowel.
D. provide a means of ventilating the patient.

_____ **32.** When you are unable to adequately ventilate the pediatric patient due to distention of the stomach, you should consider the use of a
    A. nasotracheal tube.
    B. nasogastric tube.
    C. shunt.
    D. tracheal tube.

_____ **33.** The major contraindication for a nasogastric tube placement in the infant or child is
    A. pulmonary edema.
    B. an inflated stomach.
    C. trauma to the chest.
    D. head or major facial trauma.

_____ **34.** The nasogastric tube should be measured from the
    A. tip of the nose around the ear to below the xiphoid process.
    B. bottom of the earlobe to the stomach.
    C. tip of the nose and directly to the xiphoid process.
    D. nose to the angle of the jaw and then to the umbilicus.

_____ **35.** Once the nasogastric tube is passed gently downward along the nasal floor, the EMT-B should do all of the following except
    A. confirm tube placement by aspirating stomach contents.
    B. secure the tube in place with tape.
    C. confirm placement by auscultating the epigastrium while injecting 10–20 cc of air.
    D. hook the tube up to the suction unit.

COMPLETE THE FOLLOWING

1. List four indications for when to perform orotracheal intubation.

    A. _____

    B. _____

    C. _____

    D. _____

2. List six complications of deep suctioning that can be avoided by hyperventilation.

    A. _____

    B. _____

    C. _____

    D. _____

    E. _____

    F. _____

VIRTUAL STREET SCENE

(First review the Street Scene on pp. 790 of the textbook. Then answer the questions below.)

1. What would you have done if the patient regained consciousness and started to gag on the tube?

   _____

   _____

2. Should ALS be requested for this patient?

   _____

   _____

3. Imagine that when you pull back on the EIDD, the tube fills with stomach contents. What should you do?

   _____

   _____

4. Suppose your patient had experienced neck trauma. Would your technique be any different?

   _____

   _____

   _____

WEB SIMULATION

For interactive. case studies that will help you review and practice basic skills, visit the *Emergency Case 9/e Companion Website* at www.bradybooks.com/emergencycare.

EMT-BASIC SKILL PERFORMANCE CHECKLISTS

▶ **VENTILATORY MANAGEMENT AND ENDOTRACHEAL INTUBATION**

❏ Take BSI precautions.

❏ Open airway manually.

❏ Elevate tongue and insert airway adjunct (oropharyngeal or nasopharyngeal airway).

❏ Ventilate the patient immediately using a BVM device unattached to oxygen.

❏ Hyperventilate the patient with room air.

- ❏ Attach the oxygen reservoir to the BVM.
- ❏ Attach BVM to high-flow oxygen.
- ❏ Ventilate patient at proper volume and rate.
- ❏ Direct assistant to hyperventilate the patient.
- ❏ Identify and select proper equipment for intubation.
- ❏ Check equipment (cuff for leaks, laryngoscope batteries, and bulb tightness).
- ❏ Position the head properly.
- ❏ Insert the laryngoscope blade with left hand while displacing the tongue.
- ❏ Elevate the mandible with laryngoscope.
- ❏ Insert the ET tube and advance it to the proper depth (until cuff is past vocal cords).
- ❏ Inflate cuff to the proper pressure (5 cc to 10 cc) and disconnect the syringe.
- ❏ Direct ventilation of the patient.
- ❏ Confirm proper placement by auscultation over the epigastrium and bilaterally over the lungs and over epigastrium.
- ❏ Secure the ET tube with a commercial tube restraint device.

Note: Some medical directors also require the use of an esophageal intubation detector device, pulse oximeter, or end-tidal CO_2 detector device to confirm and monitor tube placement.

▶ INSERTION OF THE NASOGASTRIC TUBE

- ❏ Take BSI precautions.
- ❏ Prepare and assemble the equipment.
- ❏ Oxygenate the patient.
- ❏ Measure tube from the tip of nose, over ear, to below xiphoid process.
- ❏ Lubricate end of tube and pass tube gently downward along the nasal floor into the stomach.
- ❏ To confirm correct placement, auscultate over epigastrium. Listen for bubbling while injecting 10 to 20 cc of air into tube.
- ❏ Use suction to aspirate stomach contents.
- ❏ Secure tube in place.

INSERTION OF THE LARYNGEAL MASK AIRWAY (LMA)® (OPTIONAL EMT-B SKILL)

- ❏ Ensure the AHA BLS airway maneuvers are being attempted whil preparing equipment.
- ❏ Take BSI precautions.
- ❏ Select and assemble correct equipment.
- ❏ An LMA.properly sized for the patient.
- ❏ LMA deflator tool.

- ❑ BVM with reservoir.

- ❑ 30cc syringe

- ❑ Suction unit and rigid Yankauer tip.

- ❑ Test cuff by inflation and deflation.

- ❑ Water based lubricant jel for mask tip.

- ❑ Gloves, mask, and protective eyewear.

- ❑ Have another rescuer hyperoxygenate the patient with a BVM.

- ❑ Places LMA – gently introduce in oropharynx following curvature of tube, mask is swung into place in a single circular movement ensuring pressure is maintained against palate and posterior pharynx, inflate mask without holding the tube, oxygenate the patient with the BVM.

- ❑ Confirms LMA placement – visually confirms chest rise, auscultates epigastrium for absence of breath sounds, auscultates lung fields for presence of breath sounds bilaterally, EtCO-2 monitoring, immediately removes the LMA if breath sounds are heard in epigastrium, maintain continuous ventilation during confirmation process.

- ❑ Reassess the patient – confirms placement after LMA is secured, reassesses the ventilations for adequacy of depth and rate.

- ❑ Documents the procedure on the PCR – confirmation of placement of the LMA, number of attempts.

INSERTION OF THE ESOOPHAGEAL TRACHEAL COMBITUBE® (OPTIONAL EMT-B SKILL)

- ❑ Take BSI precautions

- ❑ Position yourself at the patient's head.

- ❑ Assemble equipment.

- ❑ Insert the device blindly, watching for two black rings used for measuring depth of insertion. The teeth of their bony cavities, if teeth are missing, should be positioned between these rings.

- ❑ Use the large syringe to inflate the pharyngeal cuff with 100 cc of air. On infation, the device will seat itself in the posterior pharynx behind the hard palate.

- ❑ Use the smaller syringe to fill the distal cuff with 10 cc to 15 cc of air.

- ❑ Usually (90–95 percent of the time), the tube will have been placed in the esophagus. On this assumption, ventilate through the esophageal connector (the external tube that is the longer of the two and is marked #1). You must listen for the presence of breath sounds in the lungs and the absence of sounds from the epigastrium in order to be sure that the tube is, in fact, placed in the esophagus.

- ❑ If there is an absence of lung sounds and presence of sounds in the epigastrium, the tube has been placed in the trachea. In this case, change the ventilator to the shorter tracheal connector, which is marked #2.

- ❑ Listen again to be sure of proper placement of the tube.

ALS-ASSIST SKILLS

MATCH TERMINOLOGY/DEFINITIONS

A. Drip chamber used when minimal flow of fluid is needed (with children, for example)

B. Stop cock located below the drip chamber that can be pushed up or down to start, stop, or control the flow rate

C. Chamber from which the drops of IV fluid flow

D. Drip chamber used when a higher flow of fluid is needed (for a multi-trauma victim in shock, for example)

E. Measurement of the electrical activity of the heart on a graph

F. When an IV needle has either punctured a vein and exited the other side or has pulled out of the vein and the fluid is flowing into the surrounding tissues instead of into the vein

G. Gently pressing the thumb and index finger just to either side of the medial throat and over the cricoid cartilage to bring the patient's vocal cords into view

H. Intravenous line inserted into a vein so that blood, fluids, or medications can be administered directly into a patient's circulation

I. Opening below the flow regulator on an IV set into which medication is injected

_____ **1.** Cricoid pressure

_____ **2.** Drip chamber

_____ **3.** ECG

_____ **4.** Flow regulator

_____ **5.** Infiltration

_____ **6.** IV

_____ **7.** Macro drip

_____ **8.** Mini drip

_____ **9.** Needle port

MULTIPLE-CHOICE REVIEW

_____ **1.** The "gold standard" of airway care is the
 A. jaw-thrust maneuver. **C.** endotracheal tube.
 B. ATV. **D.** nasal airway.

_____ **2.** Typical patients who need an endotracheal tube inserted include all of the following <u>except</u>
 A. pulmonary or cardiopulmonary arrest patients.
 B. trauma patients in need of airway control.
 C. patients with respiratory failure due to overdose.
 D. patients with full-thickness burns to the extremities.

_____ **3.** Prior to an intubation attempt, you may be asked to
 A. hyperventilate the patient. **C.** flex the neck.
 B. insert a gastric tube. **D.** press on the neck.

_____ 4. During the intubation attempt, you may be asked to do any of the following <u>except</u>
   A. shock the patient.
   B. stand by and be prepared to begin ventilations.
   C. gently press on the sides of the cricoid cartilage.
   D. maintain neck stabilization.

_____ 5. Once the endotracheal tube is inserted in the trachea and the cuff is inflated, the paramedic should
   A. extend the patient's neck.
   B. use an esophageal intubation detector.
   C. tape the endotracheal tube in place.
   D. insert an oral airway as a bite block.

_____ 6. After inserting the tube, the intubator should listen with a stethoscope in all of the following locations <u>except</u> the
   A. left lung.   C. epigastrium.
   B. right lung.   D. lower abdomen.

_____ 7. If, during the movement of the patient, the ET tube is moved, you should
   A. notify the paramedic, who will immediately recheck placement.
   B. apply the pulse oximeter to the patient.
   C. increase the oxygen concentration.
   D. quickly pull out the tube and replace it.

_____ 8. If you are ventilating a breathing patient with a BVM, you should
   A. increase the liter flow to at least 25 liters per minute.
   B. time your ventilations with the patient's respiratory efforts.
   C. decrease the oxygen concentration.
   D. ventilate at a faster rate than you normally would.

_____ 9. If, when ventilating, you feel a sudden change in the resistance, this could be caused by
   A. shock.
   B. anaphylaxis.
   C. air escaping through a hole in the lungs.
   D. a sucking chest injury.

_____ 10. When ventilating a patient in cardiac arrest with a BVM, with each defibrillation attempt you should
   A. drop the bag and move back.   C. lower the ventilation rate.
   B. remove the bag from the tube.   D. continue ventilations.

_____ 11. Why is it important to note the mental status changes of patients who are intubated?
   A. They may not be getting enough oxygen.
   B. They may wake up and bite on the tube.
   C. They may need to be hypoventilated.
   D. They may need a larger tube.

_____ 12. After the paramedic injects some medication down the tube, if you are assigned to ventilations, you may be asked to
   A. hyperventilate the patient.
   B. turn up the oxygen concentration.
   C. reassess the tube placement.
   D. hyperventilate the neck.

_____ 13. If the patient has a suspected cervical-spine injury, your role will be to
   A. hold the patient's chin forward during the intubation attempt.
   B. hand the paramedic the equipment for intubation.
   C. maintain in-line spinal stabilization throughout the procedure.
   D. place your fingers on the patient's throat throughout the procedure.

_____ **14.** A standard procedure used to alert EMS personnel to life-threatening heart rhythm disturbances is the
  A. myelogram.   **C.** ECG.
  B. EEG.   **D.** AED.

_____ **15.** The EMT-B should know how to turn on the ECG monitor and do all of the following <u>except</u>
  A. change the battery.   **C.** record an ECG strip.
  B. change the roll of paper. **D.** interpret the ECG.

_____ **16.** When assisting with an ECG, you should try to get in the habit of applying the
  A. electrode to the patient right away.
  B. leads to the electrode and then to the patient.
  C. electrode to the patient and then the leads to the electrodes.
  D. defibrillator to the patient to monitor the ECG.

_____ **17.** Which of the following is <u>not</u> part of preparing the patient's skin for ECG electrodes?
  A. drying the area   **C.** shaving excessive hair
  B. removing oil   **D.** applying alcohol

_____ **18.** In the most common electrode configuration, the red electrode is placed
  A. under the center of the left lower chest.
  B. under the center of the left clavicle.
  C. on the right lower chest.
  D. on the left lower chest.

_____ **19.** In the most common electrode configuration, the green or black electrode is placed
  A. under the center of the left lower chest.
  B. under the center of the left clavicle.
  C. on the right clavicle.
  D. on the left lower chest.

_____ **20.** A mini drip IV administration set produces _____ drops for every cc.
  A. 15   **C.** 45
  B. 30   **D.** 60

_____ **21.** A macro drip IV administration set produces _____ drops for every cc.
  A. 10 to 15   **C.** 30 to 40
  B. 20 to 30   **D.** 40 to 50

_____ **22.** When inspecting an IV fluid bag, always check for
  A. expiration date.   **C.** leaks in the bag.
  B. clarity of the fluid. **D.** all of the above.

_____ **23.** When removing the protective covering from the port of the fluid bag and the protective covering from the spiked end of the tubing,
  A. be very careful to maintain sterility.
  B. only touch the ends with gloves.
  C. hold the bag lower than the tubing.
  D. it is not necessary to protect the end of this tubing.

_____ **24.** Why is the IV line flushed prior to using it on a patient?
  A. It prevents the patient from developing a blood clot.
  B. It prevents introducing an air embolism.
  C. It helps to maintain sterility of the entire system.
  D. The fluid will run much faster without air in the line.

_____ **25.** Interruptions in the flow of an IV can be caused by each of the following <u>except</u>
   A. a closed flow regulator.
   B. a constricting band left on the patient's arm.
   C. a rise in the patient's blood pressure.
   D. kinked tubing.

COMPLETE THE FOLLOWING

List four steps that you may be asked to perform in the process of applying electrodes.

A. _____

B. _____

C. _____

D. _____

EMT-BASIC SKILL PERFORMANCE CHECKLIST

▶ ## SETTING UP AND RUNNING AN IV LINE

❑ Take BSI precautions.

❑ Inspect fluid bag for clarity, expiration date, and leaks. Remove outer wrapper and gently squeeze bag.

❑ Select proper administration set, uncoil tubing, and keep ends sterile.

❑ Connect an extension set if using a mini drip. (Macro drips should not have an extension set.)

❑ Make sure flow regulator is closed by rolling stopcock away from direction of fluid bag.

❑ Remove the protective coverings from the port of fluid bag and spiked end of tubing. Insert spiked end of tubing into fluid bag with a quick twist.

❑ Hold fluid bag higher than drip chamber. Squeeze drip chamber one or two times to start flow. Fill chamber to marker line (one-third full).

❑ Open flow regulator, and allow fluid to flush all the air from tubing. You may need to loosen cap at lower end to get fluid to flow. Be very careful to maintain sterility and to replace cap.

STRESS IN EMS

MATCH TERMINOLOGY/DEFINITIONS

A. State of physical and/or psychological arousal to a stimulus

B. Hormone that influences your metabolism and your immune response

C. Any situation that triggers a strong emotional response

D. Posttraumatic stress disorder, which may occur at any time, days to years, following a critical incident; also called PTSD

E. Reaction that is a result of prolonged recurring stressors in our work or private lives

F. First stage of the body's response to stress in which the sympathetic nervous system increases its activity in what is known as the "fight or flight" syndrome

G. Shorter and less structured form of debriefing usually led by a peer support member

H. Formal, highly structured process employed to assist individuals who are experiencing acute stress reactions; it includes six phases: fact, thought, reaction, symptom, teaching, and re-entry.

I. During this phase of grief, the dying person comes to peace with impending death.

J. Emotional reaction to a loss that includes the process of recovery and adjustment to the loss

_____ **1.** Acceptance

_____ **2.** Alarm reaction

_____ **3.** Cortisol

_____ **4.** Critical incident

_____ **5.** Cumulative stress reaction

_____ **6.** Debriefing

_____ **7.** Defusing

_____ **8.** Delayed stress reaction

_____ **9.** Grief

_____ **10.** Stress

MULTIPLE-CHOICE REVIEW

_____ **1.** Stressors that you are exposed to as an EMT-B may be the result of any of the following <u>except</u>
   A. environmental factors.
   B. predictable factors that can be avoided.
   C. your dealings with other people.
   D. your self-image or performance expectations.

_____ **2.** The three stages of the general adaptation syndrome as described by Dr. Hans Selye include alarm reaction, resistance, and
   A. exhaustion.   **C.** denial.
   B. acceptance.   **D.** bargaining.

_____ **3.** Cortisol, which influences your metabolism and immune response under stress, is produced by which body system?
   A. respiratory
   B. digestive
   C. endocrine
   D. nervous

_____ **4.** The stress triad, which occurs late in the exhaustion phase, involves all of the following <u>except</u>
   A. enlargement of the adrenal glands.
   B. wasting of the lymph nodes.
   C. development of cancer.
   D. bleeding gastric ulcers.

_____ **5.** What is another term for burnout?
   A. PTSD
   B. cumulative stress reaction
   C. delayed stress reaction
   D. acute stress reaction

_____ **6.** Which of the following signs and symptoms of acute stress reaction is unlikely to require intervention?
   A. acute chest pain
   B. long periods of uncontrollable crying
   C. continuous abnormal heart rhythms
   D. overeating for a 24-hour period

_____ **7.** The late signs of cumulative stress reaction include all of the following <u>except</u>
   A. headaches and stomach ailments.
   B. sleep disturbances.
   C. loss of emotional control.
   D. boredom or apathy.

_____ **8.** The ultimate key to preventing or managing cumulative stress lies in
   A. ongoing psychological help.
   B. seeking balance in one's life.
   C. replacing EMS with another career.
   D. drugs and alcohol use.

_____ **9.** Which of the following statements does <u>not</u> support the viewpoint that critical incidents can be developmental rather than pathogenic?
   A. People come out of incidents just as they were when going into them.
   B. A sound, routine incident command structure can prevent many critical incidents.
   C. Informal critiques should be conducted following every incident.
   D. Organizational and functional factors have minimal effect on job-related stress.

_____ **10.** The phases of grief generally follow which order?
   1. anger,
   2. bargaining,
   3. depression,
   4. denial and isolation,
   5. acceptance
   A. 1, 2, 3, 4, 5
   B. 5, 4, 1, 2, 3
   C. 4, 1, 2, 3, 5
   D. 3, 2, 1, 4, 5

COMPLETE THE FOLLOWING

1. List five of the signs and symptoms associated with an acute stress reaction that may require intervention.

   A. _____

   B. _____

   C. _____

   D. _____

   E. _____

2. List the six phases of a CISD.

   A. _____

   B. _____

   C. _____

   D. _____

   E. _____

   F. _____

BASIC CARDIAC LIFE SUPPORT REVIEW

Before beginning your EMT-B course, you are required to have completed a course in cardiopulmonary resuscitation. The elements of CPR are tested here as "extra value" for your review.

MATCH TERMINOLOGY/DEFINITIONS

A. Providing artificial ventilations to a person who has stopped breathing or whose breathing is inadequate

B. Manual thrusts to the abdomen used to dislodge an airway obstruction

C. When breathing and heartbeat stop

D. Pulse felt between the groove of the Adam's apple and the muscles located along the side of the neck

E. Requirement that the amount of time you spend compressing the patient's chest should be the same as the time spent for release

F. Bulging of the stomach that may be caused by forcing air into the patient's stomach during rescue breathing

G. When brain cells die

H. Short triangular piece of cartilage (tough, elastic gristle) that extends from the bottom of the sternum

I. General term for the area of the lower border of the sternum

J. Maneuver that provides for maximum opening of the airway

K. Pulse measured by feeling the major artery of the arm; the absence of this pulse is used as a sign, in infants, that heartbeat has stopped and CPR should begin.

L. Actions you take to revive a person—or at least temporarily prevent biological death—by keeping the person's heart and lungs working

M. Maneuver used to open the airway of a patient with a suspected spine injury

N. Red or purple skin discoloration that occurs when gravity causes the blood to sink to the lowest parts of the body and collect there

O. Lying the patient on his/her side to allow for drainage from the mouth and to prevent the tongue from falling backward

_____ **1.** Biological death

_____ **2.** Brachial pulse

_____ **3.** Cardiopulmonary resuscitation

_____ **4.** Carotid pulse

_____ **5.** Clinical death

_____ **6.** 50 : 50 rule

_____ **7.** Gastric distention

_____ **8.** Head-tilt, chin-lift maneuver

_____ **9.** Heimlich maneuver

_____ **10.** Jaw-thrust maneuver

_____ **11.** Line of lividity

_____ **12.** Recovery position

_____ **13.** Rescue breathing

_____ **14.** Substernal notch

_____ **15.** Xiphoid process

_____ 1. When a patient's breathing and heartbeat stop, the _____ cells will begin to die after 4 to 6 minutes.
    A. heart   **C.** liver
    B. brain   **D.** kidney

_____ 2. Once clinical death occurs, how long does it usually take for biological death to occur?
    A. 4 minutes   **C.** 8 minutes
    B. 6 minutes   **D.** 10 minutes

_____ 3. In the ABC method of cardiopulmonary resuscitation, the "A" stands for
    A. air flow.   **C.** airway.
    B. arterial pulse.   **D.** aorta.

_____ 4. In the ABC method of cardiopulmonary resuscitation, the "C" stands for
    A. cardiac.   **C.** circulation.
    B. compression.   **D.** carotid.

_____ 5. To determine if an adult or a child is pulseless, the EMT-B should check for a pulse at the _____ artery.
    A. femoral   **C.** radial
    B. brachial   **D.** carotid

_____ 6. To determine pulselessness in an infant, the EMT-B should use the _____ artery.
    A. brachial   **C.** femoral
    B. carotid   **D.** apical

_____ 7. If you are alone, and do not have an AED, after determining unresponsiveness in the adult the next thing you should do before starting CPR is
    A. reposition the patient.   **C.** establish an open airway.
    B. activate EMS.   **D.** check for breathing.

_____ 8. When an unconscious patient's head flexes forward, the _____ could cause an airway obstruction.
    A. hypopharynx   **C.** tongue
    B. uvula   **D.** larynx

_____ 9. One of the best methods to relieve an airway obstruction due to the positioning of the patient's tongue is the
    A. jaw-thrust maneuver.   **C.** head-tilt, chin-lift maneuver.
    B. abdominal-thrust maneuver.   **D.** jaw-lift maneuver.

_____ 10. The head-tilt, chin-lift maneuver should <u>not</u> be used on a
    A. stroke victim.
    B. diabetic patient.
    C. diving accident victim.
    D. patient who had a seizure in bed.

_____ 11. The recommended maneuver for opening the airway of a patient with possible cervical-spine injury is the _____ maneuver.
    A. jaw-thrust   **C.** head-tilt, chin-lift
    B. mouth-to-nose   **D.** jaw-lift

_____ 12. After opening the airway in a patient who requires rescue breathing, the EMT-B should inflate the patient's lung with
    A. one quick, full breath.   **C.** one-half breath.
    B. two slow breaths.   **D.** four slow breaths.

_____ **13.** Initial ventilations did not result in chest rise. Your next step is to
   A. continue standard mouth-to-mask ventilations.
   B. administer oxygen.
   C. perform airway clearance techniques.
   D. deliver four quick breaths.

_____ **14.** A common problem in the resuscitation of infants and children caused by improper head position or too quick ventilations is
   A. spinal injury.   **C.** pulmonary trauma.
   B. gastric distention.   **D.** airway injury.

_____ **15.** Adult rescue breathing should be provided at a rate of _____ breaths per minute.
   A. 5–7   **C.** 15–20
   B. 10–12   **D.** 21–25

_____ **16.** Infants should be ventilated at the rate of one breath every _____ seconds.
   A. 3   **C.** 8
   B. 5   **D.** 10

_____ **17.** When a patient has a distended abdomen due to air being forced into the stomach, the EMT-B should
   A. manually press on the abdomen to relieve the distention.
   B. decrease the oxygen concentration being administered to the patient.
   C. be prepared to suction should the patient vomit.
   D. increase the force of the ventilation.

_____ **18.** Why is the recovery position used?
   A. It protects the airway and allows for drainage from the mouth.
   B. It forces the mouth to remain open at all times.
   C. It protects the patient's head during a seizure.
   D. It makes oxygen administration possible in the unconscious patient.

_____ **19.** When delivering chest compressions during CPR, which of the following is not correct?
   A. Keep your elbows straight.
   B. Keep your hands on the sternum.
   C. Deliver compressions with a stabbing motion.
   D. Move from your hips.

_____ **20.** The CPR compression point is located on the lower half of the _____ , centered between the nipples.
   A. clavicle   **C.** ribs
   B. substernal notch   **D.** sternum

_____ **21.** Before beginning artificial ventilation, assess the patient's breathing for _____ seconds.
   A. 5   **C.** 15
   B. 10   **D.** 20

_____ **22.** For an adult, the one-rescuer compressions-to-ventilations ratio is
   A. 5 : 1.   **C.** 10 : 2.
   B. 5 : 2.   **D.** 15 : 2.

_____ **23.** The adult CPR compression rate in one-rescuer CPR is _____ times a minute.
   A. 60   **C.** 100
   B. 80   **D.** 120

_____ **24.** The adult CPR compressions rate in two-rescuer CPR is _____ times a minute.
   A. 60   **C.** 100
   B. 80   **D.** 120

_____ **25.** In two-rescuer CPR, the ratio of compressions to ventilations is
  A. 5 : 1.   **C.** 10 : 1.
  B. 15 : 20.   **D.** 10 : 2.

_____ **26.** When performing CPR on an adult, the sternum is depressed
  A. 1/2 to 3/4 inch.   **C.** 1 1/2 to 2 inches.
  B. 3/4 to 1 inch.   **D.** 2 1/2 to 3 inches.

_____ **27.** When performing CPR on an infant, the sternum is depressed
  A. 1/4 to 1/2 inch.   **C.** 3/4 to 1 1/2 inches.
  B. 1/2 to 1 inch.   **D.** 1 to 1 1/2 inches.

_____ **28.** When performing CPR on a child, the sternum is compressed
  A. 1/4 to 1/2 inch.   **C.** 3/4 to 1 1/2 inches.
  B. 1/2 to 1 inch.   **D.** 1 to 1 1/2 inches.

_____ **29.** The compression rate when performing CPR on an infant is at least
  _____ times a minute.
  A. 70   **C.** 90
  B. 80   **D.** 100

_____ **30.** When opening the airway of an infant, use a
  A. full head-tilt method.   **C.** slight head-tilt.
  B. jaw-thrust method.   **D.** neck hyperextension method.

_____ **31.** With effective CPR, the patient's pupils may
  A. dilate.
  B. constrict.
  C. assume a ground-glass appearance.
  D. begin to move.

_____ **32.** CPR compressions are delivered to children
  A. in the same manner as to adults.
  B. with the fingertips of index and middle fingers.
  C. with the palm of one hand.
  D. with the heel of one hand.

_____ **33.** With the exceptions of endotracheal tube placement or defibrillation,
  CPR should not be interrupted for more than _____ seconds.
  A. a few   **C.** 15
  B. 10   **D.** 20

_____ **34.** If you are treating a patient with a partial airway obstruction, poor air
  exchange, and gray skin, you should
  A. wait for the patient to stop breathing, then ventilate.
  B. treat the patient for a complete airway obstruction.
  C. increase the delivered oxygen concentration.
  D. do none of the above.

_____ **35.** Complete airway obstruction in a conscious patient is indicated by
  A. crowing sounds.   **C.** gurgling sounds.
  B. an inability to speak.   **D.** snoring sounds.

_____ **36.** When you recognize complete airway obstruction in a conscious adult
  patient, you should immediately
  A. place the patient in the supine position.
  B. deliver four back blows in rapid succession.
  C. deliver the Heimlich maneuver five times.
  D. attempt to ventilate the patient.

_____ **37.** To deliver abdominal thrusts to an unconscious patient, place the patient
  in the _____ position.
  A. upright   **C.** coma
  B. prone   **D.** supine

_____ 38. You are treating an unresponsive adult patient with a complete airway obstruction. You have been unsuccessful in your initial attempts to ventilate the patient. Which is the correct sequence to continue your effort?
   A. finger sweeps, back blows, adominal thrusts
   B. adominal thrusts, finger sweeps, back blows
   C. ventilations, finger sweeps, adominal thrusts
   D. adominal thrusts, finger sweeps, ventilations

_____ 39. When treating an 8-month pregnant woman who has a complete airway obstruction, the EMT-B should
   A. use the Heimlich maneuver.
   B. only use the back blows.
   C. use chest thrusts.
   D. start CPR immediately.

_____ 40. If a patient has a partial airway obstruction and is able to speak and cough forcefully, you should
   A. perform the Heimlich maneuver.
   B. carefully watch the patient.
   C. perform the chest thrust.
   D. position the patient on the floor.

_____ 41. A major difference between the adult and child obstructed airway procedure is
   A. chest thrusts are used with children.
   B. back blows are administered to adults.
   C. blind finger sweeps are not used with children.
   D. the number of abdominal thrusts is greater in the adult.

_____ 42. While you are trying to clear an adult's obstructed airway, the patient loses consciousness. You open the airway, perform a finger sweep, open the airway and attempt to ventilate. If this fails,
   A. deliver five chest thrusts.
   B. retilt the head and again attempt to ventilate.
   C. deliver four back blows.
   D. attempt another finger sweep.

_____ 43. You have been unsuccessful in initially ventilating an unconscious infant. You reposition the infant's head and attempt to ventilate again but are unsuccessful. Your next step is to perform
   A. a series of chest thrusts.   C. the Heimlich maneuver.
   B. back blows and chest thrusts.   D. a tongue-jaw lift.

_____ 44. Which of the following is not a sign of choking in an infant?
   A. ineffective cough   C. wheezing
   B. agitation   D. strong cry

_____ 45. To correct a complete airway obstruction in an infant, position the patient in the _____ position.
   A. upright   C. head-down
   B. supine   D. prone

COMPLETE THE FOLLOWING

1. List the special circumstances in which the EMT-B should not initiate CPR even though the patient is pulseless.

   _____

   _____

   _____

   _____

   _____

2. List situations in which the EMT-B may stop CPR.

   _____

   _____

   _____

   _____

   _____

EMT-BASIC CHECKLISTS

▶ MOVING WHILE DOING CPR

❑ Take BSI precautions.

❑ Begin CPR immediately.

❑ Place a long backboard under the patient, interrupting CPR for a maximum of 7 seconds.

❑ Resume CPR, and prepare to lift on signal.

❑ On signal, quickly transfer patient and spine board to litter.

❑ Move litter slowly so CPR can continue.

❑ Before moving down stairs, pause briefly at landing, continuing CPR.

❑ On signal, stop CPR and move quickly to next landing and resume CPR for a maximum of 30 seconds.

❑ Move safely down stairs.

❑ Begin CPR again.

NOTE: If the patient has an IV or ET tube, be extemely careful when moving patient.

▶ USING THE THUMPER

❑ Take BSI precautions.

❑ Assure CPR is in progress and effective.

❑ Attach the Thumper base plate to long backboard.

❑ Stop CPR momentarily to slide the long backboard under the patient.

❑ Restart CPR and attach shoulder straps to patient.

❑ Slide the Thumper piston plate into position on the base plate (away from the chest).

❑ Stop CPR and quickly pivot the piston arm into place, measuring the anterior/posterior and middle sternum placement.

❑ Slowly adjust the depth of compression to the appropriate diagram.

❑ Adjust the ventilations.

❑ Demonstrate the procedure for pulse check, a defibrillation, and how to power down the unit. (Always remember to store the unit with the compression depth turned down to the minimum setting.)

NATIONAL REGISTRY SKILL SHEETS

The National Registry of Emergency Medical Technicians is an organization founded in 1970, one of whose goals is to establish nationwide professional standards for EMTs. Many state EMS systems use examinations developed by the National Registry to establish certification of EMTs.

The National Registry has prepared a certification examination correlated to the 1994 Department of Transportation "Emergency Medical Technician-Basic: National Standard Curriculum." The examination includes both a written portion and a practical portion that consists of a series of performance-based skill stations.

To assist students in preparing for the skill stations that are part of the EMT-B examination, as well as to establish guidelines and parameters for those who will evaluate students' performance at the skill stations, the National Registry has developed a series of skill sheets. Each skill sheet contains a set of directions, the skill criteria, and the critical criteria that, if not met by the student, result in immediate failure of the station.

In studying for the National Registry examination, you should use these skill sheets in conjunction with the material presented in the textbook and not as the sole means of learning the individual skills. The skill sheets will aid you in organizing the steps necessary to perform each skill and in identifying the criteria that will be used to evaluate your performance. You can use these sheets to evaluate your own performance when practicing these skills and preparing for your practical skills evaluation.

Note: Three skill sheets regarding advanced airway management are included. The use of these skills will vary based on your medical director, training program, and local protocol.

ORGANIZATION OF THE NATIONAL REGISTRY EXAMINATION

The practical examination consists of six stations, five mandatory stations and one random basic skill station, consisting of both skill-based and scenario-based testing. The random skill station is conducted so the candidate is totally unaware of the skill to be tested until he or she arrives at the test site.

The candidate will be tested individually in each station and will be expected to direct the actions of any assistant EMTs who may be present in the station. The candidate should pass or fail the examination based solely on his or her actions and decisions.

On the next page is a list of the stations and their established time limits. The maximum time is determined by the number and difficulty of tasks to be completed.

INSTRUCTIONS TO THE CANDIDATE

▶ PATIENT ASSESSMENT/MANAGEMENT— TRAUMA

This station is designed to test your ability to perform a patient assessment of a victim of multi-system trauma and voice-treat all conditions and injuries discovered. You must conduct your assessment as you would in the field, including communicating with your patient. You may remove the patient's clothing down to shorts or swimsuit if you feel it is necessary. As you conduct your assessment, you should state everything you are assessing. Clinical information not obtainable by visual or physical inspection, for example, blood pressure, will be given to you after you demonstrate how you would normally gain that information. You may assume that you have two EMTs working with you and that they are correctly carrying out the verbal treatments you indicate. You have ten (10) minutes to complete this skill station. Do you have any questions?

▶ PATIENT ASSESSMENT/MANAGEMENT— MEDICAL

This station is designed to test your ability to perform a patient assessment of a victim with a chief complaint of a medical nature and voice-treat all conditions and injuries discovered. You must conduct your assessment as you would in the field, including communicating with your patient. As you conduct your assessment, you should state everything you are assessing. Clinical information not obtainable by visual or physical inspection, for

Station 1:	Patient Assessment/Management—Trauma	10 min
Station 2:	Patient Assessment/Management—Medical	10 min
Station 3:	Cardiac Arrest Management/AED	15 min
Station 4:	Bag-Valve Mask Apneic Patient	10 min
Station 5:	Spinal Immobilization Station	
	Spinal Immobilization—Supine Patient	10 min
	Spinal Immobilization—Seated Patient	10 min
Station 6:	Random Basic Skill Verification	
	Long Bone Injury	5 min
	Joint Injury	5 min
	Traction Splint	10 min
	Bleeding Control/Shock Management	10 min
	Upper Airway Adjuncts and Suction	5 min
	Mouth-to-Mask with Supplemental Oxygen	5 min
	Supplemental Oxygen Administration	5 min

example, blood pressure, will be given to you after you demonstrate how you would normally gain that information. You may assume that you have two EMTs working with you and that they are correctly carrying out the verbal treatments you indicate. You have ten (10) minutes to complete this skill station. Do you have any questions?

▶ CARDIAC ARREST MANAGEMENT/AED

This station is designed to test your ability to manage a prehospital cardiac arrest by integrating CPR skills, defibrillation, airway adjuncts, and patient/scene management skills. There will be an EMT assistant in this station. The EMT assistant will only do as you instruct him. As you arrive on the scene, you will encounter a patient in cardiac arrest. A First Responder will be present performing single rescuer CPR. You must immediately establish control of the scene and begin resuscitation of the patient with an automated external defibrillator. At the appropriate time, you must control the airway and ventilate the victim using adjunctive equipment. You may not delegate this action to the EMT assistant. You may use any of the supplies available in this room. You have fifteen (15) minutes to complete this skill station. Do you have any questions?

▶ AIRWAY, OXYGEN, VENTILATION SKILLS BAG-VALVE MASK APNEIC PATIENT WITH PULSE

This station is designed to test your ability to ventilate a patient using a bag-valve mask. As you enter the station, you will find an apneic patient with a palpable central pulse. There are no bystanders and artificial ventilation has not been initiated. The only patient intervention required is airway management and ventilatory support using a bag-valve mask. You must initially ventilate the patient for a minimum of 30 seconds. You will be evaluated on the appropri-

ateness of ventilator volumes. I will inform you that a second rescuer has arrived and will instruct you that you must control the airway and the mask seal while the second rescuer provides ventilation. You may use only the equipment available in this room. You have ten (10) minutes to complete this procedure. Do you have any questions?

▶ SPINAL IMMOBILATION—SUPINE PATIENT

This station is designed to test your ability to provide spinal immobilization on a patient using a long spine immobilization device. You arrive on the scene with an EMT assistant. The assistant EMT has completed the scene size-up as well as the initial and focused assessments. As you begin the station, there are no airway, breathing, or circulatory problems. You are required to treat the specific, isolated problem of an unstable spine using a long spine immobilization device. When moving the patient to the device, you should use the help of the assistant EMT and the evaluator. The assistant EMT should control the head and cervical spine of the patient while you and the evaluator move the patient to the immobilization device. You are responsible for the direction and subsequent action of the EMT assistant. You may use any equipment available in this room. You have ten (10) minutes to complete this procedure. Do you have any questions?

▶ SPINAL IMMOBILIZATION—SEATED PATIENT

This station is designed to test your ability to provide spinal immobilization on a patient using a half spine immobilization device. You arrive on the scene with an EMT assistant. The assistant EMT has completed the scene size-up, and initial and focused assessments. As you begin the station, there are no airway, breathing, or circulatory problems. You are required to treat the specific, isolated problem of an unstable spine using a half spine immobilization device.

Continued assessment of airway, breathing, and central circulation is not necessary. You are responsible for the direction and subsequent actions of the EMT assistant.

Transferring the patient to the long spine board should be accomplished verbally. You may use any equipment available in this room. You have ten (10) minutes to complete this procedure. Do you have any questions?

▶ IMMOBILIZATION—LONG BONE INJURY

This station is designed to test your ability to properly immobilize a closed, non-angulated long bone injury. You are required to treat only the specific, isolated injury. The scene size-up and initial assessment have been completed, and during the focused assessment a closed, non-angulated injury of the _____ (radius, ulna, tibia, fibula) was detected. Ongoing assessment of the patient's airway, breathing, and central circulation is not necessary. You may use any equipment available in this room. You have five (5) minutes to complete this procedure. Do you have any questions?

▶ IMMOBILIZATION—JOINT INJURY

This station is designed to test your ability to properly immobilize a non-complicated shoulder injury. You are required to treat only the specific, isolated injury. The scene size-up and initial assessment have been accomplished on the victim, and during the focused assessment a shoulder injury was detected. Ongoing assessment of the patient's airway, breathing, and central circulation is not necessary. You may use any equipment available in this room. You have five (5) minutes to complete this procedure. Do you have any questions?

▶ IMMOBILIZATION—TRACTION SPLINTING

This station is designed to test your ability to properly immobilize a mid-shaft femur injury with a traction splint. You will have an EMT assistant to help you in the application of the device by applying manual traction when directed to do so. You are required to treat only the specific, isolated injury. The scene size-up and initial assessment have been accomplished on the victim, and during the focused assessment a mid-shaft femur deformity was detected. Ongoing assessment of the patient's airway, breathing, and central circulation is not necessary. You may use any equipment available in this room. You have ten (10) minutes to complete this procedure. Do you have any questions?

▶ BLEEDING CONTROL/SHOCK MANAGEMENT

This station is designed to test your ability to control hemorrhage. This is a scenario-based testing station. As you progress through the scenario, you will be offered various signs and symptoms appropriate for the patient's condition. You will be required to manage the patient based on these signs and symptoms. A scenario will be read aloud to you, and you will be given an opportunity to ask clarifying questions about the scenario; however, you will not receive answers to any questions about the actual steps of the procedures to be performed. You may use any of the supplies and equipment available in this room. You have ten (10) minutes to complete this skill station. Do you have any questions?

▶ AIRWAY, OXYGEN, VENTILATION SKILLS UPPER AIRWAY ADJUNCTS AND SUCTION

This station is designed to test your ability to properly measure, insert, and remove an oropharyngeal and a nasopharyngeal airway as well as suction a patient's upper airway. This is an isolated skills test comprised of three separate skills. You may use any equipment available in this room. You have five (5) minutes to complete this skill station. Do you have any questions?

▶ AIRWAY, OXYGEN, VENTILATION SKILLS MOUTH-TO-MASK WITH SUPPLEMENTAL OXYGEN

This station is designed to test your ability to ventilate a patient with supplemental oxygen using a mouth-to-mask technique. This is an isolated skills test. You may assume that mouth-to-mouth ventilation is in progress and that the patient has a central pulse. The only patient management required is ventilatory support using a mouth-to-mask technique with supplemental oxygen. You must ventilate the patient for at least 30 seconds. You will be evaluated on the appropriateness of ventilatory volumes. You may use any equipment available in this room. You have five (5) minutes to complete this skill station. Do you have any questions?

▶ AIRWAY, OXYGEN, VENTILATION SKILLS SUPPLEMENTAL OXYGEN ADMINISTRATION

This station is designed to test your ability to correctly assemble the equipment needed to administer supplemental oxygen in the prehospital setting. This is an isolated skills test. You will be required to assemble an oxygen tank and regulator and administer oxygen to a patient using a nonrebreather mask. At this point, you will be instructed to discontinue oxygen administration by the nonrebreather mask, because the patient cannot tolerate the mask, and start oxygen administration using a nasal cannula. Once you have initiated oxygen administration using a nasal cannula, you will be instructed to discontinue oxygen administration completely. You may use only the equipment available in this room. You have five (5) minutes to complete this skill station. Do you have any questions?

PATIENT ASSESSMENT/MANAGEMENT—TRAUMA

		Points Possible	Points Awarded
Takes or verbalizes body substance isolation precautions		1	
SCENE SIZE-UP			
Determines the scene is safe		1	
Determines the mechanism of injury		1	
Determines the number of patients		1	
Requests additional help if necessary		1	
Considers stabilization of spine		1	
INITIAL ASSESSMENT			
Verbalizes general impression of patient		1	
Determines responsiveness		1	
Determines chief complaint/apparent life threats		1	
Assesses airway and breathing	Assessment	1	
	Initiates appropriate oxygen therapy	1	
	Assures adequate ventilation	1	
	Injury management	1	
Assesses circulation	Assesses for and controls major bleeding	1	
	Assesses pulse	1	
	Assesses skin (color, temperature, and condition)	1	
Identifies priority patients/makes transport decision		1	
FOCUSED HISTORY AND PHYSICAL EXAM/RAPID TRAUMA ASSESSMENT			
Selects appropriate assessment (focused or rapid assessment)		1	
Obtains or directs assistant to obtain baseline vital signs		1	
Obtains SAMPLE history		1	
DETAILED PHYSICAL EXAMINATION			
Assesses the head	Inspects and palpates the scalp and ears	1	
	Assesses the eyes	1	
	Assesses the facial area including oral and nasal area	1	
Assesses the neck	Inspects and palpates the neck	1	
	Assesses for JVD	1	
	Assesses for tracheal deviation	1	
Assesses the chest	Inspects	1	
	Palpates	1	
	Auscultates the chest	1	
Assesses the abdomen/pelvis	Assesses the abdomen	1	
	Assesses the pelvis	1	
	Verbalizes assessment of genitalia/perineum as needed	1	
Assesses the extremities	1 point for each extremity	4	
	includes inspection, palpation, and assessment of pulses, sensory and motor activity		
Assesses the posterior	Assesses thorax	1	
	Assesses lumbar	1	
Manages secondary injuries and wounds appropriately **1 point for appropriate management of secondary injury/wound**		1	
Verbalizes reassessment of the vital signs		1	
	TOTAL:	40	

CRITICAL CRITERIA

___ Did not take or verbalize body substance isolation precautions
___ Did not assess for spinal protection
___ Did not provide for spinal protection when indicated
___ Did not provide high concentration of oxygen
___ Did not find or manage problems associated with airway, breathing, hemorrhage, or shock (hypoperfusion)
___ Did not differentiate patients needing transportation versus continued on scene assessment
___ Did other detailed physical examination before assessing airway, breathing, and circulation
___ Did not transport patient within ten (10) minute time limit

PATIENT ASSESSMENT/MANAGEMENT—MEDICAL

		Points Possible	Points Awarded
Takes or verbalizes body substance isolation precautions		1	
SCENE SIZE-UP			
Determines the scene is safe		1	
Determines the mechanism of injury/nature of illness		1	
Determines the number of patients		1	
Requests additional help if necessary		1	
Considers stabilization of spine		1	
INITIAL ASSESSMENT			
Verbalizes general impression of patient		1	
Determines responsiveness/level of consciousness		1	
Determines chief complaint/apparent life threats		1	
Assesses airway and breathing	Assessment	1	
	Initiates appropriate oxygen therapy	1	
	Assures adequate ventilation	1	
Assesses circulation	Assesses/controls major bleeding	1	
	Assesses pulse	1	
	Assesses skin (color, temperature, and condition)	1	
Identifies priority patients/makes transport decision		1	
FOCUSED HISTORY AND PHYSICAL EXAM/RAPID ASSESSMENT			
Signs and Symptoms (Assesses history of present illness)		4	

Respiratory	Cardiac	Altered Mental Status	Allergic Reaction	Poisoning/ Overdose	Environmental Emergency	Obstetrics	Behavioral
•Onset? •Provokes? •Quality? •Radiates? •Severity? •Time? •Interventions?	•Onset? •Provokes? •Quality? •Radiates? •Severity? •Time? •Interventions?	•Description of the episode •Onset? •Duration? •Associated symptoms? •Evidence of trauma? •Interventions? •Seizures? •Fever?	•History of allergies? •What were you exposed to? •How were you exposed? •Effects? •Progression? •Interventions?	•Substance? •When did you ingest/become exposed? •How much did you ingest? •Over what time period? •Interventions? •Estimated weight? •Effects?	•Source? •Environment? •Duration? •Loss of consciousness? •Effects— General or local?	•Are you pregnant? •How long have you been pregnant? •Pain or contractions? •Bleeding or discharge? •Do you feel the need to push? •Last menstrual period? •Crowning?	•How do you feel? •Determine suicidal tendencies •Is the patient a threat to self or others? •Is there a medical problem? •Interventions?

		Points Possible	Points Awarded
Allergies		1	
Medications		1	
Past pertinent history		1	
Last oral intake		1	
Events leading to present illness (rule out trauma)		1	
Performs focused physical examination Assesses affected body part/system or, if indicated, completes rapid assessment		1	
VITALS (Obtains baseline vital signs)		1	
INTERVENTIONS Obtains medical direction or verbalizes standing order for medication interventions and verbalizes proper additional intervention/treatment		1	
TRANSPORT (Re-evaluates transport decision)		1	
Verbalizes the consideration for completing a detailed physical examination		1	
Ongoing ASSESSMENT (verbalized)			
Repeats initial assessment		1	
Repeats vital signs		1	
Repeats focused assessment regarding patient complaint or injuries		1	
Checks interventions		1	
CRITICAL CRITERIA **TOTAL:**		34	

CRITICAL CRITERIA

___ Did not take or verbalize body substance isolation precautions if necessary
___ Did not determine scene safety
___ Did not obtain medical direction or verbalize standing orders for medication interventions
___ Did not provide high concentration of oxygen
___ Did not evaluate and find conditions of airway, breathing, circulation
___ Did not find or manage problems associated with airway, breathing, hemorrhage, or shock (hypoperfusion)
___ Did not differentiate patients needing transportation versus continued assessment at the scene
___ Did detailed or focused history/physical examination before assessing airway, breathing, and circulation
___ Did not ask questions about the present illness
___ Administered a dangerous or inappropriate intervention

CARDIAC ARREST MANAGEMENT/AED

	Points Possible	Points Awarded
ASSESSMENT		
Takes or verbalizes body substance isolation precautions	1	
Briefly questions rescuer about arrest events	1	
Directs rescuer to stop CPR	1	
Verifies absence of spontaneous pulse *(skill station examiner states "no pulse")*	1	
Turns on defibrillator power	1	
Attaches automated defibrillator to patient	1	
Ensures all individuals are standing clear of the patient	1	
Initiates analysis of rhythm	1	
Delivers shock (up to three successive shocks)	1	
Verifies absence of spontaneous pulse *(skill station examiner states "no pulse")*	1	
TRANSITION		
Directs resumption of CPR	1	
Gathers additional information on arrest event	1	
Confirms effectiveness of CPR (ventilation and compressions)	1	
INTEGRATION		
Directs insertion of a simple airway adjunct (oropharyngeal/nasopharyngeal)	1	
Directs ventilation of patient	1	
Assures high concentration of oxygen connected to the ventilatory adjunct	1	
Assures CPR continues without unnecessary/prolonged interruption	1	
Re-evaluates patient/CPR in approximately one minute	1	
Repeats defibrillator sequence	1	
TRANSPORTATION		
Verbalizes transportation of patient	1	
TOTAL:	20	

CRITICAL CRITERIA

____ Did not take or verbalize body substance isolation precautions
____ Did not evaluate the need for immediate use of the AED
____ Did not direct initiation/resumption of ventilation/compressions at appropriate times
____ Did not assure all individuals were clear of patient before delivering each shock
____ Did not operate the AED properly (inability to deliver shock)

BAG-VALVE MASK
APNEIC PATIENT

	Points Possible	Points Awarded
Takes or verbalizes body substance isolation precautions	1	
Voices opening the airway	1	
Voices inserting an airway adjunct	1	
Selects appropriate size mask	1	
Creates a proper mask-to-face seal	1	
Ventilates patient at no less than 800 ml volume *(The examiner must witness for at least 30 seconds)*	1	
Connects reservoir and oxygen	1	
Adjusts liter flow to 15 liters/minute or greater	1	
The examiner indicates the arrival of second EMT. The second EMT is instructed to ventilate the patient while the candidate controls the mask and the airway.		
Voices re-opening the airway	1	
Creates a proper mask-to-face seal	1	
Instructs assistant to resume ventilation at proper volume per breath *(The examiner must witness for at least 30 seconds)*	1	
TOTAL:	11	

CRITICAL CRITERIA

___ Did not take or verbalize body substance isolation precautions
___ Did not immediately ventilate the patient
___ Interrupted ventilations for more than 20 seconds
___ Did not provide high concentration of oxygen
___ Did not provide or direct assistant to provide proper volume/breath
  (more than 2 ventilations per minute are below 800 ml)
___ Did not allow adequate exhalation

SPINAL IMMOBILIZATION
SUPINE PATIENT

	Points Possible	Points Awarded
Takes or verbalizes body substance isolation precautions	1	
Directs assistant to place/maintain head in neutral in-line position	1	
Directs assistant to maintain manual stabilization of the head	1	
Assesses motor, sensory, and distal circulation in extremities	1	
Applies appropriate size extrication collar	1	
Positions the immobilization device appropriately	1	
Directs movement of the patient onto device without compromising the integrity of the spine	1	
Applies padding to voids between the torso and the board as necessary	1	
Immobilizes the patient's torso to the device	1	
Evaluates the pads behind the patient's head as necessary	1	
Immobilizes the patient's head to the device	1	
Secures the patient's legs to the device	1	
Secures the patient's arms to the device	1	
Reassesses motor, sensory, and distal circulation in extremities	1	
TOTAL:	14	

CRITICAL CRITERIA

___ Did not immediately direct or take manual stabilization of the head
___ Released or ordered release of manual stabilization before it was maintained mechanically
___ Patient manipulated or moved excessively, causing potential spinal compromise
___ Patient moves excessively up, down, left, or right on the device
___ Head immobilization allows for excessive movement
___ Upon completion of immobilization, head is not in the neutral in-line position
___ Did not reassess motor, sensory, and distal circulation after immobilization to the device
___ Immobilized head to the board before securing torso

SPINAL IMMOBILIZATION
SEATED PATIENT

	Points Possible	Points Awarded
Takes or verbalizes body substance isolation precautions	1	
Directs assistant to place/maintain head in neutral in-line position	1	
Directs assistant to maintain manual stabilization of the head	1	
Reassesses motor, sensory, and distal circulation in extremities	1	
Applies appropriate size extrication collar	1	
Positions the immobilization device behind the patient	1	
Secures the device to the patient's torso	1	
Evaluates torso fixation and adjusts as necessary	1	
Evaluates and pads behind the patient's head as necessary	1	
Secures the patient's head to the device	1	
Verbalizes moving the patient to a long board	1	
Reassesses motor, sensory, and distal circulation in extremities	1	
TOTAL:	12	

CRITICAL CRITERIA

____ Did not immediately direct or take manual stabilization of the head
____ Released or ordered release of manual stabilization before it was maintained mechanically
____ Patient manipulated or moved excessively, causing potential spinal compromise
____ Device moves excessively up, down, left, or right on patient's torso
____ Head immobilization allows for excessive movement
____ Torso fixation inhibits chest rise, resulting in respiratory compromise
____ Upon completion of immobilization, head is not in the neutral position
____ Did not reassess motor, sensory, and distal circulation after voicing immobilization to the long board
____ Immobilized head to the board before securing the torso

IMMOBILIZATION SKILLS
LONG BONE

	Points Possible	Points Awarded
Takes or verbalizes body substance isolation precautions	1	
Directs application of manual stabilization	1	
Assesses motor, sensory, and distal circulation	1	
NOTE: The examiner acknowledges present and normal.		
Measures splint	1	
Applies splint	1	
Immobilizes the joint above the injury site	1	
Immobilizes the joint below the injury site	1	
Secures the entire injured extremity	1	
Immobilizes hand/foot in the position of function	1	
Reassesses motor, sensory, and distal circulation	1	
NOTE: The examiner acknowledges present and normal.		
TOTAL:	10	

CRITICAL CRITERIA

___ Grossly moves injured extremity

___ Did not immobilize adjacent joints

___ Did not assess motor, sensory, and distal circulation before and after splinting

IMMOBILIZATION SKILLS
JOINT INJURY

	Points Possible	Points Awarded
Takes or verbalizes body substance isolation precautions	1	
Directs application of manual stabilization of the injury	1	
Assesses motor, sensory, and distal circulation	1	
NOTE: The examiner acknowledges present and normal.		
Selects proper splinting material	1	
Immobilizes the site of the injury	1	
Immobilizes bone above injured joint	1	
Immobilizes bone below injured joint	1	
Reassesses motor, sensory, and distal circulation	1	
NOTE: The examiner acknowledges present and normal.		
TOTAL:	8	

CRITICAL CRITERIA

___ Did not support the joint so that the joint did not bear distal weight

___ Did not immobilize bone above and below injured joint

___ Did not reassess motor, sensory, and distal circulation before and after splinting

IMMOBILIZATION SKILLS
TRACTION SPLINTING

	Points Possible	Points Awarded
Takes or verbalizes body substance isolation precautions	1	
Directs application of manual stabilization of the injured leg	1	
Directs the application of manual traction	1	
Assesses motor, sensory, and distal circulation	1	
NOTE: The examiner acknowledges present and normal.		
Prepares/adjusts splint to the proper length	1	
Positions the splint on the injured leg	1	
Applies the proximal securing device (e.g., ischial strap)	1	
Applies the distal securing device (e.g., ankle hitch)	1	
Applies mechanical traction	1	
Positions/secures the support straps	1	
Re-evaluates the proximal/distal securing devices	1	
Reassesses motor, sensory, and distal circulation	1	
NOTE: The examiner acknowledges present and normal.		
NOTE: The examiner must ask candidate how he/she would prepare the patient for transportation.		
Verbalizes securing the torso to the long board to immobilize the hip	1	
Verbalizes securing the splint to the long board to prevent movement of the splint	1	
TOTAL:	14	

CRITICAL CRITERIA

____ Loss of traction at any point after it is assumed
____ Did not reassess motor, sensory, and distal circulation before and after splinting
____ The foot is excessively rotated or extended after splinting
____ Did not secure the ischial strap before taking traction
____ Final immobilization failed to support the femur or prevent rotation of the injured leg
____ Secured leg to splint before applying mechanical traction

NOTE: If the Sager splint or Kendrick Traction Device is used without elevating the patient's leg, application of manual traction is not necessary. The candidate should be awarded 1 point as if manual traction were applied.

NOTE: If the leg is elevated at all, manual traction must be applied before elevating the leg. The ankle hitch may be applied before elevating the leg and used to provide manual traction.

BLEEDING CONTROL/SHOCK MANAGEMENT

	Points Possible	Points Awarded
Takes or verbalizes body substance isolation precautions	1	
Applies direct pressure to the wound	1	
Elevates the extremity	1	
NOTE: The examiner must now inform the candidate that the wound continues to bleed.		
Applies an additional dressing to the wound	1	
NOTE: The examiner must now inform the candidate that the wound still continues to bleed. The second dressing does not control the bleeding.		
Locates and applies pressure to appropriate arterial pressure point	1	
NOTE: The examiner must now inform the candidate that the bleeding is controlled.		
Bandages the wound	1	
NOTE: The examiner must now inform the candidate that the patient is showing signs and symptoms indicative of hypoperfusion.		
Properly positions the patient	1	
Applies high-concentration oxygen	1	
Initiates steps to prevent heat loss from the patient	1	
Indicates need for immediate transportation	1	
TOTAL:	10	

CRITICAL CRITERIA

___ Did not take or verbalize body substance isolation precautions
___ Did not apply high concentration of oxygen
___ Applied tourniquet before attempting other methods of bleeding control
___ Did not control hemorrhage in a timely manner
___ Did not indicate a need for immediate transportation

OROPHARYNGEAL AIRWAY

	Points Possible	Points Awarded
Takes or verbalizes body substance isolation precautions	1	
Selects appropriate size airway	1	
Measures airway	1	
Inserts airway without pushing the tongue posteriorly	1	
NOTE: The examiner must advise the candidate that the patient is gagging and becoming conscious.		
Removes oropharyngeal airway	1	

SUCTION

	Points Possible	Points Awarded
NOTE: The examiner must advise the candidate to suction the patient's oropharynx/nasopharynx.		
Turns on/prepares suction device	1	
Assures presence of mechanical suction	1	
Inserts suction tip without suction	1	
Applies suction to the oropharynx/nasopharynx	1	

NASOPHARYNGEAL AIRWAY

	Points Possible	Points Awarded
NOTE: The examiner must advise the candidate to insert a nasopharyngeal airway.		
Selects appropriate airway	1	
Measures airway	1	
Verbalizes lubrication of the nasal airway	1	
Fully inserts the airway with the bevel facing toward the septum	1	
TOTAL:	13	

CRITICAL CRITERIA

___ Did not take or verbalize body substance isolation precautions
___ Did not obtain a patent airway with the oropharyngeal airway
___ Did not obtain a patent airway with the nasopharyngeal airway
___ Did not demonstrate an acceptable suction technique
___ Inserted any adjunct in a manner dangerous to the patient

MOUTH-TO-MASK WITH SUPPLEMENTAL OXYGEN

	Points Possible	Points Awarded
Takes or verbalizes body substance isolation precautions	1	
Connects one-way valve to mask	1	
Opens patient's airway or confirms patient's airway is open (manually or with adjunct)	1	
Establishes and maintains a proper mask-to-face seal	1	
Ventilates the patient at the proper volume and rate *(800–1200 ml per breath/10–20 breaths per minute)*	1	
Connects mask to high-concentration oxygen	1	
Adjusts flow rate to 15 liters per minute or greater	1	
Continues ventilation at proper volume and rate *(800–1200 ml per breath/10–20 breaths per minute)*	1	
NOTE: *The examiner must witness ventilations for at least 30 seconds.*		
TOTAL:	8	

CRITICAL CRITERIA

____ Did not take or verbalize body substance isolation precautions

____ Did not adjust liter flow to 15 liters per minute or greater

____ Did not provide proper volume per breath
  (more than 2 ventilations per minute are below 800 ml)

____ Did not ventilate the patient at 10–20 breaths per minute

____ Did not allow for complete exhalation

	Points Possible	Points Awarded
Takes or verbalizes body substance isolation precautions	1	
Assembles regulator to tank	1	
Opens tank	1	
Checks for leaks	1	
Checks tank pressure	1	
Attaches nonrebreather mask	1	
Prefills reservoir	1	
Adjusts liter flow to 12 liters per minute or greater	1	
Applies and adjusts mask to the patient's face	1	
NOTE: The examiner must advise the candidate that the patient is not tolerating the nonrebreather mask. Medical direction has ordered you to apply a nasal cannula to the patient.		
Attaches nasal cannula to oxygen	1	
Adjusts liter flow to 6 liters per minute or less	1	
Applies nasal cannula to the patient	1	
NOTE: The examiner must advise the candidate to discontinue oxygen therapy.		
Removes the nasal cannula	1	
Shuts off the regulator	1	
Relieves the pressure within the regulator	1	
TOTAL:	15	

CRITICAL CRITERIA

___ Did not take or verbalize body substance isolation precautions
___ Did not assemble the tank and regulator without leaks
___ Did not prefill the reservoir bag
___ Did not adjust the device to the correct liter flow for the nonrebreather mask
       (12 liters per minute or greater)
___ Did not adjust the device to the correct liter flow for the nasal cannula (up to 6 liters per minute)

VENTILATORY MANAGEMENT
ENDOTRACHEAL INTUBATION

NOTE: If a candidate elects to initially ventilate with a BVM attached to a reservoir and oxygen, full credit must be awarded for steps denoted by "**" if the first ventilation is delivered within the initial 30 seconds.

	Points Possible	Points Awarded
Takes or verbalizes body substance isolation precautions	1	
Opens airway manually	1	
Elevates tongue and inserts simple airway adjunct (oropharyngeal or nasopharyngeal airway)	1	
NOTE: The examiner now informs the candidate no gag reflex is present and the patient accepts the adjunct.		
**Ventilates the patient immediately using a BVM device unattached to oxygen	1	
**Hyperventilates the patient with room air	1	
NOTE: The examiner now informs the candidate that ventilation is being performed without difficulty.		
Attaches the oxygen reservoir to the BVM	1	
Attaches BVM to high-flow oxygen	1	
Ventilates the patient at the proper volume and rate (800–1200 ml per breath/10–20 breaths per minute)	1	
NOTE: After 30 seconds, the examiner auscultates and reports breath sounds are present and equal bilaterally and medical direction has ordered intubation. The examiner must now take over ventilation.		
Directs assistant to hyperventilate patient	1	
Identifies/selects proper equipment for intubation	1	
Checks equipment — Checks for cuff leaks	1	
Checks laryngoscope operation and bulb tightness	1	
NOTE: The examiner must remove the OPA and move out of the way when the candidate is prepared to intubate.		
Positions the head properly	1	
Inserts the laryngoscope blade while displacing the tongue	1	
Elevates the mandible with the laryngoscope	1	
Introduces the ET tube and advances it to the proper depth	1	
Inflates the cuff to the proper pressure	1	
Disconnects the syringe from the cuff inlet port	1	
Directs ventilation of the patient	1	
Confirms proper placement by auscultation bilaterally and over the epigastrium	1	
NOTE: The examiner must ask, "If you had proper placement, what would you expect to hear?"		
Secures the ET tube *(may be verbalized)*	1	
TOTAL:	21	

CRITICAL CRITERIA

____ Did not take or verbalize body substance isolation precautions
____ Did not initiate ventilations within 30 seconds after applying gloves or interrupts ventilations for greater than 30 seconds at any time
____ Did not voice or provide high-oxygen concentrations (15 liters per minute or greater)
____ Did not ventilate patient at a rate of at least 10/minute
____ Did not provide adequate volume per breath (maximum of 2 errors/minute permissible)
____ Did not hyperventilate the patient prior to intubation
____ Did not successfully intubate within 3 attempts
____ Used the patient's teeth as a fulcrum
____ Did not assure proper tube placement by auscultation bilaterally and over the epigastrium
____ If used, the stylette extended beyond the end of the ET tube
____ Inserted any adjunct in a manner that would be dangerous to the patient
____ Did not disconnect syringe from cuff inlet port

VENTILATORY MANAGEMENT
DUAL LUMEN AIRWAY DEVICE (PTL OR COMBI-TUBE) INSERTION
FOLLOWING AN UNSUCCESSFUL ENDOTRACHEAL INTUBATION ATTEMPT

	Points Possible	Points Awarded
Continues body substance isolation precautions	1	
Confirms the patient is being properly ventilated with high-percentage oxygen	1	
Directs assistant to hyperventilate the patient	1	
Checks/prepares airway device	1	
Lubricates distal tip of the device *(may be verbalized)*	1	
Removes the oropharyngeal airway	1	
Positions the head properly	1	
Performs a tongue-jaw lift	1	
Inserts airway device to proper depth	1	
COMBI-TUBE / PTL		
Inflates pharyngeal cuff and removes syringe / Secures strap	1	
Inflates distal cuff and removes syringe / Blows into tube #1 to inflate both cuffs	1	
Ventilates through proper first lumen	1	
Confirms placement by observing chest rise and auscultating over the epigastrium and bilaterally over the chest	1	
NOTE: *The examiner states: "You do not see rise and fall of the chest and hear sounds only over the epigastrium."*		
Ventilates through the alternate lumen	1	
Confirms placement by observing chest rise and auscultating over the epigastrium and bilaterally over the chest	1	
NOTE: *The examiner confirms adequate chest rise, bilateral breath sounds, and absent sounds over the epigastrium.*		
Secures tube at appropriate step in sequence	1	
TOTAL:	16	

CRITICAL CRITERIA

___ Did not take or verbalize body substance isolation precautions

___ Interrupted ventilation for greater than 30 seconds

___ Did not direct hyperventilation of the patient prior to placement of the device

___ Did not assure proper placement of the device

___ Did not successfully ventilate patient

___ Did not provide high-flow oxygen (15 liters per minute or greater)

___ Inserted any adjunct in a manner that would be dangerous to the patient

	Points Possible	Points Awarded
Continues body substance isolation precautions	1	
Confirms the patient is being properly ventilated	1	
Directs assistant to hyperventilate the patient	1	
Identifies/selects proper equipment	1	
Assembles airway	1	
Tests cuff	1	
Inflates mask	1	
Lubricates tube *(may be verbalized)*	1	
Removes the oropharyngeal airway	1	
Positions head properly with neck in the neutral or slightly flexed position	1	
Grasps and elevates tongue and mandible	1	
Inserts tube in the same direction as the curvature of the pharynx	1	
Advances tube until the mask is sealed against the face	1	
Ventilates the patient while maintaining a tight mask seal	1	
Confirms placement by observing chest rise and auscultating over the epigastrium and bilaterally over the chest	1	
NOTE: The examiner confirms adequate chest rise, bilateral breath sounds, and absent sounds over the epigastrium.		
Inflates the cuff to the proper pressure	1	
Disconnects the syringe	1	
Continues ventilation of the patient	1	
TOTAL:	18	

CRITICAL CRITERIA

____ Did not take or verbalize body substance isolation precautions
____ Interrupted ventilation for more than 30 seconds
____ Did not direct hyperventilation of the patient prior to placement of the device
____ Did not assure proper placement of the device
____ Did not successfully ventilate the patient
____ Did not provide high-flow oxygen (15 liters per minute or greater)
____ Inserted any adjunct in a manner that would be dangerous to the patient

Answer Key

Note: Page numbers in parentheses ( ) refer to page numbers in the textbook where answers can be found or supported.

Chapter 1: Introduction to Emergency Medical Care

MATCH TERMINOLOGY/DEFINITIONS

1. **(I)** Designated agent—an EMT-B or other person authorized by a Medical Director to give medications and provide emergency care

2. **(D)** EMS System—a system designed to get trained personnel to the patient as quickly as possible and to provide emergency care on the scene, en route to the hospital, and in the hospital

3. **(A)** Enabling legislation—state laws that allow an EMS system to exist

4. **(G)** Enhanced 9-1-1—a communications system that has the capability of automatically identifying the caller's phone number and location

5. **(C)** Medical direction—the provision for physician input and direction of patient care, training, and quality assurance of an emergency medical service or system

6. **(J)** Medical Director—a physician who assumes the ultimate responsibility for the patient care aspects of the EMS system

7. **(H)** 9-1-1 system—a system for telephone access to report emergencies in which a dispatcher answers the call, takes the information, and alerts EMS or the fire or police departments as needed

8. **(F)** Protocols—lists of steps, such as assessment and interventions, to be taken in different situations that are developed by the Medical Director of an EMS system

9. **(B)** Quality improvement—an all out effort by EMS personnel to improve the service provided from the moment of contact to the moment of delivery to the most appropriate medical facility and personnel

10. **(E)** Standing order—policy or protocol issued by a Medical Director that authorizes EMT-Bs or others to perform particular skills in certain situations

MULTIPLE-CHOICE REVIEW

1. **(B)** In the 1790s, France began to transport wounded soldiers so they could be cared for by physicians away from the scene of the battle. (p. 3)

2. **(C)** In 1966, the National Highway Safety Act charged the United States Department of Transportation with developing EMS standards. (p. 3)

3. **(B)** Computerization is helpful, but is not considered a major NHTSA EMS system assessment standard. (p. 4)

4. **(C)** "Specialty" hospitals include poison control centers, trauma centers, burn centers, and pediatric centers. Most hospitals have an Emergency Department. Correctional facilities and primary care centers are not considered EMS specialty care units. (p. 5)

5. **(A)** The U.S. Department of Transportation publishes curricula for the First Responder, EMT-Basic, EMT-Intermediate, and EMT-Paramedic levels. (pp. 6–7)

6. **(C)** The EMT-B curriculum deals with basic assessment and care of the patient. The EMT-B course is not limited to immediate life-threatening care. Electrocardiograms are beyond the scope of the EMT-B curriculum, and advanced airway techniques are optional, not a major emphasis, in the EMT-B curriculum. (p. 6)

7. **(B)** The care provided by the EMT-B is based upon your assessment findings. It is not delayed until transportation, nor should it be guided by attorneys. EMT-Bs do not make a diagnosis; rather treatment is based upon patient complaints. (p. 7)

8. **(A)** During the transfer of care, continuity of care can be improved by providing pertinent patient information to the hospital staff. This includes information on the patient's condition and your observation of the scene. (p. 7)

9. **(D)** While patient advocacy—speaking up for your patient—is one of the important roles of the EMT-B, it is not your primary responsibility. Your first responsibility is keeping yourself safe. (p. 7)

10. **(A)** Good personality traits of the EMT-B include: pleasant, cooperative, resourceful, a self-starter, emotionally stable, able to lead, neat and clean, of good moral character, having respect for others, in control of personal habits, and controlled in conversation. (pp. 8–9)

11. **(D)** An EMT-B should be in control of personal habits such as smoking, drinking, and using inappropriate language in order to avoid contaminating the patient's wounds, making inappropriate decisions, and rendering improper care. (pp. 8–9)

12. **(C)** Avoiding inappropriate conversation is paramount in protecting a patient's confidentiality. (p. 9)

13. **(C)** Continuing education includes attending conferences and watching training videos that further your education. Since procedures often change, rereading your old textbook or repeating the EMT-B course cannot keep you up-to-date on these changes. (p. 9)

14. **(C)** By definition, quality improvement is a process of continuous self-review with the purpose of identifying and correcting aspects of the EMS system that require improvement. (p. 9)

15. **(B)** Additional ways of providing quality improvement are listed in answer #16 below. (p. 10)

16. **(C)** Participating in continuing education and keeping careful written documentation are just two of the ways EMT-Bs can work toward quality care. Others include becoming involved in the quality improvement process, maintaining your equipment, and obtaining feedback from patients and the hospital staff. (p. 10)

17. **(D)** Each EMS system should have a Medical Director to provide oversight of patient care procedures. (p. 10)

18. **(C)** As an EMT-B, you often act as an extender, or designated agent, of the Medical Director. (p. 10)

19. **(D)** On-line medical direction involves talking to a physician over the telephone or radio. Off-line medical direction includes the physician developing protocols and policies,

Chapter 1 (continued)

advising the EMS service, and reviewing quality assurance issues. (p. 10)

20. **(B)** Activated charcoal is one of the medications for which EMT-Bs need on-line medical approval in order to give to a patient. (p. 10)

COMPLETE THE FOLLOWING

1. The categories and standards of an EMS system established by the National Highway Traffic Safety Administration are: (any six) (p. 4)
   - regulation and policy
   - resource management
   - human resources and training
   - trauma systems
   - public information and education
   - communications
   - transportation
   - facilities
   - evaluation
   - medical direction

2. Four types of specialty hospitals are: (p. 5)
   - trauma centers
   - burn centers
   - pediatric centers
   - poison control centers

3. Four levels of EMS certification are: (pp. 6–7)
   - First Responder
   - EMT-Basic
   - EMT-Intermediate
   - EMT-Paramedic

VIRTUAL STREET SCENES

Scene safety, patient assessment (first), (and then) patient care, lifting and moving patients, and patient transport.

Chapter 2: The Well-being of the EMT-B

MATCH TERMINOLOGY/DEFINITIONS

1. **(J)** Anger—when a patient gets upset and questions, "Why me?"

2. **(G)** Bargaining—when a patient mentally tries to postpone death for a short time

3. **(M)** Biohazard—a potentially infectious material

4. **(A)** Body substance isolation (BSI)—infection control based on the presumption that all body fluids are infectious

5. **(B)** Critical incident stress debriefing (CISD) teams—mental health professionals and peer counselors who work as a team to provide emotional and psychological support to EMS personnel who are or have been involved in a highly stressful incident

6. **(C)** Decontamination—the removal or cleansing of dangerous chemicals or other dangerous or infectious materials

7. **(L)** Denial—when the patient puts off dealing with the inevitable end of the process of dying

8. **(I)** Distress—when a rescuer becomes overwhelmed by the stress of a scene

9. **(H)** Hazardous material incident—the release of a harmful substance into the environment

10. **(N)** HEPA—a High Efficiency Particulate Air respirator or mask designed to reduce the spread of TB

11. **(K)** Immunizations—injections given to a rescuer that are designed to prevent him/her from getting a disease

12. **(F)** MCI—an emergency involving multiple patients

13. **(E)** Pathogens—the organisms that cause infection, such as viruses and bacteria

14. **(D)** Personal protective equipment—equipment such as eyewear, mask, gloves, gown, turnout gear, or helmet that protect the EMS worker from infection and/or from hazardous materials and the dangers of rescue operations

15. **(O)** PPD test—purified protein derivative test that determines if a person has been exposed to TB

MULTIPLE-CHOICE REVIEW

1. **(A)** The best EMT-B can be of no help to the patient if he/she is injured during a rescue situation or becomes ill. (p. 15)

2. **(D)** By definition, a pathogen is an organism that causes infection, such as a virus or bacteria. (p. 15)

3. **(C)** Since the EMT-B cannot identify patients who carry infectious diseases just by looking at them, all body fluids must be considered infectious and body substance isolation (BSI) precautions must be taken all the time. (p. 15)

4. **(C)** BSI involves handwashing, disposable gloves, and eye protection. A HEPA mask is used to protect against airborne particles that may cause TB. Leather gloves are helpful in a rescue to protect the EMT-B from cutting his/her hands but are not useful for BSI. (pp. 16–18)

5. **(B)** Surgical masks are routinely used for treating patients with a potential for blood or fluid spatter. If TB is suspected, a HEPA mask should be used. (p. 17)

6. **(A)** Whenever a mask is placed on a patient, the EMT-B will need to monitor the patient to assure respirations are adequate and the airway is open. Check often to ensure the patient doesn't vomit into the mask. If you think the patient has TB, you should wear a HEPA mask, not a surgical mask. (p. 17)

7. **(B)** In some states, keeping lists of certain types of patients, such as AIDS patients, may be a violation of the law. All other responses listed are ways to plan safety precautions. Since you never know which of your patients may have a communicable disease, you need to treat them all as if they do and take BSI precautions. (pp. 19–20)

8. **(C)** The purified protein derivative (PPD) is a test for tuberculosis and is not a vaccine. (p. 23)

9. **(C)** The employee safety regulations come under the Occupational Safety and Health Administration (OSHA). The FDA regulates drugs and foods; the FCC regulates radio equipment; and the Public Health Service provides regulations and educational efforts to assure children are immunized, water is clean, and so on. (pp. 19–20)

10. **(C)** Employers of EMT-Bs must make available the hepatitis B vaccination series as outlined in the OSHA standards on bloodborne pathogens, which took effect in March 1992. Employers must also provide training and personal protective equipment. (pp. 20–22)

11. **(B)** The Ryan White CARE Act provides two different systems for infectious disease exposure—airborne disease exposure and bloodborne disease exposure. Ensure that you understand these notification procedures since treatment must be timely in order to be effective. (pp. 20–22)

12. **(C)** The designated officer is responsible for gathering facts surrounding emergency responder airborne or bloodborne infectious disease exposures. Be sure you know who the designated officer is in your organization. (pp. 20–22)

13. **(B)** It is safest to assume that any person with a productive cough may be infected with TB. Since there are rising cases of multi-drug resistant TB, you should learn to recognize situations in which the potential of TB exposure exists, as well as the signs and symptoms of TB patients. (p. 22)

14. **(D)** An EMT-B should never treat a contaminated patient. If you treated the patient in an ambulance, it would be contaminated. If you took the contaminated patient to the hospital, you could effectively close it down. (p. 26)

15. **(D)** The well-being of the EMT-B involves dealing with job stress, ensuring scene safety, and taking BSI precautions to avoid contracting diseases. (pp. 24–25)

16. **(B)** An adult cardiac arrest is considered a "routine" EMS call. Calls involving a higher potential for causing excess stress on EMS providers include calls involving infants and children, elder abuse, death or injury of a coworker, plus severe injuries and MCIs. (p. 23)

17. **(C)** The warning signs that an EMT-B is being affected by stress include irritability with family, friends, and coworkers; inability to concentrate; changes in daily activities; difficulty sleeping or nightmares; loss of appetite; loss of interest in sexual activity; anxiety; indecisiveness; guilt; isolation; and loss of interest in work. (p. 24)

18. **(D)** Talking about your feelings with your partners is healthy. (p. 24)

19. **(C)** By definition, a critical incident stress debriefing is a process in which a team of trained peer counselors and mental health professionals meet with rescuers and health care providers who have been involved in a major incident. (p. 24)

20. **(D)** All are true. Also the normal reactions to stress should be discussed and provisions for follow-up set up for those who may need it. (pp. 24–25)

21. **(D)** The CISD is effective in accelerating the recovery process for the participants because it is nonthreatening and avoids performance review. It should never be combined with an incident critique or investigation. (pp. 24–25)

22. **(C)** The emotional stages that patients go through when they find out they are dying include denial, anger, bargaining, depression, and acceptance. (p. 25)

23. **(B)** The emotional stages have differing duration and magnitude but generally occur in the following order: denial, anger, bargaining, depression, and acceptance. (p. 25)

24. **(B)** All responses are correct except lying to the patient by saying everything will be all right when it will not. (pp. 25–26)

25. **(B)** It is not an EMT-B's responsibility to respond to dangerous situations. Rather, you should retreat, radio to police for assistance, and reevaluate the scene once it has been secured by the police. (pp. 27–29)

COMPLETE THE FOLLOWING

1. Types of calls with high potential of stress for EMS personnel include: (p. 23)
   * MCIs
   * infants and children
   * severe injuries
   * abuse and neglect
   * death of a coworker

2. Signs and symptoms of stress include: (any five) (p. 24)
   * irritability with family and friends and coworkers
   * inability to concentrate
   * changes in daily activities
   * loss of interest in sexual activity
   * anxiety
   * isolation
   * loss of interest in work

3. The critical elements of the infection control plan required by Title 29 Code of Federal Regulation 1910.1030 are: (any five) (p. 20)
   * infection exposure control plan
   * adequate education and training
   * hepatitis B vaccination
   * personal protective equipment
   * methods of control
   * housekeeping
   * labeling
   * post-exposure evaluation and follow-up

VIRTUAL STREET SCENES

1. Hepatitis B, C, or D, or HIV

2. AZT, safe sex with a condom, and regular blood tests

3. Yes, by being inoculated for hepatitis B, he may have prevented contraction of the disease.

4. Hepatitis B is a very hardy virus that kills approximately 200 health-care workers each year.

Chapter 3: Medical/Legal and Ethical Issues

MATCH TERMINOLOGY/DEFINITIONS

1. **(M)** Abandonment—leaving a patient after care has been initiated and before the patient has been transferred to someone with equal or greater medical training

2. **(B)** Advance directive—a written order given by the physician based upon a decision by a patient prior to his demise

3. **(O)** Battery—subjecting a patient to unwanted care and transport can be considered this in a court of law

4. **(I)** Breach of duty—not providing the standard of care

5. **(L)** Confidentiality—the obligation not to reveal information about a patient except to other health-care professionals involved in the patient's care, or under subpoena, or in a court of law

6. **(F)** Consent—permission from the patient to treat him/her

7. **(K)** DNR order—a legal document, usually signed by the patient and his/her physician, to "do not resuscitate"

8. **(D)** Duty to act—an obligation to provide emergency care to a patient

9. **(N)** Emancipated minor—child who is married or of a specific age who, in certain states, can make his/her own legal decisions

10. **(E)** Expressed consent—permission given by adults who are of legal age and mentally competent to make a rational decision in regard to their medical well-being

11. **(G)** Good Samaritan laws—a series of laws, varying in each state, designed to provide immunity from liability to individuals trying to help in emergencies

12. **(A)** Implied consent—permission to treat an unconscious patient until he/she becomes conscious

13. **(C)** Liability—being held legally responsible

14. **(J)** Negligence—a finding of failure to act properly in a situation in which there was a duty to act

15. **(H)** Scope of practice—the collective medical, legal, and ethical guidelines that govern the EMT-B

MULTIPLE-CHOICE REVIEW

1. **(B)** The collective set of regulations and ethical considerations governing the EMT-B's responsibilities is called the scope of practice. Duty to act is an obligation to provide care to the patient. Advance directives are the written and signed wishes of the patient in advance of any event where resuscitation might be undertaken. The Good Samaritan laws vary by state and often do not cover the EMT-B. (p. 33)

2. **(B)** Legislation that governs the skills and medical interventions that an EMT-B may perform not only differ from state to state, but may even vary from region to region within the state. (p. 33)

3. **(C)** Making the physical/emotional needs of the patient a priority is considered an ethical responsibility of the EMT-B. A legal responsibility would be assuring consent was gained prior to treating a patient. Advance directives involve orders on how a patient wants to be treated in the event resuscitation is needed. Protocols are models of care that an EMT-B follows in treating patients. (p. 33)

4. **(C)** Applied consent is a meaningless term that is often put on exams to test the student's understanding of consent terminology. The types of consent include consent for a minor or child, consent for a mentally incompetent adult, expressed consent (see answer #5), and implied consent (see answer #6). (pp. 33–34)

5. **(A)** Expressed consent is obtained by informing an adult patient of a procedure you are about to perform and its associated risks, then gaining his/her permission to proceed. Negligence is a finding of failure to act properly in a situation where there was a duty to act. Implied consent is defined in answer #6, and applied consent is a meaningless term. (pp. 33–34)

6. **(C)** Consent that is based on the assumption that an unconscious patient would approve the EMT-B's life-saving interventions is called implied consent. Expressed consent, negligence, and applied consent are explained in answer #5. (pp. 33–34)

7. **(C)** A patient refusal of medical aid or transport does not require any physician's signature. Your official record of a patient's refusal to accept medical aid must carefully and completely document the attempts you made to get the patient to accept care. Include the names of any witnesses to your attempts, and include the patient's "release" form with the patient's witnessed signature. (pp. 34–35)

8. **(B)** Forcing a competent adult patient to go to the hospital against his will may result in assault and battery charges against the EMT-B. You could also be charged with kidnapping the patient. Both implied consent and negligence are discussed above in answers #5 and #6. (pp. 34–35)

9. **(C)** All choices are correct except C. In all cases of refusal, you should advise patients to call back at any time if there is a problem or they wish to be cared for or transported. While there may be patients who legitimately refuse care, such as for minor wounds, patients with any significant medical condition should be transported to the hospital. (pp. 34–35)

10. **(D)** A "DNR order" is a physician's order to "do not resuscitate" a patient. This is also referred to as an advance directive. (pp. 35, 37–38)

11. **(A)** There are varying degrees of DNR orders, expressed through a variety of detailed instructions that may be part of the order, such as allowing for CPR only if cardiac or respiratory arrest was observed. Comfort care measures such as intravenous feeding, administering pain medications, and the long-term use of a respirator are a part of a living will and are not part of a DNR order. These orders generally do not specify procedures that are improper, such as specifying that only five minutes of artificial respiration will be attempted. (pp. 35, 37–38)

12. **(B)** In a hospital, long-term life-support and "comfort care" measures would consist of intravenous feeding and the use of a respirator. Once a patient is considered terminal, routine inoculations would not be needed. Infection control by the health-care providers is a given. Documentation needs to be the same as it would be had the patient not had an advance directive. (p. 37)

13. **(B)** In order to prove negligence, an attorney must prove the EMT-B had a duty to the patient, failed to provide the standard of care or breached his/her duty, and this failure caused harm to the patient. (p. 38)

14. **(C)** Termination of care of the patient without assuring the continuation of care at the same level or higher is called abandonment. Liability is being held legally responsible. Battery is attacking someone physically; and a breach of duty is not acting when you have an obligation to act. (pp. 38–39)

15. **(D)** Information considered confidential includes patient history gained through interview, assessment findings, and treatment rendered. The release of this information can cause embarrassment as well as potential harm to the patient. In the past, when the public was uninformed about the causes and consequences of AIDS, release of a patient's HIV positive status caused cross burnings and sick graffiti on the property of patients' homes. (p. 39)

16. **(D)** The only times an EMT-B may release confidential patient information is to inform other health-care professionals who need to know the information to continue care, to report incidents required by state law, such as rape or abuse, and to comply with a legal subpoena. It is not your responsibility to release confidential patient information in an effort to protect the other victims of a motor-vehicle collision. (p. 39)

17. **(D)** Medical identification insignia that indicate serious patient medical conditions come in the form of bracelets, necklaces, and cards because patients wear/carry these all the time and they are easily located. Patches are not medical IDs. (pp. 39–40)

18. **(B)** The patient is "not dead yet" so treat the critical patient who has an organ donor card the same as any other patient and inform the ED physician. Withholding oxygen therapy from the critically ill patient will just speed up his/he demise. (pp. 39–40)

19. **(A)** At a crime scene, the EMT-B should avoid disturbing any evidence unless emergency care requires. The patient himself provides valuable information. The position the patient is found in, condition of the clothing, and injuries are all pieces of evidence. Do not move obstacles from around the patient to make more room to work; this may destroy evidence. Leave the search of the house for clues to the police. It is not your responsibility. (pp. 40, 42)

20. **(B)** Commonly required reporting situations include sexual assault, domestic abuse, and child and elder abuse. A crime in a public place does not require the EMT-B to report the crime to the authorities. (p. 42)

COMPLETE THE FOLLOWING

1. In order for a patient to refuse care or transport, these three conditions must be fulfilled: (pp. 34–35)
   - The patient must be mentally competent and oriented.
   - The patient must be fully informed.
   - The patient must sign a "release" form.
   - The patient must be 18 years old or an emancipated minor.

2. Negligence, or failure to act properly, requires all of the following circumstances in order to be proven: (p. 38)
   - The EMT had a duty to the patient.
   - The EMT did not provide the standard of care.
   - The actions of the EMT in not providing the standard of care caused harm to the patient.

3. Four examples of conditions that may be listed on a medical identification device (such as a necklace, bracelet, or card) include: (p. 40)
   - Heart conditions
   - Allergies
   - Diabetes
   - Epilepsy

VIRTUAL STREET SCENES

1. Not really. This is not a confidentiality issue. It is more of an ethical issue and a matter of professional behavior in any conversation you have about any patient's residence. If, however, there are hazards observed while treating the patient in his residence (e.g., fire hazards, uncaged dangerous animals, explosives, dangerous conditions to future responders as well as to the patient), you should seriously consider notifying the appropriate authorities in your community.

2. Yes, it is medical documentation. You can always write things that the patient says in quotes in the narrative section of the PCR, too.

3. The appropriate BSI equipment would be gloves, and because the patient was vomiting, a mask and eye shield.

CASE STUDY—A Witnessed Collision: First on the Scene

1. No, except if your state law requires you must stop. You should, however, understand that once you do stop, you should not leave the patient except in the hands of another EMT-B or advanced EMT. Leaving a patient is considered abandonment, an example of "gross negligence."

2. Yes and No! Anyone can be sued. Most states do have some form of Good Samaritan laws or laws dealing specifically with EMS personnel that protect you in this situation provided you do not render treatment that is grossly negligent.

3. Yes, in most states.

4. Nine-One-One (9-1-1).

5. A) What is the exact location of the sick or injured person?
   B) What is your call back number?
   C) How old is the patient?
   D) What's the problem?
   E) What's the patient's sex?
   F) Is the patient breathing?

6. The police, the fire department, and the ambulance service.

7. Assign them to perform manual stabilization of the head and neck and to help with lifting the patient once the ambulance arrives.

8. The patient could have additional broken bones, internal bleeding, a head or neck injury to name a few.

9. No permission is needed as consent is implied because the patient is unconscious.

10. He could have a ruptured spleen, fractured ribs, back and neck injuries, as well as the obvious fractured leg.

11. Assign someone to lift the patient's injured leg and hold it as still as possible.

12. Yes, he is conscious and must give actual consent.

13. No, not until you check with the EMT-B or paramedic in charge to be sure your assistance is no longer needed.

14. Gross negligence due to abandonment.

Chapter 4: The Human Body

MATCH TERMINOLOGY/DEFINITIONS

▶ **Part A**

1. **(O)** Arteries—vessels that carry blood away from the heart
2. **(B)** Atria—upper chambers of the heart
3. **(I)** Brachial pulse—pulse in the arm used to take a blood pressure
4. **(A)** Bronchi—main branch of the respiratory system that enters each of the lungs
5. **(E)** Capillaries—tiny blood vessels
6. **(G)** Cardiovascular system—body system that transports blood throughout the body
7. **(F)** Carotid pulse—pulse in the neck at the side of the larynx
8. **(K)** Cricoid cartilage—ring-shaped structure that forms the lower larynx
9. **(C)** Diaphragm—muscle that divides the chest cavity from the abdominal cavity
10. **(N)** Dorsalis pedis pulse—pulse on the top of the foot
11. **(M)** Epiglottis—structure that closes to prevent food from going into the trachea during swallowing
12. **(D)** Femoral pulse—the carotid and this pulse are considered central pulses
13. **(L)** Larynx—structure that contains the vocal cords
14. **(J)** Nasopharynx—area directly posterior to the nose
15. **(H)** Oropharynx—area directly posterior to the mouth

▶ **Part B**

1. **(I)** Acetabulum—socket that holds the ball of the femur
2. **(M)** Femur—long bone in the upper leg

3. **(O)** Fibula—bone at the back of the lower leg

4. **(K)** Involuntary muscle—muscle type that works without the patient thinking about its operation

5. **(A)** Pharynx—area that includes the oropharynx and nasopharynx

6. **(B)** Platelets—parts of the blood needed to form blood clots

7. **(C)** Plasma—watery, salty fluid that makes up over one-half of the blood's volume

8. **(D)** Posterior tibial pulse—pulse that may be palpated on the posterior aspect of the medial malleolus

9. **(N)** Radial pulse—pulse on the thumb side of the wrist

10. **(H)** Respiratory system—body system that takes in oxygen and eliminates carbon dioxide

11. **(G)** Systolic—blood pressure created in the arteries when the left ventricle contracts and forces blood into circulation

12. **(E)** Trachea—structure that carries inhaled air from the larynx to the bronchi; also called the windpipe

13. **(F)** Veins—vessels that carry blood from the capillaries back to the heart

14. **(L)** Venae cavae—two large veins that return blood to the heart

15. **(J)** Ventricles—lower chambers of the heart

▶ **Part C**

1. **(C)** Anatomical position—standing face forward with palms forward

2. **(M)** Cervical spine—seven vertebrae in the neck

3. **(D)** Coccyx—inferior most division of the spine that is referred to as the tailbone

4. **(H)** Iliac crest—wide bony ring that can be felt near the waist

5. **(J)** Lateral malleolus—round ball of bone on the outside of the ankle

6. **(F)** Mandible—lower jaw bone

7. **(E)** Medial—towards or closer to the midline

8. **(G)** Medial malleolus—round ball of bone on the inside of the ankle

9. **(K)** Orbit—facial bone that surrounds each of the eyes

10. **(I)** Peripheral nervous system—system that consists of sensory and motor nerves

11. **(A)** Pubis—medial anterior portion of the pelvis

12. **(B)** Sacral spine—vertebrae that form the back of the pelvis

13. **(L)** Sternum—breastbone

14. **(N)** Tarsals—bones of the ankle

15. **(O)** Tibia—medial and larger of the two bones of the lower leg

▶ **Part D**

1. **(M)** Anterior—front side of the torso

2. **(N)** Calcaneus—heel bone

3. **(J)** Dermis—layer of the skin in which the hair follicles, sweat glands, and oil glands are located

4. **(G)** Distal—when two points on the extremities are compared, the point further away from the torso

5. **(L)** Elbow—joint where three bones of the upper arm and forearm are connected

6. **(F)** Epidermis—outermost layer of the skin

7. **(B)** Humerus—upper arm bone

8. **(C)** Lateral—away from the midline

9. **(H)** Motor nerves—nerves that carry messages from the brain to the body

10. **(K)** Phalanges—bones in the fingers and toes

11. **(O)** Posterior—back side of the torso

12. **(E)** Proximal—when two points on the extremities are compared, the point closer to the torso

13. **(D)** Sensory nerves—nerves that transmit information from the body to the spinal cord and brain

14. **(I)** Superior—above or towards the head end of the torso

15. **(A)** Xiphoid process—inferior tip of the sternum

▶ **Part E**

1. **(E)** Acromion process—highest portion of the shoulder

2. **(N)** Bilaterally—similar on both sides of the body

3. **(G)** Carpals—bones that make up the wrist

4. **(I)** Clavicle—bone in the front of the shoulder

5. **(A)** Endocrine system—body system that regulates metabolic functions such as sugar absorption by the cells

6. **(M)** Fowler's—sitting position on a stretcher with the body at a 45-to-60-degree angle

7. **(D)** Metacarpals—bones that make up the hand

8. **(L)** Mid-clavicular—an imaginary line drawn vertically from the center of the clavicle to the nipple below

9. **(B)** Nervous system—body system that governs sensations, movement, and thought

10. **(C)** Radius—lateral bone of the forearm aligned with the thumb

11. **(H)** Scapula—shoulder blade

12. **(K)** Supine—lying on the back

13. **(J)** Torso—the body less the extremities and the head

14. **(O)** Trendelenburg—lying supine with the legs elevated a few inches

15. **(F)** Ulna—medial bone of the forearm

▶ **Part F**

1. **(B)** Abdominal quadrants—four divisions of the abdomen used to pinpoint the location of pain

2. **(M)** Axilla—anatomical term for the armpit

3. **(D)** Coronary arteries—blood vessels that supply the muscle of the heart

4. **(H)** Diastolic—blood pressure in the arteries when the left ventricle is refilling

5. **(E)** Dorsal—referring to the back of the body

6. **(N)** Left side—patient's left side

7. **(J)** Lumbar spine—vertebrae of the lower back

8. **(F)** Maxilla—upper jaw bone

9. **(L)** Midline—imaginary line drawn vertically through the middle of the body

10. **(G)** Musculoskeletal system—body system that provides protection and movement

11. **(I)** Patella—kneecap

12. **(C)** Plantar—referring to the sole of the foot

13. **(O)** Prone—lying on the stomach or face down

14. **(K)** Thoracic spine—rib area of the spinal column

15. **(A)** Voluntary muscle—muscle under conscious control of the brain

MULTIPLE-CHOICE REVIEW

1. **(C)** The abdomen is a cavity of the body containing hollow and solid organs. Body systems include: respiratory, cardiovascular, musculoskeletal, skin (integumentary), nervous, endocrine, and digestive (not discussed in this chapter). (p. 48)

2. **(B)** If a patient is lying on his left side, this position is called the recovery, or left lateral recumbent, position. Fowler's position is sitting on a stretcher, supine is lying on the back, and prone is lying on the stomach. (p. 48)

3. **(C)** When a patient is placed in a sitting-up position on a stretcher, this position is called Fowler's. Lying on the stomach is prone; lying on the back is supine. Trendelenburg is defined below in answer #4. (p. 48)

4. **(D)** When a patient is lying flat with head lower than legs, this position is called Trendelenburg. For an explanation of the other choices, see answer #3. (pp. 48–49)

5. **(B)** The musculoskeletal system has three main functions: It gives the body shape, provides for body movements, and protects vital internal organs. Body sensation is a function of the nervous system. The skin, or integumentary, system is the body's outer covering. The cardiovascular system, working along with the respiratory system, transports oxygen into the cells. (p. 49)

6. **(C)** The upper jaw is also called the maxillae. The way to remember which of the two jaw bones is which, maxillae or mandible, is to use the rhyme "the mandible is moveable." The orbit is the area around the eyes, and the nasal bone protects the nose. (p. 49)

7. **(A)** The spinal column consists of the 7 cervical, 12 thoracic, 5 lumbar, 5 sacral, and 4 coccyx bones. (p. 52)

8. **(C)** An injury to the cervical spine may be fatal because control of the muscles of breathing arise from the spinal cord at this level. The lumbar region is also subject to injury because it is not supported by other parts of the skeleton. The thoracic spine, as well as the sacral spine and coccyx, are less easily injured. (p. 52)

9. **(A)** Bones in the lower extremities include the femur, tibia, fibula, patella, tarsals, metatarsals, calcaneus, and phalanges. The ischium is a pelvic bone. The ulna and radius are bones in the forearm. The orbit is the area around the eyes in the face. (p. 53)

10. **(A)** Bones in the upper extremities include the humerus, ulna, radius, carpals, metacarpals, and phalanges. The cervical bones are in the neck, and the tibia and calcaneus are in the lower extremities. (p. 53)

11. **(D)** The types of muscle tissue include voluntary, involuntary, and cardiac. Cardiac muscle has a specific quality called "automaticity," or the ability to generate and conduct electrical impulses on its own. (p. 54)

12. **(A)** The type of muscle that allows body movement such as walking is called voluntary. Involuntary and cardiac muscles are described in answers #11 and #13. Smooth is the same as involuntary. (p. 54)

13. **(B)** Involuntary, or smooth, muscle is found in the blood vessels, gastrointestinal system, lungs, and urinary system and controls the flow of materials through these systems. The heart has a special type of muscle (cardiac), and the quadriceps and biceps have voluntary, or striated, muscle. (p. 54)

14. **(B)** The larynx is the structure in the throat that is commonly known as the voice box. The pharynx is the area directly posterior to the mouth and nose; the trachea is the windpipe; and the sternum is the breastbone. (p. 54)

15. **(B)** The epiglottis is a leaf-shaped valve that prevents food and foreign objects from entering the trachea. The bronchi are the two major tubes that allow air to enter each of the two lungs. The pharynx and larynx are defined above in answer #14. (p. 54)

16. **(C)** The normal order of passage of oxygen from the environment to the lungs is through mouth and nose to the pharynx, through the larynx, through the trachea, into the bronchi, then down into the bronchioles, and then into the alveoli. Normally air does not go into the esophagus, which is a tube that brings food into the stomach. (p. 55)

17. **(C)** When the diaphragm and intercostal muscles relax, the size of the chest cavity decreases, causing exhalation. When the diaphragm contracts, it moves down, enlarging the chest cavity; the intercostal muscles pull the chest upward and outward to enlarge the cavity. This rapid pressure change accounts for air moving from the outside environment to fill the cavity. (p. 55)

18. **(D)** The difference between the adult airway and the pediatric airway is that all structures are smaller and more easily obstructed in a child. Actually, the adult's tongue takes up proportionately less space in the mouth than the child's. The trachea and cricoid cartilage is softer and more flexible in a child. (pp. 55–56)

19. **(A)** The right atrium receives blood from the venae cavae. It then pumps the blood into the right ventricle and then on to the pulmonary artery (only artery that carries deoxygenated blood) to the lungs. (p. 56)

20. **(A)** The aorta is the major artery originating from the heart. It lies in front of the thoracic spine. It divides at the level of the navel into the iliac arteries and supplies all the vessels of the upper and lower body with blood. (p. 56)

21. **(B)** The major artery in the thigh is called the femoral artery. The carotid is in the neck, radial is in the wrist, and brachial is in the arm. (p. 58)

22. **(C)** The vessel that carries oxygen-poor blood from the portion of the body below the heart and back to the right atrium is called the inferior vena cava. The posterior tibial is a pulse that can be palpated on the posterior aspect of the medial malleolus. The internal jugular is a vein that drains blood from the head. The aorta is the largest artery, which carries oxygen-rich blood away from the left ventricle. (p. 58)

23. **(B)** The left atrium receives blood from the pulmonary veins (the only veins that contain oxygenated blood). The left atrium then pumps the blood into the left ventricle, where it is then pumped out to the rest of the body. (pp. 56, 59)

24. **(C)** The fluid that carries the blood cells and nutrients is called plasma. Platelets are defined in answer #25. Urine is a waste product of the body excreted by the kidneys and held in the urinary bladder prior to being excreted from the body. (p. 59)

25. **(B)** The blood component that is essential to the formation of blood clots is called platelets. Plasma is the fluid part of the blood that carries blood cells and nutrients. The white blood cells fight infection, and the red cells carry oxygen to or carbon dioxide away from tissues. (p. 59)

26. **(A)** The pressure on the walls of an artery when the left ventricle contracts is called the systolic pressure. The pressure upon relaxation is the diastolic pressure. Residual and arterial pressures are utilized in critical care monitoring. (p. 60)

27. **(A)** The two main divisions of the nervous system are the central and peripheral nervous systems. The bones, muscles, and spinal column are parts of the musculoskeletal system. The spinal cord and brain are major components of the central nervous system. (p. 60)

28. **(D)** Nerves that carry information from throughout the body to the brain are sensory nerves. The motor nerves allow for movement. Spinal nerves, along with the brain, are actually a part of the central nervous system. There is no specific category called cardiac nerves. (p. 60)

29. **(C)** One of the functions of the skin is to protect the body from the environment, bacteria, and other organisms. Other functions of the skin include water balance, temperature regulation, excretion, and shock absorption. The respiratory system eliminates excess oxygen into the atmosphere. The nervous system regulates the diameter of the blood vessels in the circulation. The skin prevents environmental water from entering the body. (p. 62)

30. **(C)** The system that secretes hormones, such as insulin and adrenaline, and which is responsible for regulating body activities, is called the endocrine system. The skin provides covering, and the nervous system provides overall control. The gastrointestinal system digests food. (p. 63)

COMPLETE THE FOLLOWING

1. Arteries in the body include: (p. 58)
   - Coronary
   - Aorta
   - Pulmonary
   - Carotid
   - Femoral
   - Brachial
   - Radial
   - Posterior tibial
   - Dorsalis pedis

2. Functions of the skin include: (pp. 60, 62)
   - Protection
   - Water balance
   - Temperature regulation
   - Excretion
   - Shock absorption

LABEL THE DIAGRAMS

▶ Anatomical Postures (pp. 48–49)

1. Supine
2. Prone
3. Recovery

▶ Anatomical Position (pp. 48–49)

Diagram 1
1. Distal
2. Proximal
3. Midline
4. Mid-clavicular line
5. Medial
6. Lateral
7. Palmar
8. Left
9. Dorsal
10. Right

Diagram 2
11. Anterior (ventral)
12. Posterior (dorsal)
13. Superior
14. Mid-axillary line
15. Inferior

▶ Topography of the Torso (pp. 73–74)

1. Scapular region
2. Lumbar region
3. Iliac crest
4. Pubis
5. Costal arch (margin)
6. Xiphoid process
7. Pectoral region
8. Sternoclavicular joints
9. Suprasternal (jugular) notch
10. Clavicle
11. Sternum
12. Diaphragm
13. Umbilicus

VIRTUAL STREET SCENES

1. Manual stabilization is needed because the slightest movement of the neck could cause serious, permanent damage—or death—if in fact there is an actual injury to the spine.

2. As an EMT-B who was dispatched to the scene, you clearly have a duty to act. That means, yes, he is a patient in need of evaluation.

Chapter 5: Lifting and Moving Patients

MATCH TERMINOLOGY/DEFINITIONS

1. **(A)** Basket stretcher—stretcher, made of steel wire mesh and tubular steel rim or plastic and steel rim, used to transport patients from one level to another or over rough terrain

2. **(H)** Body mechanics—proper use of the body to facilitate lifting and moving and to prevent injury

3. **(D)** Direct carry—method of transferring a patient from bed to stretcher in which two or more rescuers curl the patient to their chests, then reverse the process to lower the patient to the stretcher

4. **(M)** Direct ground lift—method of lifting and carrying a patient from ground level to a stretcher in which two or more rescuers kneel, curl the patient to their chests, stand, then reverse the process to lower the patient to the stretcher

5. **(K)** Draw-sheet method—method of transferring a patient from bed to stretcher by gasping and pulling the loosened bottom sheet of the bed

6. **(N)** Emergency move—removal of a patient from a hazardous environment in which safety is the first priority and spinal integrity is second priority

7. **(F)** Extremity lift—method of lifting and carrying a patient in which one rescuer slips hands under the patient's armpits and grasps the wrists, while another rescuer grasps the patient's knees

8. **(O)** Log roll—procedure done by three or four rescuers that is designed to move a patient onto a long backboard without compromising spinal integrity

9. **(L)** Long axis—line that runs down the center of the body from the top of the head and along the spine

10. **(E)** Non-urgent move—patient move that may be made if speed is not priority

11. **(I)** Power grip—gripping with as much hand surface as possible the object being lifted, with all fingers bent at the same angle

12. **(G)** Power lift—also called the squat-lift position; a lift is made from a squatting position with weight to be lifted close to the body, feet apart and flat on the ground, body weight on or just behind the balls of the feet, back locked in.

13. **(C)** Scoop (orthopedic) stretcher—aluminum stretcher that splits in halves, which can be pushed together under the patient

14. **(B)** Stair chair—portable folding chair with wheels used to transport patient in a sitting position up or down stairs

15. **(J)** Urgent move—patient move that should be done quickly yet without any compromise of spinal integrity

MULTIPLE-CHOICE REVIEW

1. **(C)** To assure your own safety when lifting a patient, it is important to use your legs, not your back, to lift. Some EMT-Bs use a soft back brace when they lift. These devices should only be used if your physician suggests you do so. When lifting, keep the weight as close to your body as possible. Consider the weight of the patient you are lifting: be realistic about your limitations and ask for help. (p. 81)

2. **(B)** Avoid twisting motions while you are lifting; such motions can lead to a back injury. When lifting a patient, you should communicate clearly and frequently with your partner and know your limitations. (p. 81)

3. **(A)** When lifting a cot or stretcher, use an even number of people so that balance of the device is maintained. Your feet should be a comfortable distance apart so you can maintain balance. If a third person is positioned on the heaviest side, he or she stands a greater chance of being injured. If you must use only one hand to carry a piece of equipment, never compensate by using your back. (p. 82)

4. **(A)** When placing all fingers and the palm in contact with the object being lifted, you are using a power grip. A power lift involves squatting and using the legs. The lock grip and grip lift are inventive distracters for this question. (pp. 82–83)

5. **(A)** When you must push an object, keep the line of pull through the center of your body by bending your knees. Also keep the weight as close to your body as possible, avoid pushing or pulling overhead, and keep elbows bent with arms close to your sides. (p. 83)

6. **(D)** The fact that the dispatcher has another more serious call is not an appropriate reason to compromise the patient's spine. The situations in which an emergency move would be used include fire or danger of fire, explosives or other hazardous chemicals, and inability to protect the patient from other hazards at the scene. (p. 84)

7. **(C)** If the patient is on the floor or ground and the EMT-B has decided that an emergency move is appropriate, the patient can be moved by pulling on his/her clothing in the neck and shoulder area, which maintains some spinal integrity and doesn't require additional equipment or other rescuers. (p. 84)

8. **(B)** If the patient has an altered mental status, the EMT-B should consider an urgent move. The emergency move is used in situations where there is a real danger to rescuer or patient, such as a fire. (p. 84)

9. **(C)** When doing a log roll, lean from your hips and use your shoulder muscles to help with the roll. Also try to keep your back straight and position yourself right next to the patient. Maintaining spinal integrity is more important than speed. (p. 84)

10. **(A)** The final step in packaging a patient on a wheeled stretcher is securing the patient to the stretcher. The particulars about using towels under the head and top sheets are specific to the standard operating procedures of your service. Adjusting the back rest is optional depending on the patient's condition. (p. 89)

11. **(D)** If you are carrying a patient down stairs, when possible use a stair chair since it weighs less than a stretcher. Do not flex at the waist with or without bent knees. Both hands should be used to carry the stair chair. (pp. 89, 92)

12. **(B)** A scoop stretcher does not offer any support directly under the spine. It does work well for non-spinal injured patients found in narrow places like bathrooms or hallways that will not accommodate the wheeled stretcher. (p. 92)

13. **(A)** You have a patient positioned on a scoop-style stretcher and wish to lower the patient from a roof top. You should place the stretcher and patient in a plastic basket stretcher. Make sure the basket is rated for the lift and you have the appropriate training in high-angle rescue techniques. It is not necessary to take the patient out of the scoop to place him into the wire basket. Never lower the patient in the scoop alone, as this could lead to serious injury or death. (p. 92)

14. **(A)** To avoid trauma to an injured spine, the best patient-carrying device would be the long spine board for immobilization. Then place the patient on the wheeled stretcher to move him. (p. 92)

15. **(D)** The direct ground lift is an example of a non-urgent move for a patient who has no spine injury. (p. 92)

COMPLETE THE FOLLOWING

1. Seven patient carrying devices include: (pp. 89, 92)
   - wheeled ambulance stretcher
   - portable ambulance stretcher
   - stair chair
   - scoop stretcher
   - spine board
   - basket stretcher
   - flexible stretcher

2. Body mechanic principles include: (any four) (p. 81)
   - Position your feet properly.
   - When lifting, use your legs, not your back, to do the lifting.
   - When lifting, never twist or attempt to make any moves other than the lift.
   - When lifting with one hand, do not compensate.
   - Keep the weight as close to your body as possible.
   - When carrying a patient on stairs, use a stair chair instead of a stretcher when possible.

LABEL THE PHOTOGRAPHS (pp. 85–87)

1. Shoulder Drag
2. Incline Drag
3. Foot Drag
4. Clothes Drag

5. Firefighter's Drag
6. Blanket Drag
7. One-Rescuer Assist
8. Cradle Carry
9. Pack Strap Carry
10. Piggy Back Carry
11. Firefighter's Carry
12. Two-Rescuer Assist

VIRTUAL STREET SCENES

1. You can try to use the vest type immobilization device if she fits into it.

2. Just as long as the chest straps connect, the device should work to get her out of the car if you and your partners move her carefully. If the leg straps do not reach, you may need to omit them.

3. Obese people do not like to lie down because it makes breathing difficult. Once she is on a long backboard, the vest can be loosened and 10 foot straps can be used around the long backboard to secure her chest, pelvis, and legs.

Chapter 6: Airway Management

MATCH TERMINOLOGY/DEFINITIONS

▶ Part A

1. (D) Bronchi—the two large tubes that bring air to and from the lungs

2. (F) Cricoid cartilage—the ring-shaped structure that forms the lower portion of the trachea

3. (H) Diaphragm—the muscle of breathing that separates the abdomen from the thorax

4. (A) Epiglottis—the flap of tissue that caps the trachea as you swallow

5. (I) Exhalation—the process of breathing out

6. (B) Head-tilt, chin-lift maneuver—a means of correcting blockage of the airway by the tongue by tilting the head back and lifting the chin

7. (G) Inhalation—the process of breathing in

8. (J) Jaw-thrust maneuver—a means of correcting blockage of the airway by moving the jaw forward without tilting the head or neck

9. (E) Larynx—the voicebox, which contains the epiglottis and vocal cords

10. (C) Pharynx—the area inside the mouth joining the nasal passageways and the throat

▶ Part B

1. (G) Airway—the passageway by which air enters or leaves the body

2. (H) Artificial ventilation—forcing air or oxygen into the lungs when a patient has stopped breathing or has inadequate breathing

3. (B) Bag-valve mask (BVM)—a hand-held device with a face mask and self-refilling bag that can be squeezed to provide artificial ventilations to a patient

4. (I) Cyanosis—a blue or gray skin color resulting from lack of oxygen in the body

5. (A) Flow-restricted, oxygen-powered ventilation device—a device that uses oxygen under pressure to deliver artificial ventilation

6. (C) Gastric distention—expansion of the stomach caused by too forceful ventilation pressures, which cause excess air to enter the stomach instead of the lungs

7. (F) Humidifier—a device connected to the flowmeter to add moisture to the dry oxygen coming from an oxygen cylinder

8. (D) Respiration—another word for breathing

9. (E) Stoma—permanent surgical opening in the neck through which the patient breathes

10. (J) Ventilation—the breathing in of air or oxygen

▶ Part C

1. (N) Flowmeter—a valve that indicates the flow of oxygen in liters per minute

2. (K) Gag reflex—vomiting or retching that results when something is placed in the pharynx

3. (G) Hyperventilate—to provide ventilations at a higher rate to compensate for oxygen not delivered during suctioning

4. (M) Hypoxia—an insufficiency of oxygen in the body's tissues

5. (C) Nasal cannula—a device that delivers low concentrations of oxygen through two prongs that rest in the patient's nostrils

6. (A) Nasopharyngeal airway—a flexible breathing tube inserted through the patient's nose into the pharynx to help maintain an open airway

7. (B) Nonrebreather mask—a face mask and reservoir bag device that delivers high concentrations of oxygen. The patient's exhaled air escapes through a valve.

8. (J) Oropharyngeal airway—a rigid curved device inserted through the patient's mouth into the pharynx to help maintain an open airway

9. (H) Oxygen cylinder—container filled with oxygen under pressure

10. (E) Pocket face mask—a device, usually with a one-way valve, to aid in artificial ventilation. A rescuer breathes through the valve when the device is placed over the patient's face. It also acts as a barrier to prevent contact with a patient's breath or body fluids and can be used with supplemental oxygen when fitted with an oxygen inlet.

11. (O) Pop-off valve—a valve on a BVM designed to blow off excessive pressure; this valve is no longer allowed per AHA standards on any BVM due to the danger of underinflation of the lungs.

12. (D) Pressure regulator—a device connected to an oxygen cylinder to reduce cylinder pressure to a safe pressure for delivery of oxygen to a patient

13. (F) Respiratory arrest—when breathing completely stops

14. (L) Respiratory failure—the reduction of breathing to the point where not enough oxygen is being taken in to sustain life

15. (I) Suctioning—use of vacuum device to remove blood, vomitus, and other secretions or foreign materials from the airway

MULTIPLE-CHOICE REVIEW

1. (A) When we breathe in, or inspire, 21% oxygen enters the body (lungs); when we breathe out, or expire, carbon dioxide, the major waste product of respiration, and 16% oxygen exits the body. (p. 106)

2. **(B)** Respiratory failure is the reduction of breathing to a point where it is not sufficient to support life. Electrocution causes respiratory arrest, which is the cessation of breathing. (p. 106)

3. **(C)** Abdominal breathing, a sign of inadequate breathing, is the result of a patient using the abdomen to push up on the diaphragm in an effort to force air out of the lungs. Remember, however, infants and children normally use their abdominal muscles more than adults do. Look, listen, and feel for air exchange to determine adequate breathing; if air is entering and leaving the nose, mouth, and chest without abnormal sounds, and at a regular rate, the patient has adequate breathing. (p. 107)

4. **(D)** All are signs of inadequate breathing. Cyanosis is common in both adults and children. Retractions (a pulling in of muscles) above the clavicles and between and below the ribs, as well as nasal flaring, occur especially in children. (p. 107)

5. **(B)** In an adult, the normal respirations (in Table 6-1) are 12 to 20 a minute; therefore 14–18 is normal. (p. 108)

6. **(B)** When air can be felt at the mouth and nose, it may be a sign of adequate breathing. Remember, even if air can be felt at the mouth and nose, the respiratory rate must still be adequate for the breathing to be considered adequate. All other choices indicate signs of inadequate breathing. (pp. 106–107)

7. **(C)** When breathing is too slow or too fast, it can be inadequate. According to Table 6-1, for a child, that would be less than 15 per minute or greater than 30 per minute. (p. 108)

8. **(A)** According to Table 6-1, the normal adult breathing rate is 12 to 20 times a minute. (p. 108)

9. **(D)** All of the locations listed are correct, as well as the skin and lips. (p. 107)

10. **(C)** The short, choppy sentences are due to the patient being short of breath, therefore forcing him/her to take a breath between syllables. (p. 107)

11. **(D)** An open airway is paramount, since the patient who is not breathing deteriorates rapidly. This is a life-threatening situation. Open the airway, then clear the mouth and administer oxygen. (p. 107)

12. **(B)** Trauma victims require the jaw-thrust maneuver to open the airway. (p. 111)

13. **(B)** The head-tilt, chin-lift maneuver provides for the maximum opening of the airway on a patient with no suspected head, neck or spine injury. (p. 110)

14. **(A)** Do not allow the mouth to close when using a head-tilt, chin-lift or you will have difficulty ventilating the patient. (p. 110)

15. **(D)** Do not tilt or rotate the patient's head. All other choices are steps to perform the jaw-thrust maneuver. In addition, you will need to retract the patient's lower lip with your thumb to keep the mouth open. (p. 110)

16. **(B)** The jaw-thrust is used when you suspect possible neck, head, or spinal trauma. (p. 111)

17. **(C)** BVM is more effective with two rescuers. (p. 111)

18. **(C)** The patient's color would not improve if artificial ventilations were inadequate. (pp. 111–112)

19. **(A)** Each ventilation should be delivered over 1 to 1¹/₂ seconds for an adult. When oxygen is supplemented. (pp. 112–113)

20. **(B)** The BVM should have a self-refilling bag, a standard 15/22 mm fitting, and a non-jam valve with an oxygen inlet. Studies show that pop-off valves prevent adequate ventilations. (pp. 113–114)

21. **(A)** It is important for the BVM to perform in cold temperatures. High pressure in the chest and airway is not desirable as it increases gastric distention. As noted above, a pop-off (blow off) valve is also undesirable. The oxygen inlet flow should be 15 liters per minute. (pp. 113–114)

22. **(D)** When trauma is suspected, you should always use the jaw-thrust maneuver. All other answer choices are correct. Also make sure you use an airway and 100% oxygen reservoir system. (pp. 114–115)

23. **(D)** To be complete, all items listed must be used with the BVM when ventilating an unconscious patient. (pp. 113–114)

24. **(D)** Increasing the rate at which the bag is squeezed will <u>not</u> help. All other answer choices are correct. Also check for airway obstruction or obstruction in the BVM system. If all else fails, try a pocket mask. (pp. 114–115)

25. **(C)** Of the choices listed, the BVM is the best to use on a stoma, which is a surgical hole in the neck that creates an opening to the airway. (pp. 115–116)

26. **(D)** All are correct. In addition, the FROPVD should have a peak flow of 100% oxygen at up to 40 liters per minute. (p. 116)

27. **(C)** The main function of oral or nasal airways is to keep the tongue from blocking the airway. These airways are not reusable. A patient with an amputated hand is critically injured yet probably does not need an airway. When an airway adjunct is in place, you must still remain ready to suction the patient's airway. (pp. 116–117)

28. **(C)** A gag reflex causes vomiting or retching but not deep breaths or passing out. (pp. 116–117)

29. **(A)** The oropharyngeal airway is measured from the corner of the patient's mouth to the tip of the earlobe on the same side of the face. (pp. 117, 120)

30. **(C)** Both methods are acceptable, but the first method is preferred for adults. (pp. 117, 120)

31. **(B)** A nasopharyngeal airway should be measured from the patient's nostril to the earlobe (or angle of the jaw), which assures a proper diameter. Most nasopharyngeal airways are designed to be placed in the right nostril. The bevel should face toward the base of the nostril or toward the septum, which is in the medial portion of the nose. (p. 120)

32. **(D)** Always use a water-based lubricant. Petroleum and oil-based or silicone-based lubricants could cause aspiration pneumonia. (p. 120)

33. **(C)** The purpose of suctioning is to remove blood, vomitus, and other secretions. Teeth and large pieces need to be scooped out with a gloved hand. We try not to remove excess oxygen while suctioning. (p. 122)

34. **(A)** The suction unit is helpful in case the airway needs to be cleared. (p. 122)

35. **(C)** The Yankauer is most successfully used with an <u>unresponsive</u> patient, especially if the patient is not completely unresponsive or may be regaining consciousness. But caution must be used with rigid-tip suction; when the tip is placed into the pharynx, the gag reflex may be activated, producing additional vomiting. (pp. 122–123)

36. **(D)** All choices are incorrect. The length of the catheter that should be inserted into the patient's mouth is equal to the

distance between the corner of the patient's mouth and the earlobe. (p. 126)

37. **(C)** Never suction for longer than 15 seconds at a time, since supplemental oxygen or ventilations cease during suctioning. (p. 123)

38. **(A)** It is not necessary to measure when using a rigid-tip suction catheter. Rather, you should be sure not to lose sight of the tip when inserting it. (p. 126)

39. **(C)** The atmosphere provides 21% oxygen. Exhaled air has an oxygen concentration of 16%. (p. 126)

40. **(C)** Fully pressurized, a tank holds approximately 2,000 to 2,200 psi. (p. 127)

41. **(B)** An E cylinder is the largest portable cylinder of those listed, having 625 liters when full. The M cylinder is not a portable cylinder. (p. 127)

42. **(B)** Before connecting the regulator to the tank, the EMT-B should stand to the side and crack the valve slightly. This will clean the opening prior to attaching the regulator. Opening the valve before attaching the regulator will cause uncontrolled rushing of oxygen and is dangerous. Attach the nonrebreather mask to the regulator after it has been attached to the tank. (pp. 128–129)

43. **(C)** In short term use, the dryness of the oxygen is not a problem; however, the patient is usually more comfortable when given humidified oxygen. This is true if the patient has COPD or is a child. (p. 130)

44. **(A)** It is now widely believed that more harm is done by withholding high-concentration oxygen from COPD patients than could be done by administering it. (pp. 131–132)

45. **(D)** The nonrebreather mask provides oxygen concentrations from 80% to 100%. The nasal cannula and venturi are low concentration; the simple face mask is a medium concentration device. (pp. 132, 138)

46. **(D)** As noted above, the nonrebreather mask will provide concentrations of oxygen ranging from 80% to 100%. (pp. 132, 138)

47. **(B)** The maximum flow can range from 12 to 15 liters per minute. The reservoir bag must always contain enough oxygen so that it does not deflate by more than one-third when the patient takes his deepest inspiration. (pp. 132, 138)

48. **(C)** A nasal cannula provides low concentrations of oxygen between 24% and 44%. (p. 138)

COMPLETE THE FOLLOWING

1. The signs of inadequate breathing are: (any six) (p. 107)
   - Chest movements are absent, minimal, or uneven.
   - Movements associated with breathing are limited to the abdomen (abdominal breathing).
   - No air can be felt or heard at the nose or mouth, or the amount of air exchanged is below normal.
   - Breath sounds are diminished or absent.
   - Noises such as wheezing, crowing, stridor, snoring, gurgling, or gasping are heard during breathing.
   - The rate of breathing is too rapid or slow—above or below normal rates.
   - Breathing is very shallow, very deep, or appears labored.
   - The patient's skin, lips, tongue, earlobes, or nail beds are blue or gray.
   - Inspirations are prolonged or expirations are prolonged.
   - The patient is unable to speak, or the patient cannot

speak in full sentences because of shortness of breath.
   - In children, there may be retractions above the clavicles and between and below the ribs.
   - Nasal flaring may be present, especially in infants and children.

2. In order of preference, the four techniques available to the EMT-B to provide artificial ventilations are: (p. 111)
   - Mouth-to-mask (preferably with high-flow supplemental oxygen at 15 liters per minute).
   - Two-rescuer bag-valve mask (preferably with high-flow supplemental oxygen at 15 liters per minute).
   - Flow restricted, oxygen-powered ventilation device.
   - One-rescuer bag-valve mask.

LABEL THE DIAGRAM (p. 108)

1. Pharynx
2. Nasopharynx
3. Oropharynx
4. Epiglottis
5. Larynx
6. Thyroid cartilage
7. Cricoid cartilage
8. Trachea
9. Bronchiole
10. Left main bronchus
11. Right main bronchus
12. Diaphragm
13. Lungs

VIRTUAL STREET SCENES

1. An oropharyngeal (oral) airway. Try inserting one of the appropriate size straight in with a tongue depressor.

2. Quickly turn the patient onto his side, remove the airway adjunct and BVM, and allow him to vomit. Make sure you clear out the airway so he does not aspirate vomitus into his lungs.

3. Yes, consider an ALS unit. If one is not on scene when you are ready to transport, arrange an intercept en route to the hospital. ALS providers can intubate the patient and administer medication as needed.

CASE STUDY—The Complicated Airway: The Self-Inflicted Shooting

1. Open the patient's airway by jutting the jaw, if possible, or pulling the tongue forward away from the back of the throat.

2. **A)** Yes! The patient needs to be suctioned.

   B) The maximum time is about 15 seconds per attempt. Keep in mind, however, that you must adequately clear his airway so he does not aspirate any blood.

3. Yes, an oral or nasal airway would be helpful to this patient.

4. A bag-valve mask should be used to assist this patient's ventilations.

5. Use 12 to 15 liters per minute.

6. **A)** A full D tank has about 350 liters in it.

   B) A pressure of 2,000 to 2,200 pounds per square inch (psi).

   C) It takes about 19 minutes to run the tank down to 200 psi. (This is figured out by dividing 350 liters by 15 liters per minute, which equals 23 minutes.) Then use the formula from text page 129 for cylinder D.
   $$\frac{(2,000-200) \times 0.16}{15} = \frac{288}{15} = 19.2 \text{ minutes}$$

7. **A)** Don't exceed 15 seconds.

   B) You are removing oxygen when you suction the patient.

C) A rigid Yankauer suction tip is most appropriate in this patient.

8. **A)** This patient is a high priority.

   B) His complicated airway is the major problem making him a priority patient.

   C) He should be transported right away.

   D) Take him to a trauma center if there is one in your region.

9. The ALS (advanced life support) treatment that might be most helpful to this patient, if you can arrange for an ALS intercept, is endotracheal intubation.

10. If you hear hissing or bubbling around the mask as you ventilate, you should check the seal on the mask and reposition the mask if necessary. Also check the jutting of the jaw since it is possible the airway is not fully opened due to the presence of partial airway obstruction noises.

Interim Exam 1

1. **(C)** Most EMT-B courses today are based on models developed by the United States Department of Transportation (DOT). The American Red Cross (ARC) is involved in disaster relief and basic first aid and CPR training. The American Heart Association (AHA) is involved in basic and advanced cardiac life support as well as cardiovascular research. The National Institutes of Health (NIH) provides grants for health research. (p. 3)

2. **(D)** Being pleasant, cooperative, sincere, and a good listener inspires confidence in patients and bystanders. Do not put patient safety above your own, and do not lie to the patient by telling him/her everything is all right. (p. 8)

3. **(C)** Negligence is a failure to act properly in a situation in which there was a duty to act, needed care as would reasonably be expected of the EMT-B was not provided, and harm was caused to the patient as a result. Assault means you struck someone. Abandonment means you left the patient in no one's care. Breach of promise is a distracter. (p. 38)

4. **(D)** In order for a patient to refuse care or transport, he/she must be mentally competent, oriented fully, and informed of potential consequences of refusing care. Document the refusal on a release form. (pp. 34–35)

5. **(B)** In the case of an unconscious patient, consent may be assumed. This is known as implied consent. Triage is a French word that means "to sort." Immunity is a protection from lawsuits. Applied is a distracter. (pp. 33–34)

6. **(D)** Since the child's injury is not described as life-threatening, parental consent is still required. A minor cannot give actual consent. Only life-threatening situations involve implied consent. (pp. 33–34)

7. **(C)** Good Samaritan laws (in a number of states) grant immunity from liability to off-duty rescuers who act in good faith to provide care to the level of his training. (p. 39)

8. **(A)** Entering hazmat scenes with SCBA is not the responsibility of an EMT-B. Protecting yourself and others, recognizing potential problems, and notifying the hazardous-materials response team are the responsibilities of an EMT-B at a hazardous-materials incident. (p. 26)

9. **(B)** The form of infection control based on the presumption that all body fluids are infectious is called body substance isolation. Universal precautions are taken only in certain circumstances. An infectious disease is a reason to take BSI precautions. (p. 15)

10. **(D)** While the distance the object is to be carried is a consideration when planning to lift, it is not as important as the other factors. (p. 81)

11. **(C)** Use the leg muscles. Do not twist or use your back muscles while lifting; both may cause injury. (p. 81)

12. **(C)** Use the stair chair whenever possible. (pp. 89, 92)

13. **(C)** Keep your arms bent, <u>not</u> fully extended, when pushing or pulling objects. (p. 83)

14. **(D)** Unconsciousness is not a reason to use an emergency move. Use an urgent move for an unconscious patient. (pp. 84, 89)

15. **(A)** The greatest danger of an emergency move is that a spinal injury may be aggravated. (p. 84)

16. **(B)** This is an extremity lift. The draw-sheet method involves a sheet. The direct ground lift requires lifting the patient from a supine position onto the rescuer's knees and then to the stretcher. The direct carry involves two rescuers lifting and curling the patient into their chests, then returning to a standing position, and then walking together with the patient. (pp. 92, 96–98)

17. **(B)** When moving a patient from the ambulance stretcher to the hospital stretcher, you probably will use the modified draw sheet method. (pp. 99, 100)

18. **(A)** The EMT-Bs should move to opposite sides of the stretcher to load it into the ambulance. (p. 89)

19. **(B)** Patients without spinal injury or fractures can be moved to a stretcher, using the extremity lift. A slide transfer is from a bed to a bed. Chair lift and indirect carry are distracters. (p. 92)

20. **(A)** Drags are used only for emergencies because they do not protect the neck and spine. (p. 84)

21. **(B)** Use an even number of rescuers to lift patient carrying devices. Odd numbers will create an imbalance. (p. 82)

22. **(B)** In order to control the patient's airway and bleeding, use an urgent move, the rapid extrication procedure. Taking time to apply a short backboard may cause a deadly delay in removing the patient. (p. 84)

23. **(D)** The piggyback carry requires that the patient be conscious so he can hold on to the rescuer. (p. 86)

24. **(C)** The firefighter's carry is generally done in one sweeping motion. (p. 86)

25. **(C)** A flexible stretcher is used in narrow hallways or restricted areas to remove a patient without spinal injuries. (p. 92)

26. **(B)** Carefully drag the patient's clothing, trying to minimize further spinal injury. The other moves would not be used on a patient with a spinal injury. (p. 84)

27. **(C)** If the patient has no spinal injury and there are no space restrictions, then move the patient on the wheeled-ambulance stretcher. (p. 89)

28. **(D)** Proper personal protective equipment can prevent injuries to you and your crew. (p. 15)

29. **(A)** When a threat presents itself, retreat to a safe area. (p. 28)

30. **(B)** Eustress is positive stress. Distress is negative, can be cumulative, and may require a critical incident debriefing. (p. 24)

31. **(C)** When responding to a violent situation, observation begins when you enter the neighborhood or immediate area of the scene. (pp. 27–28)

32. **(B)** One crew member should always carry a portable radio to enable him to call for police assistance. (p. 27)

33. **(B)** Quickly control bleeding; then have the dog locked in another room so it doesn't try to protect its owner by attacking you. (p. 28)

34. **(C)** Treat life-threatening problems and transport a patient who refuses care and then becomes unconscious. (p. 35)

35. **(B)** An advance directive is the expressed wishes of the patient or family in writing. If one of these documents is signed and at the patient's side, it can simplify resuscitation situations. (pp. 35, 37–38)

36. **(C)** The oral wishes of the patient's family are not a reason to withhold medical care. (pp. 35, 37–38)

37. **(D)** Providing care within the scope of your practice, using proper documentation, and being courteous and respectful can prevent lawsuits. (p. 38)

38. **(D)** If you are proven negligent, you may be required to pay for the patient's lost wages, medical expenses, and pain and suffering. Generally, insurance costs would not be your responsibility. (p. 38)

39. **(D)** The skin, not the musculoskeletal system, regulates body temperature. The musculoskeletal system gives the body shape, protects internal organs, and provides for body movement. (pp. 60–62)

40. **(C)** The superior portion of the sternum is called the manubrium. (p. 53)

41. **(B)** The protrusion on the inside of the ankle is called the medial malleolus. The lateral malleolus is on the outside of the ankle. (p. 53)

42. **(B)** Automaticity is the ability of the heart to generate and conduct electrical impulses on its own. (p. 54)

43. **(A)** The autonomic nervous system, a division of the peripheral nervous system, controls involuntary motor functions. (p. 60)

44. **(B)** The anatomical position is a standard reference position for the body in which the body is standing erect, facing the observer. The arms are down at the sides, and the palms of the hands are forward. (p. 47)

45. **(A)** See answer #44. (p. 47)

46. **(D)** Plantar refers to the sole of the foot. (p. 48)

47. **(C)** The zygomatic bones are the cheekbones. (pp. 49, 52)

48. **(D)** The heart is superior, or above, the stomach. (p. 47)

49. **(B)** Knees are proximal, or closer, to the torso as compared to the toes. The toes are distal, or farther away, from the torso than are the knees. (pp. 47–48)

50. **(C)** Supine means lying on the back. Prone means lying face down. (p. 48)

51. **(C)** The abdomen is divided into four parts, or quadrants. (p. 48)

52. **(A)** The torso consists of the abdomen, pelvis, and thorax. (pp. 47–48)

53. **(A)** The heart is located in the center of the thoracic cavity. There is no such thing as the cardiac cavity. (p. 53)

54. **(C)** The structure that divides the chest from the abdominal cavity is the diaphragm. (p. 54)

55. **(C)** The kneecap is the patella. The ilium is a pelvic bone; the malleolus is in the ankle; and the phalanges are fingers and toes. (p. 53)

56. **(C)** The cranium is the skull minus the facial bones. (p. 49)

57. **(A)** The acromion process of the scapula is the highest portion of the shoulder. (p. 53)

58. **(C)** Good Samaritan Laws provide some limited immunity to EMS personnel in some states. (p. 39)

59. **(B)** Unconsciousness in adults or children allows implied consent, thus allowing for care to begin. (pp. 33–34)

60. **(C)** For negligence, three actions must be proved: the EMT had a duty to act; the EMT breached that duty; this breach of duty caused harm (physical or psychological) to the patient. (p. 38)

61. **(B)** Lying on the stomach face down is a prone position; recovery is on the side; and supine is lying face up. Coma is a distracter. (p. 48)

62. **(C)** In a trauma center, surgery teams are available all the time. (p. 5)

63. **(B)** The National Registry of Emergency Medical Technicians has established professional standards for EMS since 1970. (p. 9)

64. **(D)** Most patients are transported by ground ambulance. (p. 4)

65. **(B)** EMT-Intermediates are trained to start IVs, perform advanced airway procedures, and administer some medications beyond the EMT-B. (pp. 6–7)

66. **(B)** Quality improvement is a continuous self-review of the EMS system or service. (pp. 9–11)

67. **(B)** The Medical Director assumes the ultimate responsibility for the patient care aspects of the EMS system. (pp. 11–12)

68. **(A)** A common cause of lawsuits against EMS agencies is patients who refuse care. (pp. 34–35)

69. **(D)** The scope of practice defines the legal limits of the EMT-B's job. (p. 33)

70. **(A)** Decisiveness is not a sign of stress. (p. 24)

71. **(D)** Most motor-vehicle collisions don't result in excessive stress reactions. (pp. 23–24)

72. **(B)** Increasing consumption of fatty foods is the wrong reaction to stress. (p. 24)

73. **(A)** If you want to reduce stress, request a change in shift or work location. Increasing your workload in any way will further increase your stress level. (p. 24)

74. **(D)** After a CISD, a member of the peer team offers support and referrals to assist in coping and recovering. (pp. 24–25)

75. **(C)** After a major EMS incident, stress is normal and expected. (pp. 23–24)

76. **(B)** The five stages of grief include a stage where the patient may retreat to a world of his own. This is called depression. (p. 25)

77. **(D)** PPD (purified protein derivative) is a test that will detect exposure to tuberculosis; it is not a disease. EMS providers should be concerned with hepatitis B, tuberculosis, and HIV/AIDS. (p. 23)

78. **(C)** A disease spread by exposure to an open wound or sore of an infected individual is caused by a bloodborne pathogen. (p. 15)

79. **(D)** Hepatitis is an infection that causes inflammation of the liver. (p. 18)

80. **(C)** Airborne diseases are spread by inhaling or absorbing droplets from the air through the eyes, nose, or mouth. (p. 15)

81. **(D)** Hepatitis B virus kills approximately 200 health workers every year in the United States. (p. 18)

82. **(B)** Assume that a patient with a productive cough has TB. (p. 18)

83. **(D)** HIV is not an airborne disease; it is a bloodborne disease. (p. 18)

84. **(C)** There is about a 30% chance of spreading hepatitis B with an infected needle. (p. 19)

85. **(A)** There is about a 0.5% chance of spreading HIV with an infected needle. (p. 19)

86. **(C)** To protect yourself from TB, wear BSI equipment as well as a HEPA respirator. A surgeon's mask will not protect you from this airborne disease. (p. 22)

87. **(A)** Use a pocket mask with one-way valve when you are confronted with a nonbreathing patient and you are alone. The bag-valve mask needs two rescuers in order to be used effectively. You do not blow directly into the ET tube or the one-way valve. (p. 111)

88. **(C)** Handwashing after each patient contact is an effective method of infection control and will reduce others' exposure risks. (p. 17)

89. **(B)** The Ryan White CARE Act establishes procedures for emergency response workers to find out if they have been exposed to life-threatening infectious diseases. OSHA does not require this. There is no such thing as an AIDS protection act. (pp. 20–22)

90. **(A)** OSHA 1910.1030 requires an exposure control plan and annual training. (p. 20)

91. **(D)** The OSHA regulation requires that every employer of EMT-Bs provide hepatitis B vaccination. Insurance or annual physicals are not required. (p. 20)

92. **(D)** Engineering controls to prevent spread of infectious diseases include all those listed. (p. 20)

93. **(C)** The bloodborne pathogen OSHA standard does not address the use of HEPA respirators since they are used for an airborne disease (e.g. TB). (p. 20)

94. **(B)** High-risk locations for TB do not include day care centers since children are not prone to TB. (p. 22)

95. **(D)** Avoid approaching a scene with your lights and sirens on, since this attracts a crowd, which you wish to avoid. (p. 27)

96. **(A)** Notify police immediately if there may be any weapons at the scene. The police are responsible for weapons control; your responsibility is patient care. (p. 27)

97. **(A)** Respiratory failure is the reduction of breathing to the point where oxygen intake is not sufficient to support life. Respiratory support is what you provide. Respiratory arrest is when breathing stops. Anoxic metabolism occurs in the absence of breathing. (p. 106)

98. **(C)** Cyanosis, or blue or gray skin, is not a sign of adequate breathing. (pp. 106–107)

99. **(B)** Widening of the nostrils with respirations is called nasal flaring. Increased breathing rate is hyperventilation. Wheezes are a musical tone caused by spasms of the small airways. (p. 107)

100. **(B)** Blue or gray skin is called cyanosis. Anemia is a disease in which the patient has too few red blood cells. (p. 106)

101. **(C)** Inability to speak in full sentences is a sign of shortness of breath. Snoring is a noise made from a partial airway obstruction caused by the tongue. (p. 107)

102. **(B)** EMT-Bs do not routinely insert ET tubes. All other answers listed are principle procedures used by the EMT-B to treat life-threatening respiratory problems. (p. 107)

103. **(A)** The tongue causes most airway problems. (p. 110)

104. **(D)** If the unconscious patient was found at the bottom of a stairwell, you will need to assume a neck or spine injury and use the jaw-thrust maneuver. (p. 111)

105. **(B)** Since the one-rescuer bag-valve mask is the least effective in creating a seal, it would be the last choice. (p. 111)

106. **(C)** A ventilation rate that is too fast or too slow may result in inadequate artificial ventilation. (p. 112)

107. **(A)** The standard respiratory fitting on a bag-valve mask is 15/22 mm. (p. 113)

108. **(D)** A bag-valve mask should not have a pop-off valve. (p. 113)

109. **(C)** The proper bag-valve mask oxygen flow rate is 15 liters per minute. (p. 113)

110. **(A)** The American Heart Association guidelines state a minimum of 400 milliliters of air must be delivered to a patient when ventilating with the bag-valve mask supplemented with oxygen (p. 114)

111. **(C)** The first step in artificial ventilation of a stoma breather is to clear any mucus or secretions that may be obstructing the stoma. (p. 115)

112. **(A)** The audible alarm on the flow-restricted, oxygen-powered ventilation device should go off when the relief valve is activated but not when ventilation is activated. (p. 116)

113. **(B)** The oropharangeal and nasopharyngeal airways are the most common airway adjuncts. (p. 116)

114. **(D)** Use an oropharangeal airway on all unconscious patients with no gag reflex. Airway usage is not restricted to only medical or only trauma patients. (p. 117)

115. **(C)** When suctioning a patient, never suction for longer that 15 seconds. You do not hypoventilate, but do hyperventilate the patient prior to and after suctioning. Always wear eye protection and a mask when suctioning. Suction on the way out. (pp. 123, 126)

116. **(C)** The emergency situation in which there is a failure of the cardiovascular system to provide sufficient blood to all the vital tissues is called shock. (p. 126)

117. **(C)** Insufficiency in the supply of oxygen to the body's tissues is called hypoxia. Anoxia means no oxygen is being supplied to the cells. No-oxia is a distracter. Cyanosis is a result of hypoxia. (p. 127)

118. **(A)** Change the oxygen cylinder before the pressure gauge reads 200 psi, otherwise you may damage the inside of the tank. (p. 128)

119. **(C)** Store cylinders in a cool, dry area, not in a warm, humid room. (p. 128)

120. **(A)** Use a nonrebreather mask for high-concentration oxygen delivery to the breathing patient. We do not use partial rebreather masks in the field. A nasal cannula is a low-concentration device. (pp. 132, 138)

121. **(B)** The concentration of oxygen administered by a nasal cannula is between 24% and 44%. (p. 138)

122. **(B)** Do not remove the dentures unless they are loose. Dentures allow for an improved seal between the patient's face and mask. (p. 138)

123. **(A)** A child's mouth and nose are smaller and more easily obstructed than an adult's. The child's chest wall is softer. The trachea is narrower, so it is more easily obstructed. (p. 139)

124. **(A)** Respiratory arrest is complete breathing stoppage. (p. 106)

125. **(C)** The flow-restricted, oxygen-powered ventilation device is usually not used in children. Other devices listed are. (p. 116)

126. **(A)** A flowmeter allows the control of oxygen in liters per minute. A humidifier helps prevent the oxygen from being so dry. A reservoir is used on the BVM to increase the oxygen concentration. (pp. 129–130)

127. **(B)** The constant flow selector valve flowmeter allows for the control of the flow of oxygen in liters per minute in stepped increments. The Bourdon gauge and pressure compensated flowmeters are adjustable without stepped increments. (pp. 129–130)

128. **(A)** Some systems use oxygen humidification to prevent drying out the patient's mucous membranes. These devices actually increase the potential for infection spread and are usually not used in systems with short transports. (p. 130)

129. **(C)** Patients in the end stage of a respiratory disease are often on hypoxic drive. Carbon dioxide drive is the normal drive mechanism for healthy people. (p. 131)

130. **(D)** COPD is chronic obstructive pulmonary disease. (p. 131)

Chapter 7: Scene Size-up

MATCH TERMINOLOGY/DEFINITIONS

1. **(H)** Blunt-force trauma—injury caused by a blow that does not penetrate through the skin or body tissue

2. **(G)** CHEMTREC—agency that provides advice on hazardous materials via a hotline

3. **(D)** Danger zone—area around the wreckage of a vehicle collision or other incident within which special safety precautions should be taken

4. **(J)** Domestic violence—violence in the home

5. **(F)** High index of suspicion—keen awareness that a person may have injuries

6. **(E)** Law of inertia—principle that a body in motion will remain in motion unless acted on by an outside force

7. **(A)** Mechanism of injury—force or forces that may have caused injury

8. **(I)** *North American Emergency Response Guidebook*—material available for rescuers to obtain quick information about hazardous materials

9. **(B)** Penetrating trauma—injury caused by an object that passes through the skin and other body tissues

10. **(C)** Scene size-up—steps taken by an EMS crew when approaching, arriving, and attending at the scene of an emergency call to ensure the safety of the crew, the patient, and bystanders

MULTIPLE-CHOICE REVIEW

1. **(B)** Personal safety is your top priority. Determine dangers to yourself or other EMS providers from sources such as unstable vehicles, machinery, toxic exposure, or violence. If you and other crew members are not safe, you will be unable to continue with other steps in the scene size-up. (p. 145)

2. **(D)** Scene size-up is an ongoing process throughout the call. Emergencies are dynamic; events may change without warning. For example, family members who were docile when you first arrived could turn hostile; structures that were stable could become unstable. Keep alert at all times! (p. 145)

3. **(B)** Always conduct your own scene size-up, no matter how many rescue vehicles or personnel are at the scene when you arrive. Never assume a scene is safe because others may have taken care of the hazards. (p. 145)

4. **(D)** Always try to park your vehicle uphill from a collision scene. This way your ambulance will be out of the path of dense smoke if fuel ignites. The other actions listed are appropriate and necessary actions to take as you near a collision scene. (pp. 146, 149)

5. **(A)** When you are in sight of the collision scene, you should watch for the signals of police officers and other emergency service personnel because they may have information about hazards or the location of injured persons. Who is in charge depends on the type of incident. The police are not the medical care experts in most communities. (p. 146)

6. **(B)** When there are no apparent hazards, consider the danger zone to extend 50 feet in all directions from the wreckage. (pp. 146, 149)

7. **(C)** When a collision vehicle is on fire, consider the danger zone to extend at least 100 feet in all directions, even if the fire appears small and limited to the engine compartment. (p. 149)

8. **(A)** A good scene size-up should identify the potential for a violent situation. The name and amount of toxic substances would be difficult to determine during the scene size-up. The number of patients should be identified, but diagnosis is not the responsibility of the EMT-B. (pp. 149–150)

9. **(D)** An oxygen mask is not considered a piece of equipment used for BSI. The EMT-B's BSI equipment during the scene size-up may include eye protection, disposable gloves, and a mask. (pp. 150–151)

10. **(B)** The key element of body substance isolation is to always have personal protective equipment readily available. You only need to wear the BSI equipment when you might actually be exposed. BSI equipment is not placed on the patient. It is not practicable for the EMT-B to try to determine which body fluids are a danger. (pp. 150–151)

11. **(B)** Injuries to bones and joints are usually associated with falls and vehicle collisions. Fights usually produce blunt injuries, and drug usage often results in overdoses. Fires and explosions produce burns. Bullet wounds can cause damage to anything in their paths. (p. 151)

12. **(C)** Knowing the mechanism of injury assists the EMT-B in predicting various injury patterns. While it does not assist you in immobilizing the spine, it can tell you when immobilization may be needed. An EMT-B should always take BSI precautions. (p. 151)

13. **(C)** The law of inertia states that a body in motion will remain in motion unless acted on by an outside force. Centrifugal force is a force that explains why the faster you enter a turn the more your vehicle will be pulled straight. The formula for kinetic energy states that the mass or weight of an object is the least important contributor to the injury. (p. 151)

14. **(A)** An unrestrained driver involved in a head-on, up-and-over collision may injure his skull as well as the neck. Injuries to the fibula, knees, and femur are seen in the down-and-under pattern. (pp. 151, 153)

15. **(C)** The brake pedal is least likely to be a mechanism of injury in up-and-over and down-and-under collisions. In the up-and-over pattern, the patient commonly strikes his head on the windshield and may additionally strike his chest and abdomen on the steering wheel. In the down-and-under pattern, the patient typically strikes his knees on the dash. (pp. 151, 153)

16. **(C)** Knee, leg, and hip injuries are common in a head-on, down-and-under collision since the patient strikes the knees and the force is projected to the hips. The head-on, up-and-over collision produces head, neck, chest, and abdominal injuries. (p. 153)

17. **(D)** The roll-over collision is potentially the most serious because of the potential for multiple impacts. Roll-over collisions frequently cause ejection of anyone who is not wearing a seat belt. Expect any type of serious injury pattern. (p. 154)

18. **(D)** A patient who fell three times his height, a spiderweb crack in the windshield, or a broken steering column are examples of mechanisms of injury. A flat tire is not a mechanism of injury. (pp. 151, 153–154, 156)

19. **(A)** A severe fall for an adult is over 15 feet or three times the patient's height because a fall from this height will most likely involve a spinal injury. Falls from great heights are not always fatal because patients often strike objects that break their fall such as a canopy. (p. 156)

20. **(A)** A penetrating injury that is usually limited to the penetrated area is called a low-velocity injury. The medium- and high-velocity injuries have larger zones of damage due to cavitation in the tract of the projectile. (p. 156)

21. **(C)** The pressure wave around the bullet's tract through the body is called cavitation. Exsanguination is when a patient rapidly bleeds to death. Gas penetration can occur with air rifles. Pressure damage occurs only occasionally. (pp. 156, 157)

22. **(C)** An injury caused by a blow that strikes the body but does not penetrate the skin is called blunt-force trauma. There is no such term as inertia trauma. Cavitation is defined in answer #21. Rotational impact is a type of automobile collision. (p. 156)

23. **(B)** It would most likely be necessary for you and your partner to call for additional assistance lifting the 350-pound patient with the broken leg. Two patients with flu-like symptoms, especially if one is a child, could easily be handled in one ambulance. The patient with a deep laceration in his right forearm could be handled by you and your partner. The patient who loses consciousness while you are carrying her to the ambulance should be managed immediately by you and your partner. (pp. 157–159)

24. **(A)** While in the living room of a private house treating a patient for nausea, headache, and general body weakness, your eyes begin to tear and three family members have the same symptoms. You should immediately evacuate all people from the building. Don't automatically call for three additional ambulances until you evaluate the situation. It may be a local protocol to notify the police department, but notifying the fire department is more appropriate in this situation. Any flushing of the eyes should be done after determining the nature of the substance. (pp. 157–159)

25. **(B)** If the number of patients is more than the responding units can effectively handle, the EMT-B should call for additional EMS resources immediately. (pp. 157–159)

COMPLETE THE FOLLOWING

1. The four parts of the scene size-up include: (p. 145)
   - Scene safety
   - Mechanism of injury or nature of illness
   - Number of patients
   - Additional resources

2. The five signs of danger from violence that you may observe as you approach the scene are: (pp. 149–150)
   - Fighting or loud voices
   - Weapons visible or in use
   - Signs of alcohol or other drug use
   - Unusual silence
   - Knowledge of prior violence

3. Five types of motor vehicle collisions include: (pp. 153–154)
   - Head-on
   - Rear-end
   - Side-impact
   - Rollover
   - Rotational impact

VIRTUAL STREET SCENES

1. Try to find out what the chemical is from the driver. Let the dispatcher know right away that this is a hazardous-materials incident. (You will learn more about such incidents when you read Chapter 34.)

2. You must follow your local protocols in such a situation. In general, if you are alone, you should retreat to a position of safety, call for help, and return only after the scene has been secured by the police.

Chapter 8: The Initial Assessment

MATCH TERMINOLOGY/DEFINITIONS

1. **(H)** Alert—awake and oriented

2. **(F)** AVPU—memory aid used to keep levels of responsiveness in mind

3. **(C)** Capillary refill—method of assessing circulation in a pediatric patient

4. **(D)** Chief complaint—reason EMS was called

5. **(E)** General impression—part of the EMT-B's evaluation that includes assessment of the environment and the patient's chief complaint and appearance

6. **(A)** Initial assessment—steps taken by the EMT-B for the purpose of discovering and dealing with a patient's life-threatening problems

7. **(G)** Interventions—actions taken to correct a patient's problems

8. **(B)** Mental status—level of a patient's responsiveness

9. **(J)** Responsive—ability to respond to stimuli

10. **(I)** Unresponsive—lack of response to any stimuli

MULTIPLE-CHOICE REVIEW

1. **(D)** The assessment of blood pressure is not part of the initial assessment. It is part of taking vital signs, which is performed after the initial assessment and is discussed further in Chapter 9. (p. 163)

2. **(D)** The patient's past medical history is <u>not</u> part of the general impression. (p. 163)

3. **(C)** Drug-use paraphernalia may give clues about the cause of the patient's problem. The dark alley is not a helpful clue. The bruise is not an environmental indicator. You would not know the patient's medical history at this point. (pp. 163–164)

4. **(B)** Clinical judgment is the development of that sixth sense that provides clues to the severity of the patient's condition. EMT-Bs do not judge patients for mental status—we test it. EMT-Bs never make a diagnosis. (pp. 163–164)

5. **(D)** When forming a general impression, always look, listen, and smell. Note the patient's age and sex and look at the patient's position. Listen for sounds such as moaning or gurgling. Smell for hazardous fumes, urine, feces, vomitus, or decay. (pp. 163–164)

6. **(B)** Rubbing the patient's sternum briskly is the most common way to determine the patient's level of responsiveness. Ammonia inhalants can cause injury. The ice trick doesn't work. Pressing on the person's nail beds is a way of assessing capillary refill. (p. 164)

7. **(D)** AVPU stands for alert, verbal, painful stimuli, unresponsive. (p. 164)

8. **(C)** See answer #7. (p. 164)

9. **(B)** See answer #7. (p. 164)

10. **(B)** The unresponsive patient will be a higher priority and in need of quicker transport. The jaw-thrust maneuver is usually not used on responsive patients unless they have head, neck, or spinal injuries. (p. 169)

11. **(D)** If a patient is not alert and his breathing rate is slower than 8, provide positive-pressure ventilations with 100% oxygen. (p. 169)

12. **(B)** An alert patient with a breathing rate faster than 24 warrants high-concentration oxygen via nonrebreather. (p. 169)

13. **(D)** The circulation assessment includes evaluating pulses, skin (condition, color, and temperature), and bleeding. The blood pressure is a vital sign taken moments after the initial assessment. (p. 169)

14. **(D)** Good circulation exhibits as warm, dry, and normal in color provided the assessment is not complicated by the environment in which you find the patient (e.g., rain or cold). (p. 169)

15. **(C)** Poor circulation exhibits as cool, pale, and moist skin. Increased perfusion and high blood pressure may show as flushed colored skin. Cold exposure exhibits as red in early stages, and then pale to cyanotic in prolonged cases. (p. 169)

16. **(A)** To evaluate skin color or the presence of jaundice or cyanosis on a dark-skinned patient, look at the lips or nail beds. (p. 169)

17. **(C)** If even one large vessel or several smaller ones are bleeding, a patient can lose enough blood in a minute or two to die. Severe blood loss is life-threatening. (p. 169)

18. **(B)** Any life threats observed during the initial assessment should be treated immediately. (p. 169)

19. **(D)** High priority conditions include poor general impression, unresponsive, responsive but not following commands, difficulty breathing, shock, complicated childbirth, chest pain with systolic blood pressure less than 100, uncontrolled bleeding, severe pain anywhere. (p. 169)

20. **(C)** Uncomplicated childbirth is not a priority. See answer #19. (p. 169)

COMPLETE THE FOLLOWING

1. List the six steps of the initial assessment. (p. 163)
   - Form a general impression
   - Assess mental status
   - Assess airway
   - Assess breathing
   - Assess circulation
   - Determine priority

2. State what the letters in AVPU stand for. (p. 164)
   A = alert—awake and oriented (person, place, and day)
   V = verbal—responds to verbal stimuli
   P = painful—responds to painful stimuli
   U = unresponsive—does not respond to any stimuli

3. List five high priority conditions. (any five) (p. 169)
   - Poor general impression
   - Unresponsive
   - Responsive, but not following commands
   - Difficulty breathing
   - Shock
   - Complicated childbirth
   - Chest pain with systolic pressure less than 100
   - Uncontrolled bleeding
   - Severe pain anywhere

VIRTUAL STREET SCENES

1. The airway is always the highest priority. Suction the patient's airway while maintaining spinal stabilization. Once the airway is clear, administer high-concentration oxygen.

2. This patient is a high priority. ALS would be helpful for intubation and another set of trained hands.

3. Even though the patient seems to be okay, it is always a good idea to be checked in the hospital due to the potential for aspiration or damage to the structures of the airway.

Chapter 9: Vital Signs and SAMPLE History

▶ **Part A**

1. **(L)** Auscultation—when a stethoscope is used to listen for characteristic sounds

2. **(C)** Blood pressure—force of blood against the walls of the blood vessels

3. **(J)** Brachial artery—major artery of the arm

4. **(B)** Bradycardia—slow pulse; any pulse rate below 60 beats per minute

5. **(D)** Carotid pulse—pulse felt along the large artery on either side of the neck

6. **(N)** Constrict—to get smaller

7. **(M)** Dilate—to get larger

8. **(A)** Diastolic blood pressure—pressure remaining in the arteries when the left ventricle of the heart relaxes and refills

9. **(E)** Palpation—feeling with the fingertips

10. **(H)** Pulse—rhythmic beats felt as the heart pumps blood through the arteries

11. **(I)** Pulse quality—rhythm (regular or irregular) and force (strong or weak) of the pulse

12. **(F)** Pulse rate—number of pulse beats per minute

13. **(K)** Pupil—black center of the eye

14. **(O)** Radial pulse—pulse felt at the wrist on the lateral (thumb) side

15. **(G)** Reactivity—reacting to light by changing size such as occurs in the pupils of the eyes

▶ **Part B**

1. **(A)** Respiratory quality—normal or abnormal (shallow, labored, noisy) character of breathing

2. **(B)** Respiratory rate—number of breaths a person takes in one minute

3. **(E)** Respiratory rhythm—regular or irregular spacing of breaths

4. **(F)** SAMPLE history—information about the present problems (signs and symptoms) and past medical history of a patient

5. **(G)** Sign—an indication of a patient's condition that is objective—something you see, hear, feel, or smell

6. **(I)** Sphygmomanometer—cuff and gauge used to measure blood pressure

7. **(H)** Symptom—an indication of a patient's condition that cannot be observed but rather is subjective—something felt and reported by the patient

8. **(D)** Systolic pressure—pressure created when the heart contracts and forces blood into the arteries

9. **(C)** Tachycardia—rapid pulse; any pulse rate above 100 beats per minute

10. **(J)** Vital signs—outward signs of what is going on inside the body, including respiration; pulse; skin color, temperature, and condition; pupils; and blood pressure

MULTIPLE-CHOICE REVIEW

1. **(D)** Pulse oximetry is not officially considered a vital sign. The respiratory rate and quality, skin color and condition, and the pulse rate and quality are all vital signs. (p. 179)

2. **(B)** A sign that gives important information about the patient's condition but is <u>not</u> considered a "vital sign" is the mental status. All other signs listed are vital signs. (pp. 179–180)

3. **(B)** Vital signs should be recorded as they are obtained to prevent you from forgetting them and to note the time they were taken. The vitals can change quickly as the patient's condition changes. They are taken at least twice to develop trends in vital signs. The first measurements you take are called baseline vital signs. (pp. 179–180)

4. **(D)** When a patient's pulse rate exceeds 100 beats per minute, this is called tachycardia. See Table 9-1 for normal pulse rates and possible causes of change in pulse quality. (p. 180)

5. **(D)** Based upon the pulse alone, a sign that something may be seriously wrong with a patient could be a sustained rate below 50 beats per minute, a sustained rate above 120 beats per minute, and/or a rate above 150 beats per minute. (pp. 180–181)

6. **(B)** In addition to answer # 5, another serious indicator found in the pulse may be an irregular rhythm. An athlete with a pulse of 50 is not unusual because aerobic training will lower the at-rest pulse. Exercise normally increases the pulse rate. (p. 182)

7. **(C)** The quality of the pulse includes determining the rhythm and force. (p. 182)

8. **(C)** A patient described as having a "thready" pulse has a weak pulse. See Table 9-1. (p. 182)

9. **(C)** The normal pulse rate for a school-age child (6–10 years) is 70 to 110. See Table 9-1. (p. 181)

10. **(A)** The normal pulse rate for an adult is 60 to 100. See Table 9-1. (p. 181)

11. **(B)** The pulse at the thumb side of the wrist is referred to as the radial pulse. The femoral pulse is in the thigh. The carotid pulse is in the neck. The brachial pulse is in the arm. (p. 182)

12. **(C)** When assessing the carotid pulse, the EMT-B should be aware that excessive pressure can slow the heart, especially in older patients. Never assess the carotid pulses on both sides at the same time. (p. 182)

13. **(C)** The number of breaths a patient takes in one minute is called the respiratory rate. (p. 183)

14. **(A)** The respiratory rate is classified as normal, slow, or rapid. The respiratory <u>quality</u> is classified as normal, shallow, labored, or noisy. The pulse force is classified as weak, thready, or full. (pp. 183–184)

15. **(C)** If the EMT-B is treating a patient with a sustained respiratory rate above 24 or below 8 breaths per minute, high-concentration oxygen must be administered. Also be prepared to assist ventilations. (p. 183)

16. **(B)** The normal respiration rate for an adult at rest is 12 to 20. See Table 9-2. (p. 183)

17. **(C)** The normal respiration rate for a toddler (1–3 years) is 20 to 30. See Table 9-2. (p. 183)

18. **(A)** Shallow breathing occurs when there is only slight movement of the chest or abdomen. If there is stridor or grunting on expiration, this indicates an airway obstruction. The chest muscles normally expand fully with each breath. (p. 183)

19. **(B)** Many resting people breathe more with their diaphragm than with their chest muscles. (p. 183)

20. **(D)** Delayed capillary refill is <u>not</u> a sign of labored breathing. When a patient has labored breathing, he/she may have an increase in the work of breathing, use of accessory muscles, nasal flaring, and retractions above the collarbones. (p. 183)

21. **(C)** A harsh, high-pitched sound heard on inspiration when a patient has labored breathing is called stridor. Nasal flaring, grunting, and gurgling are signs of upper airway problems. (p. 183)

22. **(C)** When the quality of a patient's respirations are abnormal due to something blocking the flow of air, this is referred to as noisy breathing. Sounds to be concerned with are snoring, wheezing, gurgling, and crowing. (pp. 183–184)

23. **(A)** A sound made by the patient that usually indicates the need to suction the airway is called gurgling. Crowing and stridor are upper airway noises. Wheezing is usually an indication of a lower airway problem. (p. 184)

24. **(B)** The best places to assess skin color in adults are the inside of the cheek and the nail beds as well as the inside of the lower eyelids. (p. 184)

25. **(C)** Blood loss, shock, hypotension, or emotional distress may result in pale skin. Jaundiced skin is due to liver abnormalities. See Table 9-3. (p. 184)

26. **(D)** A patient with a lack of oxygen in the red blood cells resulting from inadequate breathing or heart function will exhibit cyanotic skin. Pink skin is normal; pale skin is due to shock; and flushed skin is a result of hypertension. See Table 9-3. (pp. 184–185)

27. **(D)** The skin of a patient who has liver abnormalities may appear jaundiced, or yellow tinged. See Table 9-3. (pp. 184–185)

28. **(B)** Cold, dry skin is frequently associated with exposure to cold. Shock and anxiety would result in skin that is cool and clammy. See Table 9-4. (p. 185)

29. **(A)** Hot, dry skin is frequently associated with high fever or heat exposure. See Table 9-4. (p. 185)

30. **(C)** If you notice that the patient's right arm is much cooler than the rest of the patient's body, this should lead you to consider a circulatory system problem. (p. 185)

31. **(B)** If you press on a child's nail bed and watch how long it takes for the normal pink color to return, you are testing for capillary refill. Normally, this action takes no more than 2 seconds. If it takes longer, the patient's blood is probably not circulating well. (p. 185)

32. **(B)** If a patient is in direct sunlight or very bright conditions, the EMT-B should test the pupils by covering the patient's eyes for a few moments, then uncovering one eye at a time. (pp. 185–186)

33. **(D)** A patient in shock does not normally have unequal pupils. The pupils may be unequal due to stroke, head injury, or eye injury. See Table 9-5. (pp. 185–186)

34. **(B)** Fright, blood loss, drugs, and treatment with eye drops may cause the patient's pupils to become dilated. Constricted pupils are often due to narcotics. Unequal pupils are addressed in answer #33. (pp. 185–186)

35. **(A)** When the left ventricle of the heart relaxes and refills, the pressure in the arteries is called the diastolic pressure. (p. 186)

36. **(B)** The pulse oximeter should be used with patients complaining of respiratory problems. It is inaccurate with hypothermic or shock patients, and may produce falsely high readings in patients with carbon monoxide poisoning. (p. 190)

37. **(A)** The pulse oximeter is helpful because it encourages you to be more aggressive about providing oxygen therapy. (p. 190)

38. **(C)** The oximeter will produce falsely high readings in patients with carbon monoxide poisoning. (p. 190)

39. **(B)** Chronic smokers may have a pulse oximeter reading that is higher than normal. (p. 190)

40. **(C)** The normal pulse oximeter reading for a healthy person should be between 95% and 100% (p. 190)

COMPLETE THE FOLLOWING

1. The five vital signs are: (p. 179)
   - pulse
   - respiration
   - pupils
   - blood pressure

- skin (temperature, color, condition)

2. The components of the SAMPLE history include: (p. 191)
   Signs & symptoms
   Allergies
   Medications
   Pertinent past history
   Last oral intake
   Events leading to the injury or illness

LABEL THE DIAGRAM (p. 182)

1. carotid
2. brachial
3. radial
4. femoral
5. pedal

VIRTUAL STREET SCENES

1. No. The patient had a chief complaint of abdominal pain, which cannot be diagnosed and treated in the field, especially in an elderly patient.

2. Normal ranges for an adult are respirations between 12 and 20, pulse between 60 and 100, systolic blood pressure between 90 and 150, and diastolic blood pressure between 60 and 90.

3. Yes, as you would any information pertinent to the patient's current condition. (Black, tarry stools often indicate bleeding into the intestines or lower gastrointestinal tract.)

Chapter 10: Assessment of the Trauma Patient

1. **(E)** Colostomy—surgical opening in the wall of the abdomen with a bag in place to collect excretions from the digestive system

2. **(N)** Contusion—a bruise

3. **(O)** Crepitation—grating sensation or sound made when fractured bones rub against each other

4. **(F)** DCAP-BTLS—memory aid, the initials of which stand for deformities, contusions, abrasions, punctures/penetrations, burns, tenderness, lacerations, and swelling

5. **(L)** Detailed physical exam—an assessment of the head (including face, ears, eyes, nose, and mouth), neck, chest, abdomen, pelvis, extremities, and posterior of the body to detect signs and symptoms of injury.

6. **(K)** Distention—condition of being stretched, inflated, or larger than normal

7. **(I)** Focused history and physical exam—step of patient assessment that follows the initial assessment

8. **(H)** Jugular vein distention—bulging of the neck veins

9. **(J)** Laceration—a cut

10. **(B)** Paradoxical motion—movement of part of the chest in the opposite direction from the rest of the chest during respiration

11. **(C)** Priapism—persistent erection of the penis that can result from spinal cord injury or certain medical problems

12. **(D)** Rapid trauma assessment—quick assessment of the head, neck, chest, abdomen, pelvis, extremities, and posterior body to detect signs of injury

13. **(M)** Stoma—permanent surgical opening in the neck through which the patient breathes

14. **(A)** Tenderness—found upon palpation of a body part

15. **(G)** Tracheostomy—surgical incision in the neck held open by a metal or plastic tube

MULTIPLE-CHOICE REVIEW

1. **(C)** The EMT-B inspects and palpates each body part during the focused physical exam. He/she does not auscultate, or listen, to every body part; nor does he/she percuss, or tap, to elicit a tone from each body part. (pp. 199–201)

2. **(D)** The memory aid for the physical exam is DCAP-BTLS. D = deformities, C = contusions, A = abrasions, P = punctures/perforations, B = burns, T = tenderness, L = lacerations, S = swelling. (p. 199)

3. **(B)** contusions. See answer #2. (p. 199)

4. **(D)** abrasions. See answer #2. (p. 199)

5. **(A)** punctures/penetrations. See answer #2. (p. 199)

6. **(C)** swelling. See answer #2. (p. 199)

7. **(B)** A deformity is an abnormal shaped body part. A hematoma is a collection of blood under the skin. A fracture is a broken bone. Crepitation is the sound or feel of broken bones rubbing against each other. (p. 199)

8. **(B)** Burns involve reddened, blistered, or charred looking areas. An abrasion is a scrape. A laceration is a cut, and a contusion is a bruise. (p. 199)

9. **(C)** Tenderness is usually not evident until you palpate the patient. Pain is usually present even without applying pressure, or palpation, at least until another stronger pain source overrides it. (p. 199)

10. **(A)** When capillaries bleed under the skin, this is called swelling. Punctures, lacerations, and abrasions are types of soft-tissue injuries. (p. 199)

11. **(A)** If the mechanism of injury exerts great force on the upper body, a cervical collar would be appropriate. In addition, apply a cervical collar if there is any soft-tissue damage to the head, face, or neck from trauma, if there has been a blow above the clavicles (collarbone), if the trauma patient has an altered mental status, or if injury cannot be ruled out—even if the mechanism of injury is not known. (pp. 201–202)

12. **(A)** Any blow above the clavicles may damage the cervical spine. (pp. 201–202)

13. **(B)** Experienced EMT-Bs refer to soft collars as "neck warmers" because that is about all they are good for. Soft collars are inappropriate for field use because of their inability to provide rigid support. (p. 202)

14. **(B)** A cervical collar that is the wrong size may make breathing more difficult or obstruct the airway. The collar does not cause the spine injury although mishandling it may do so. (pp. 201–202)

15. **(D)** Cervical immobilization is based upon the trauma patient's level of responsiveness, mechanism of injury, and location of injuries. (pp. 201–202)

16. **(C)** If you are applying a collar on the patient's neck, be sure to assess the neck before you cover it with the collar. (p. 202)

17. **(C)** A roll-over collision, a motorcycle collision, a pedestrian struck by a vehicle, or an adult who fell more than three times his height (which often involves a spine injury) are significant mechanisms of injury. (pp. 202, 210)

18. **(B)** When a patient is unrestrained in the front seat of an auto involved in a collision, the tell-tale sign is a spider-web crack in the windshield. This is also a sign that the patient went "up and over" to sustain the injury, rather than "down and under," which would present with leg injuries. (pp. 202, 210)

19. **(C)** Airbags minimize lacerations caused by the head striking the windshield. However, airbags can hide signs that could help you predict the severity of injuries caused by the collision. Be sure to move the collapsed bag and examine the steering wheel, which may give clues to the extent of the impact on the patient's chest. (p. 210)

20. **(C)** When assessing the head, do DCAP-BTLS and listen for crepitation, the sound or feel of broken bones rubbing against each other. (p. 212)

21. **(A)** When assessing the neck, do DCAP-BTLS and observe for jugular vein distention (JVD). The other responses are all parts of DCAP-BTLS. (p. 212)

22. **(B)** Neck veins should be flat and not visible when a patient is sitting up. Flat neck veins in a patient who is lying down, however, may be a sign of blood loss. (p. 212)

23. **(B)** When assessing the chest, in addition to DCAP-BTLS, inspect/palpate for paradoxical motion, movement of part of the chest in the opposite direction from the rest of the chest. This is a sign of serious injury since it indicates a great deal of force was applied to the patient's chest. (pp. 212–213)

24. **(B)** When assessing the abdomen, in addition to DCAP-BTLS, check to see if the patient has a colostomy and/or ileostomy, a surgical opening in the wall of the abdomen with a bag in place to collect excretions from the digestive system. (p. 213)

25. **(C)** When assessing the pelvis, in addition to DCAP-BTLS, check for priapism (persistent erection of the penis), a sign of a potential spinal-cord injury. (pp. 213, 215)

26. **(A)** The rapid trauma assessment is similar to the detailed physical exam except the rapid trauma assessment is less detailed and done more quickly. (pp. 219–220)

27. **(B)** Critical trauma patients do not always have a detailed physical exam, especially on the scene. Performing a detailed physical exam is always a lower priority than addressing life-threatening problems. (p. 219)

28. **(A)** The detailed physical exam is more specific than the rapid trauma assessment when it comes to assessing the head. You should assess the face, ears, eyes, nose, and mouth. (pp. 219–220)

29. **(B)** The final step of the detailed physical exam is to reassess the vital signs. (p. 225)

30. **(C)** A bruise behind the ear is called Battle's sign, which is indicative of a basilar skull fracture. (p. 220)

31. **(C)** Blood in the anterior chamber (front) of the eye tells you the eye is bleeding inside and that the patient's eye has sustained significant force. (p. 220)

32. **(B)** Clear fluid draining from the ears and nose is called cerebrospinal fluid. Mucous fluid lines the respiratory tract. Lymph bathes the cells and circulates throughout the body. Synovial fluid is in the joints. (p. 220)

33. **(D)** You do _not_ look for crepitation. The other choices are specific to the mouth. (p. 220)

34. **(C)** The detailed physical exam is not designed for a medical patient because there are usually few signs that an EMT-B can find in the physical exam of a medical patient that are significant or about which you can or should do anything. (p. 226)

35. **(C)** The safest and best thing to do for a patient who could

be either medical or trauma is to generally treat him/her as a trauma patient who receives the rapid trauma assessment, and if there is time, a detailed physical exam. Whenever possible, also obtain a history from any witnesses you can find. (p. 226)

COMPLETE THE FOLLOWING

1. The components of the focused history and physical exam for the trauma patient who is found with significant mechanism of injury are as follows: (p. 202)
   - Reconsider the mechanism of injury.
   - Continue spine stabilization.
   - Consider a request for advanced life-support personnel.
   - Reconsider your transport decision.
   - Reassess mental status.
   - Perform a rapid trauma assessment.
   - Assess baseline vital signs.
   - Obtain a SAMPLE history.

2. The components of the rapid trauma assessment include: (p. 212)
   - Head
   - Neck (Apply cervical collar after the neck has been assessed.)
   - Chest
   - Abdomen
   - Pelvis
   - Extremities
   - Posterior

LABEL THE PHOTOGRAPHS (p. 200)

1. Deformities
2. Contusions
3. Abrasions
4. Punctures/Penetrations
5. Burns
6. Tenderness
7. Lacerations
8. Swelling

COMPLETE THE CHART (p. 201)

1. Crepitation
2. JVD
3. Crepitation
4. Paradoxical motion
5. Crepitation
6. Breath sounds
7. Firmness
8. Softness
9. Distention
10. Pain
11. Tenderness
12. Motion
13. Distal pulse
14. Motor function
15. Sensation

VIRTUAL STREET SCENES

1. If assessment reveals respirations less than 12, greater than 28, or very shallow, you should immediately use the BVM to assist ventilation.

2. Yes, call for ALS. A patient with an open chest wound needs advanced care. If possible, arrange for ALS to intercept you en route to the hospital.

3. Emergency care priorities would be to maintain the airway and adequate ventilation of the patient.

4. If the patient is injured on the left side of the chest at the mid-clavicular line at nipple level, a lung and the heart may be injured.

CASE STUDY—Motorcycle Mishap

1. Body substance isolation—protect yourself from the blood and other body fluids found on the patient.

2. Scene safety—most notably the traffic

3. Mechanism of injury—a two-vehicle collision

4. The number of patients

5. Forming a general impression helps you to determine how serious the patient's condition is, which helps you set priorities for care and transport. The general impression is based on an immediate assessment of the environment and the patient's chief complaint and appearance. It gives you an idea of the sex and age of the patient, what happened and why EMS was called, whether the patient is injured or ill, and the severity of the patient's condition.

6. One of your partners should be holding manual stabilization of the patient's head and neck.

7. The patient appears to be alert, or "A" on the AVPU scale.

8. His broken legs may not be the worst problem, and you must assess him for life-threatening injuries first.

9. The initial assessment for Tony should consist of forming a general impression, assessing mental status (both of which you have already done), assessing his ABCs (airway, breathing, and circulation), and determining priority.

10. Signs of developing shock make Tony a high-priority patient. (You'll learn more about shock in Chapter 26.)

11. Call for ALS right away. If they are not there by the time Tony is packaged, then try to arrange a quick meeting en route to the hospital; but do not delay transport waiting for an ALS unit to arrive.

12. Deformities, Contusions, Abrasions, Punctures/penetrations, Burns, Tenderness, Lacerations, Swelling

13. Signs and symptoms, Allergies, Medications, Pertinent past medical history, Last oral intake, Events leading up to incident

14. Assess respirations, pulse, blood pressure, skin (color, condition, temperature)

15. A detailed physical exam of Tony would include an assessment of everything examined in the rapid trauma assessment, plus the face, ears, eyes, nose, and mouth.

Chapter 11: Assessment of the Medical Patient

MATCH TERMINOLOGY/DEFINITIONS

1. (I) Chief complaint—reason why EMS was called, usually in patient's own words.

2. (F) Medical identification device—necklace, bracelet or other device designed to notify emergency personnel that a patient has a specific medical history or condition

3. (H) Onset of pain— description of how fast or slow the pain came on and what the patient was doing when the pain started

4. (E) OPQRST—memory jogger designed to remind the EMT-B of what questions to ask the patient about his chief complaint.

5. (J) Prior history—history relating to the patient's chief complaint

6. (C) Provocation of pain—description of what makes the pain worse, such as sitting, standing, or eating certain foods

7. **(B)** Quality of pain—description of the pain, such as stabbing, crampy, dull, or sharp

8. **(A)** Radiation of pain—description of where pain is located and where it spreads to

9. **(D)** Severity of pain—description of how bad the pain is, often described on a scale of 1 to 10

10. **(G)** Vial of Life—medicine-like bottle kept in the patient's refrigerator that contains a listing of his past medical history

MULTIPLE-CHOICE REVIEW

1. **(D)** The rapid trauma exam is not used on a responsive medical patient. (p. 233)

2. **(B)** OPQRST is a memory aid to help the EMT-B remember questions that expand on the history of the present illness. The letters stand for onset, provides quality, radiation, severity, and time. (p. 237)

3. **(B)** Something that triggers the pain is what provokes it. Onset is when the pain started. Quality is a description of the type of pain. Radiation is where the pain is located and where it spreads. (p. 237)

4. **(B)** "How bad is the pain?" is a severity question usually evaluated on a scale of 1 to 10. (p. 237)

5. **(C)** "T" stands for time (the time the pain started). (p. 237)

6. **(A)** Vomiting is a sign of various medical illnesses. (p. 237)

7. **(B)** "P" in SAMPLE is for pertinent past history. (p. 237)

8. **(C)** "How have you felt today?" is a questions about the events leading up to the illness. (p. 237)

9. **(D)** Patients may carry an inhaler, nitroglycerin, or an epinephrine kit with them. You may need to contact the Medical Director to gain permission to assist the patient with his/her medications. (p. 237)

10. **(C)** When a medical patient complains of difficulty breathing, but does not have a prescribed medication for this condition, you should generally transport the patient to the hospital. (pp. 237–238)

11. **(B)** The main difference in approach to the focused history and physical exam for the responsive versus the unresponsive patient is that the unresponsive patient will be given a rapid physical exam first. The responsive patient would get the OPQRST questions first. Bystanders and family are more important if the patient is unresponsive, because they must supply information about the patient since the unresponsive patient is unable to do so. (pp. 234, 238)

12. **(D)** An unresponsive patient would be unable to answer the SAMPLE history questions. (p. 240)

13. **(B)** Check the medical patient's extremities for sensation and motor function as well as pulse. (p. 240)

14. **(C)** The bracelet or necklace could be a medical identification device that gives clues to the patient's medical history. (p. 240)

15. **(B)** A Vial of Life is usually stored in the refrigerator and may be helpful when treating an unconscious patient. (p. 241)

COMPLETE THE FOLLOWING

1. The components of a focused history and physical exam for an unresponsive medical patient include: (p. 238)
   - Conduct a rapid physical exam.
   - Obtain baseline vital signs.

   - Consider a request for ALS personnel.
   - Take a history of the present illness (OPQRST) and a SAMPLE history from the family or bystanders.

2. Questions to ask a bystander who witnessed a patient's medical emergency are: (any four) (pp. 240–241)
   - What is the patient's name?
   - What happened?
   - Did the bystander see anything else?
   - Did the patient complain of anything before this happened?
   - Does the patient have any known illnesses or problems?
   - Is the patient taking any medications?

COMPLETE THE CHART (p. 234)

1. Signs and symptoms
2. Allergies
3. Medications
4. Past medical history
5. Last meal
6. Events leading up to illness
7. Onset
8. Provokes
9. Quality
10. Radiation
11. Severity
12. Time

VIRTUAL STREET SCENES

1. A patient with breathing difficulty who speaks in short, choppy sentences may be breathing inadequately.

2. No. If there are no chest sounds during an asthma attack, the patient may not be moving enough air.

3. The term for lung sounds described as "noisy, like a whistling sound" is *wheezing*. A wheeze is a musical tone caused by air being forced through constricted air passageways. This is due to bronchoconstriction and the build-up of mucus.

4. Yes. If the patient has a prescribed inhaler, you may be able to assist the patient in taking the medication. This may be done only after consultation with medical direction, often during transportation to the hospital.

Chapter 12: Ongoing Assessment

MATCH TERMINOLOGY/DEFINITIONS

1. **(B)** Intervention—actions taken to prevent a patient's problems

2. **(C)** Ongoing assessment—four-step procedure for detecting changes in a patient's condition.

3. **(A)** Trending—changes in a patient's condition over time, which may show improvement or deterioration, and which can be shown by documenting repeated assessments

MULTIPLE-CHOICE REVIEW

1. **(D)** It is important to observe and re-observe the patient. Therefore, in the ongoing assessment, you need to repeat key elements of assessment procedures already performed in order to detect any changes in patient condition. (pp. 247–248)

2. **(C)** The ongoing assessment must never be omitted or skipped unless life-saving interventions prevent the EMT-B from doing it. Frequently, one partner can perform the ongoing assessment while the other performs the interventions. (p. 247)

3. **(D)** Use a quiet, reassuring voice when talking to the infant or child. Also maintain eye contact. Try to stay on the same level as the infant or child or close to or at eye level. (p. 247)

4. **(D)** The ongoing assessment does not involve repeating all interventions since some interventions may be adequate or are ongoing. However, it does involve evaluating the adequacy of your interventions more objectively and to adjust them as necessary. The ongoing assessment does include repeating the initial assessment for life-threats, the focused assessment, and the vital signs. (pp. 248, 250)

5. **(B)** The sequence for performing the ongoing assessment is: repeat the initial assessment, reassess vital signs, repeat the focused assessment, and last, check interventions. (p. 247)

6. **(D)** Applying a cervical collar is part of the rapid trauma assessment, not the initial assessment. When repeating the initial assessment, make sure that you reestablish patient priorities, monitor skin color and temperature, and maintain an open airway. (pp. 247–248)

7. **(D)** The onset of shock is signaled by rapid pulse and cool and pale skin. This is a life-threat and should be watched for continually and treated immediately. (p. 248)

8. **(C)** The mental status of an unresponsive child or infant can be checked by shouting (verbal stimulus) or by flicking the feet (painful stimulus). The parent can also be helpful by explaining how the child normally behaves. A sternal rub or pin to the foot is too aggressive and may injure the child. (p. 248)

9. **(D)** An example of checking interventions during the ongoing assessment of a medical patient is assuring adequacy of oxygen delivery. Taking a blood pressure is obtaining a vital sign and is not an intervention. Bandaging and applying a tourniquet are treatments. (pp. 248, 250)

10. **(C)** Frequent reassessment establishes trends, or changes over time, that the EMT-B needs to pay attention to. You may need to institute new treatments or adjust treatments you have already started based on these trends. (p. 250)

11. **(C)** The best way to determine if the patient is improving or deteriorating is to do frequent ongoing assessments. (p. 250)

12. **(C)** If the patient is stable, reassessment of vitals should be every 15 minutes. If the patient is not stable, the reassessment should be every 5 minutes. (p. 250)

13. **(A)** See answer #12. (p. 250)

14. **(C)** You should repeat the initial assessment whenever you believe there may have been a change in the patient's condition. This will help you determine if the patient needs to be reprioritized. (p. 250)

15. **(B)** Gurgling sounds in a patient's airway indicate the patient needs to be suctioned immediately. (p. 251)

COMPLETE THE FOLLOWING

1. The six steps involved in repeating the initial assessment involve: (pp. 247–248)
   - Reassess mental status.
   - Maintain an open airway.
   - Monitor breathing for rate and quality.
   - Reassess the pulse for rate and quality.
   - Monitor skin color and temperature.
   - Reestablish patient priorities.

2. The three steps for checking interventions are: (p. 248)
   - Assure adequacy of oxygen delivery and artificial ventilation.
   - Assure management of bleeding.
   - Assure adequacy of other interventions.

VIRTUAL STREET SCENES

1. In a stroke patient, if there is any paralysis, the patient may not be able to clear and maintain her own airway.

2. The sense of hearing is one of the last ones to go. So be very careful what you say, because the patient often can hear and understand you.

Chapter 13: Pediatric, Adolescent, and Geriatric Assessment

MATCH TERMINOLOGY/DEFINITIONS

1. **(E)** Adolescent—child from 12 to 18 years of age

2. **(M)** Alzheimer's disease—chronic disorder resulting in dementia

3. **(N)** Arrhythmia—abnormal heart rhythm

4. **(O)** Confabulation—when an elderly person replaces lost circumstances with imaginary ones

5. **(F)** Fontanelle—"soft spot" on an infant's skull

6. **(C)** Geriatric—elderly person, generally considered 65 years of age or older

7. **(K)** Hyperextension—tipping the head too far back

8. **(H)** Hypothermia—abnormally low body temperature

9. **(D)** Infant—child less than 1 year of age

10. **(J)** Obligate nose breathers—newborns and infants who do not know to open their mouths to breathe when the nose is obstructed

11. **(B)** Preschooler—child from 3 to 6 years of age

12. **(L)** Regression—when under stress, a child acts like a younger child

13. **(G)** School age—child from 6 to 12 years of age

14. **(I)** Sniffing position—chin thrust forward to maintain an open airway

15. **(A)** Toddler—child from 1 to 3 years of age

MULTIPLE-CHOICE REVIEW

1. **(C)** For the purposes of rescue breathing and CPR, a child is any patient between the ages of 1 and 8. This makes sense only for CPR and rescue breathing since the patients are unresponsive and there is no need to deal with their emotional development at this point in time. (p. 257)

2. **(D)** In general emergency care, the age categories to keep in mind are: newborns and infants: birth to 1 year; toddlers: 1 to 3 years; preschoolers: 3 to 6 years; school age: 6 to 12 years; adolescent: 12 to 18 years. (p. 257)

3. **(C)** Infants up until about 18 months will have a soft spot called a fontanelle. Avoid pressing on the soft spot since this would put pressure directly on the brain. The fontanelle is located at a suture joint of the skull that has not as yet fused. (p. 257)

4. **(A)** When an infant is crying, the fontanelle may bulge due to the temporary elevated intracranial pressure. During

dehydration, the brain shrinks and the fontanelle may be sunken, or depressed. (p. 257)

5. **(A)** Newborns usually breathe through their noses. Their breathing rate is faster than an adult's, and they are not normally on hypoxic drive. (p. 258)

6. **(B)** Hyperextension of the neck of an infant can compress the trachea and may cause an airway obstruction. Swelling is caused by anaphylaxis, infection, or neck trauma. (p. 259)

7. **(A)** Blind finger sweeps are not performed on infants with an obstructed airway because they might force an obstruction down and wedge it in the narrow trachea. Most adult fingers will fit into an infant's mouth. CPR standards prohibit the use of blind finger sweeps. (p. 260)

8. **(B)** When a child that is faced with the stress of an emergency acts like a younger child, this is called regression. (p. 261)

9. **(C)** It is always a good idea to kneel down and talk at eye level when assessing a child. Do not raise your voice or tower over a child as this can frighten him. Staring makes the child, or anyone for that matter, very nervous. (p. 261)

10. **(B)** Make all efforts to involve the parents in the care of their child. However, when you are caring for a child, if the parent is out of control, ask a friend or relative to remove him from the scene. Ignoring parents will not be effective. If you do involve them in care, make sure it is not an essential step like neck stabilization. (p. 262)

11. **(B)** When forming a general impression of a child, if the child talks in grunts only, you should assume the child has serious respiratory distress. Do not assume the child has a digestive condition, doesn't want to talk to you, or has poor language skills. (p. 263)

12. **(B)** When forming a general impression, it is most likely that a withdrawn child or one who is emotionally flat is probably sick. The child may be bored, although most children will pay a good deal of attention to a stranger who they are interested in or believe is a threat. A deaf child may use body language, rather than sound, to show excitement. (pp. 262–263)

13. **(C)** Evaluating capillary refill is part of assessing the circulation. To assess a child's breathing, observe the skin color, chest expansion, and effort of breathing. (p. 263)

14. **(A)** An infant's soft spot may bulge due to head trauma or meningitis. Dehydration would cause the soft spot to sink. Excessive eating and anaphylaxis are merely distracters. (p. 266)

15. **(C)** Starting at age 30, our organ systems lose about 1 percent function each year. This "1% rule" can make it difficult to distinguish between the normal effects of aging and the effects of disease. (p. 268)

16. **(C)** Although older patients are at least twice as likely to use EMS as younger patients, they are less likely to be involved in motor-vehicle collisions. Also, they are more likely than younger patients to have a medical problem, rather than an injury. (p. 269)

17. **(D)** Assessing the airway of an older patient is often difficult because of the patient's wearing dentures and because of arthritic changes in the bones of the neck. (p. 270)

18. **(B)** Since older patients are less likely to show severe symptoms in certain conditions, it can be difficult to determine a patient's priority. For example, when an older person is having a heart attack, rather than experiencing significant chest pain, he is more likely to have a sudden onset of weakness with no chest pain. (p. 270)

19. **(C)** When the family of an elderly patient tells you the patient was wrong with some of her responses, this can be the result of neurological problems as well as medications. (p. 270)

20. **(B)** When an elderly patient replaces lost circumstances with imaginary ones, this is known as confabulation. Confabulation can be caused by a number of neurological conditions. (p. 270)

21. **(A)** Many older people have a high threshold for pain. Be sure to keep this in mind when examining patients in order to prevent injuring a patient further. (p. 271)

22. **(B)** As a person ages, the systolic blood pressure has a tendency to increase. (p. 271)

23. **(D)** Hip fractures are common in elderly patients, especially women, due to loss of calcium. This loss of calcium weakens the bone so much that sometimes a fracture is the cause of a fall rather than the result. (p. 272)

24. **(C)** An EMT-B should consider that any injury of an elderly person could be a sign of abuse or neglect. While detecting elder abuse and neglect is difficult, many states have laws that require the reporting of such suspicions. (pp. 272–273)

25. **(A)** The EMT-B can ease the fears of a geriatric patient by understanding the effect that loss of independence has on the patient. Do not minimize the patient's fears or concerns; acknowledge them. No one expects an EMT-B to understand the proper treatment for all diseases the patient may have. (p. 273)

COMPLETE THE FOLLOWING

1. High priority patients in need of immediate transport include: (p. 263)
   - Gives a poor general impression.
   - Is unresponsive or listless.
   - Has a compromised airway.
   - Is in respiratory arrest or has inadequate breathing or respiratory distress.
   - Has a possibility of shock.
   - Has uncontrolled bleeding.

2. When dealing with a geriatric patient's fears of loss of independence, (p. 273)
   - always listen to them
   - acknowledge them
   - do not minimize their fears or concerns
   - be honest
   - try to put their fears into perspective

VIRTUAL STREET SCENES

1. If you decide that the patient's condition is serious enough to use the ambulance lights and siren, you probably should call for ALS.

2. Many elderly people are on fixed incomes. Some feel they cannot pay big heating bills, so they keep the temperature down and wear lots of clothing instead. Since older people cannot regulate their body temperature very well, this could cause medical problems.

3. The elderly patient may be afraid of losing his independence, of being left in the care of strangers, or of going to the hospital where he has lost friends and loved ones. You can help to ease this transition by treating the patient in a respectful, dignified manner, acknowledging his fears and concerns, and attempting to put them in perspective.

CASE STUDY—Abuser or Loving Parent?

1. At a motor-vehicle collision scene, traffic is usually your greatest hazard.

2. Yes, since the limping driver could change his mind. You would not want to delay transporting the child in order to call for another ambulance later in the call.

3. Your initial concerns for the child are mental status and the status of his ABCs.

4. Yes, it is a significant finding. His mental status is probably deteriorating.

5. One way to determine a child's mental status is to ask the parents what is "normal" for the child.

6. The cracks are evidence that the patients' heads impacted the windshield. This is a very significant mechanism of injury.

7. In addition to helping you determine what happened to the child, the mother's statement also tells you that the patient is normally very active and expressive. He is not now.

8. Yes. Also evaluate the need for assisting ventilation.

9. Yes, request an ALS intercept. The patient may need to be intubated and the extra hands would be helpful.

10. Just provide the facts. The mother may have broken at least two laws: she may have been driving while legally intoxicated and she did not use the proper restraints on the child. If she had followed the laws that are designed to protect children, the injuries probably would not have been so severe.

Chapter 14: Communications

MATCH TERMINOLOGY/DEFINITIONS

1. **(E)** Base station—two-way radio at a fixed site such as a hospital or dispatch center

2. **(H)** Cellular phone—phone that transmits through the air instead of over wires so that the phone can be transported and used over a wide area

3. **(I)** Digital radio equipment—equipment that permits transmission of standard messages in condensed form by punching a key

4. **(A)** FCC—(Federal Communications Commission) federal agency that regulates radio communications

5. **(G)** Mobile radio—two-way radio that is used or affixed in a vehicle

6. **(D)** Portable radio—hand-held two-way radio

7. **(J)** PTT—"press to talk" button on the EMS radio

8. **(B)** Repeater—device that picks up signals from lower-power radio units such as mobile and portable radios and retransmits them at a higher power

9. **(F)** Verbal report—update on the patient's condition given to hospital personnel either face-to-face or over the radio

10. **(C)** Watt—unit of measurement of the output power of a radio

MULTIPLE-CHOICE REVIEW

1. **(C)** As an EMT-B, your ability to communicate is very important because describing your assessment findings to the hospital may make a difference in the care the patient receives. (p. 279)

2. **(B)** EMS has progressed over the years due to the development of radio links among dispatcher, mobile units, and hospitals. (p. 279)

3. **(D)** The components of a communications system include the base station, mobile units, portable radios, repeaters, and cellular phones. (p. 279)

4. **(C)** A device that picks up a lower power signal and then retransmits it at a higher power is called a repeater. (p. 279)

5. **(A)** The Federal Communications Commission (FCC) is responsible for approving communications and maintaining order on the airwaves. The FAA is the Federal Aeronautic Administration. FEMA is the Federal Emergency Management Agency. DOT is the Department of Transportation. (p. 279)

6. **(C)** The purposes of always following the general principles of radio transmission is to allow all persons to use the frequencies and to prevent delays. EMT-Bs should request a repeat of orders from medical direction if they are unclear. The EMT-B should not use codes, but communicate in plain English. (p. 282)

7. **(C)** Of the items listed, their correct sequence in a radio report is unit identification and level of provider, chief complaint, major past illness, and emergency medical care given. (p. 283)

8. **(B)** The reason why the ambulance was called is the chief complaint. EMT-Bs do not make diagnoses. (p. 283)

9. **(D)** The fact that a patient's abdomen does not feel rigid during palpation is referred to as a pertinent finding from the physical exam and is reported to the hospital. (p. 283)

10. **(C)** Updating the physician on the patient's mental status is a way of telling him/her how the patient is responding to the emergency medical care that was given. (p. 283)

11. **(A)** Whenever the EMT-B requests an order for medical direction over the radio, it is a good practice to repeat the physician's order back word for word, question inappropriate orders, and speak slowly and clearly. (p. 283)

12. **(B)** Always question the physician about an order over the radio that you think is inappropriate or that you do not understand. The physician may have misinterpreted or misunderstood your communication. (pp. 283–284)

13. **(B)** Crossing your arms and looking down at the patient sends the message, "I am not really interested." Be aware of the nonverbal messages you may send by your body position and posture. (pp. 284–285)

14. **(D)** If a patient determines he/she has a broken leg, tell the patient the truth in a calm voice and gentle manner. (pp. 284–285)

15. **(A)** When treating a toddler, kneel down at the child's level to talk. Do not stare at the child. Never lie by saying you know his/her parents if you actually do not. The child will figure out that you are lying and will not trust you. (pp. 285–286)

COMPLETE THE FOLLOWING

1. Five components of a communications system are: (p. 279)
   - Base station
   - Mobile radios
   - Portable radios
   - Repeaters
   - Cellular phones

2. Interpersonal communication guidelines to use when dealing with patients, families, friends, and bystanders include:. (pp. 285–286)
   - Use eye contact.
   - Be aware of your position and body language.
   - Use language the patient can understand.
   - Be honest.
   - Use the patient's proper name.
   - Listen.

VIRTUAL STREET SCENES

1. Calling ahead gives hospital personnel time to prepare for the patient's arrival. This may mean calling in a surgeon or a specialist or ordering a special medication.

2. Check with your instructor for your local protocols. Generally, it is the highest medically trained rescuer on scene.

3. Other types of communication were nonverbal and face-to-face, including EMT-B to patient and other rescue personnel such as law enforcement, the extrication crew, the incident commander, and the helicopter flight crew.

Chapter 15: Documentation

MATCH TERMINOLOGY/DEFINITIONS

1. (G) Data element—each individual box on a prehospital care report

2. (C) Falsification—inaccurate entry or misrepresentation on a prehospital care report usually intended to cover up serious flaws in assessment or in care

3. (H) Minimum data set—minimum elements that are recommended by the U.S. Department of Transportation to be included in all prehospital care reports nationwide

4. (D) Objective statement—observable, measurable, and verifiable information

5. (B) PCR—report form used by EMS agencies to document prehospital assessment and care

6. (I) Electronic clipboard—clipboard-format device that is able to recognize handwriting and convert it to computer text

7. (E) Pertinent negative—exam finding that is not present or not true but is important to note (e.g., patient denies any shortness of breath)

8. (F) Special situation report—report on unusual, complex, or involved situations that is completed according to your service's standard operating procedures

9. (A) Subjective information—information from an individual point of view

10. (J) Triage tag—item affixed to a patient at a multiple-casualty-incident used to record chief complaint and injuries, vital signs, and treatment given

MULTIPLE-CHOICE REVIEW

1. (C) The prehospital care report serves as a legal document as well as an aid for research, education, and administrative efforts. We do not routinely report all calls to the local police department. Because call information is confidential, it would never be used as a press release or as a receipt for the patient. (p. 292)

2. (B) The written PCR record provides a means for the emergency department staff to review the patient's prehospital care. (pp. 291–292)

3. (C) The copy of the PCR left at the hospital should become part of the patient's permanent hospital record. (pp. 291–292)

4. (C) A complete and accurate PCR will be your best recollection of the call. (p. 292)

5. (D) The person who completed a PCR may be called to court to testify about the call in a criminal proceeding, the care provided to the patient, and the call in a civil proceeding. (p. 292)

6. (B) The routine review of PCRs for conformity to current medical and organizational standards is a process called quality improvement. (p. 292)

7. (B) Each individual box on a PCR is called a data element. The narrative is a written description. A key punch is used to input data into a computer. (p. 292)

8. (C) The patient's social security number is not part of the minimum data set. It may be collected as a part of insurance information. According to the U.S. DOT, the minimum data set on a PCR should include respiratory rate and effort; skin color and temperature; times of incident, dispatch, and arrival at the patient; and capillary refill for patients less than 6 years old. (p. 292)

9. (B) Vehicle mileage is not important data. The minimum data set includes vital signs, chief complaint, and times of the call. (p. 292)

10. (B) The time of dispatch is an example of run data on the PCR. (p. 295)

11. (A) Examples of patient data on a PCR would be date of birth and age. The other information is included elsewhere on the form. (p. 295)

12. (C) Experienced EMT-Bs consider a good PCR as one that paints a picture of the patient. Attempting to identify symptoms the patient may have overlooked is falsification. (p. 296)

13. (B) The statement "The patient has a swollen, deformed extremity" on the narrative portion of the PCR is an example of objective information. This means it is observable, measurable, or verifiable. Subjective information is information from an individual point of view. Pertinent negatives are examination findings that are negative (things that are not true), but are important to note. Nonstandard abbreviations should be avoided on PCRs. (pp. 296–297)

14. (C) Objective information is factual and need not be put in quotation marks. Subjective statements that are from an individual's point of view and that include opinions or actual statements made by bystanders, the patient, or a police officer should be in quotation marks. (pp. 296–297)

15. (B) In the narrative section of a PCR, the EMT-B should include pertinent negatives. Do not write your personal conclusions about the situation or use the radio codes for each treatment. The vital signs and times they are taken are

recorded in a different section along with additional objective information. (pp. 297–298)

16. **(C)** Medical abbreviations should be used only if they are standardized to ensure that everyone who reads them will understand them. They are not used solely to save space in the narrative section of a PCR, to replace all words you cannot spell, or to ensure correct interpretation by physicians. (p. 298)

17. **(B)** The PCR form itself and the information on it should be considered confidential information. The form is a medical document. (p. 298)

18. **(D)** When a patient refuses transport, before the EMT-B leaves the scene, he/she should document assessment findings and care given, try again to persuade the patient to go to a hospital, and ensure the patient is able to make a rational, informed decision. (pp. 298, 300–301)

19. **(D)** EMT-Bs do not make a diagnosis. When completing a PCR on a patient refusal, the EMT-B should document that he/she was willing to return if the patient changed his/her mind, a complete patient assessment, and that alternative methods of care were offered. (pp. 298, 300–301)

20. **(A)** If the EMT-B forgot to administer a treatment that is required by a state protocol, he/she should document on the PCR only treatment actually given. Never fill the form out with excuses. Recording that the patient was given the forgotten treatment would be falsification. (p. 301)

21. **(A)** Falsification of information on a prehospital care report may lead to suspension or revocation of your license or certification. (p. 301)

22. **(B)** To correct an error discovered while writing out a PCR, the EMT-B should draw a single horizontal line through the error, initial it, and write the correct information. Scribbling on the form is sloppy. You should be using a ballpoint pen to fill out the report; therefore, erasures may be looked upon by others as an attempt to cover up a mistake in patient care. (p. 301)

23. **(C)** If information was omitted on a PCR, the EMT-B should add a note with the correct information, the date, and initial it. It usually is not necessary to notify the medical director in this situation. (p. 301)

24. **(A)** An example of an instance in which it would <u>not</u> be unusual for the EMT-B to obtain only a limited amount of information is a multiple-casualty incident. An interhospital transfer and a child abuse call would probably be thoroughly documented with pertinent information. (p. 302)

25. **(A)** Special situation reports are used to document events that should be reported to local regulatory authorities. They must be accurate, neat, and submitted in a timely manner. They are reserved for special instances such as exposure to infectious disease, injury to EMT-Bs, hazardous scenes, child or elder abuse, etc. (pp. 302, 305)

COMPLETE THE FOLLOWING

Patient data on a PCR includes: (p. 295)
- the patient's name, address, date of birth, age, sex
- billing and insurance information
- nature of call
- mechanism of injury
- location where the patient was found
- treatment administered before arrival of EMT-Bs

- signs and symptoms, including baseline and subsequent vital signs
- SAMPLE history
- care administered to and effect on the patient
- changes in condition throughout the call

VIRTUAL STREET SCENES

1. If the call really does end up in court, it will be difficult to prove that the patient had distal function prior to and after immobilization. He therefore may be able to say that he lost sensation as part of the actual care you provided.

2. Sloppy documentation could lead a jury to believe the EMT-B's emergency care was sloppy, too.

3. Yes, but since it is not objective information, you should put the patient's statement in quotes.

4. The emergency department staff should place the PCR into the patient's official emergency department chart.

Chapter 16: General Pharmacology

MATCH TERMINOLOGY/DEFINITION

1. **(H)** Activated charcoal—powder, usually premixed with water, that will adsorb some poisons and help prevent them from being adsorbed by the body

2. **(F)** Epinephrine—drug that helps to constrict the blood vessels and relax airway passages; it may be used to counter a severe allergic reaction.

3. **(C)** Gel—semisolid paste form of a drug

4. **(A)** Indications—specific signs or circumstances under which it is appropriate to administer a drug to a patient

5. **(B)** Inhaler—spray device with a mouthpiece that contains an aerosol form of a medication that a patient can spray directly into his airway

6. **(D)** Oral glucose—medication given by mouth to treat a conscious patient (one who is able to swallow) with an altered mental status and a history of diabetes

7. **(I)** Oxygen—This gas, in its pure form, is used as a drug to treat any patient whose medical or traumatic condition causes them to be hypoxic, or low in oxygen.

8. **(J)** Suspension—liquid form of a drug in which a powder is mixed with a slurry or water

9. **(G)** Tablet—solid form of a drug; compressed powder

10. **(E)** Trade name—brand name of a medication

MULTIPLE-CHOICE REVIEW

1. **(D)** The study of drugs and their effects is called pharmacology. Anatomy is the study of the structure of the body. Physiology is the study of the functions of the body. Medicinology is a distracter. (p. 309)

2. **(A)** Medications that are routinely carried on the EMS unit are activated charcoal, oral glucose, and oxygen. The patients may carry nitroglycerin, epinephrine, and prescribed inhalers. (p. 309)

3. **(A)** Activated charcoal is an example of a powder, usually premixed with water. (p. 309)

4. **(B)** Activated charcoal is given to a patient because it will bind some poisons to its surface. It does not prevent vomiting. (p. 309)

5. **(B)** The brain is very sensitive to low levels of sugar in the blood, which may be caused by poorly managed diabetes; this can be a cause of a diabetic patient's altered mental status. (p. 309)

6. **(A)** Oral glucose is given between the patient's cheek and gum because this area contains many blood vessels that allow absorption into the bloodstream. It does not cause the patient to regurgitate the stomach's contents. Oral glucose does not dilate the coronary vessels. (p. 309)

7. **(C)** Examples of medications that the patient may have in his possession that the EMT-B may assist the patient in taking under the appropriate circumstances are epinephrine (Epi-Pen®), a prescribed inhaler, and nitroglycerin. Patients do not generally carry home oxygen with them. EMT-Bs do not assist patients in the administration of glucose injections, anticonvulsants, anti-inflammatories, insulin, or anti-hypertensives. (p. 309)

8. **(C)** Patients who have a medical history of asthma, emphysema, and chronic bronchitis may carry a bronchodilator. (p. 310)

9. **(C)** The drug nitroglycerin is used to dilate the coronary vessels. It is not used to constrict or dilate the peripheral vessels. (pp. 311)

10. **(C)** The government publication listing all drugs in the United States is called the *U.S. Pharmacopoeia*. (p. 312)

11. **(B)** The name that the manufacturer uses in marketing a drug is called the trade name. The generic name is used more generally by all manufacturers. (p. 312)

12. **(D)** A circumstance in which a drug should not be used because it may cause harm to the patient or offer no effect in improving the patient's condition or illness is called a contraindication. An indication is a specific sign or circumstance under which it is appropriate to administer a drug. An adverse reaction is usually not known in advance. Side effects, although not desirable, are not a reason to withhold a medication (e.g., headache from nitroglycerin). (p. 312)

13. **(A)** An action of a drug that is other than the desired action is called a side effect. See answer #12. (p. 312)

14. **(D)** Prior to administering a medication to a patient, you must know the route of administration, proper dosage, and the actions the medication will take. You should know the generic name but are not expected to know the chemical name. (p. 313)

15. **(B)** Drugs prescribed for pain relief are called analgesics. See Table 16-1. (p. 313)

16. **(D)** Drugs prescribed to reduce high blood pressure are called antihypertensives. See Table 16-1. (p. 313)

17. **(C)** Drugs prescribed for heart rhythm disorders are called antiarrhythmics. See Table 16-1. (p. 313)

18. **(B)** Drugs prescribed to relax the smooth muscles of the bronchial tubes are called bronchodilators. See Table 16-1. (p. 313)

19. **(C)** Drugs prescribed for prevention and control of seizures are called anticonvulsants. See Table 16-1. (p. 313)

20. **(A)** Drugs prescribed to help regulate the emotional activity of the patient to minimize the peaks and valleys in their psychological and emotional state are called antidepressants. See Table 16-1. (p. 313)

COMPLETE THE FOLLOWING

1. The six medications an EMT-B can administer or assist a patient in taking are: (p. 309)
   - activated charcoal
   - oral glucose
   - oxygen
   - prescribed inhalers
   - nitroglycerin
   - epinephrine auto-injectors

2. The four "rights" to adhere to when administering a medication are: (p. 313)
   - The right patient.
   - The right medication.
   - The right dose.
   - The right route.

VIRTUAL STREET SCENES

1. A side effect of nitroglycerin is a drop in blood pressure. If this should occur, you may need to lay the patient down and raise the legs as you re-contact medical direction for advice.

2. The patient expects the nitroglycerin to relieve his pain by dilating the coronary arteries, which supply the heart muscle with blood.

3. Yes. They are: "He denies any radiation down his arm or towards his jaw. He also denies any relief with the brief wait while sitting."

Chapter 17: Respiratory Emergencies

MATCH TERMINOLOGY/DEFINITION

1. **(B)** Agonal respirations—sporadic, irregular breaths that are usually seen just before respiratory arrest

2. **(C)** Bronchoconstriction—blockage of the bronchi that lead from the trachea to the lungs

3. **(E)** Expiration—passive process in which the intercostal muscles and the diaphragm relax, causing the chest cavity to decrease in size and forcing air from the lungs; also called exhalation

4. **(A)** Inspiration—active process in which the intercostal muscles and the diaphragm contract, expanding the size of the chest cavity and causing air to flow into the lungs; also called inhalation

5. **(D)** Retractions—pulling in of the accessory muscles to breathe

MULTIPLE-CHOICE REVIEW

1. **(C)** The diaphragm separates the chest from the abdomen. The intercostal muscles are between the ribs. The sternocleidomastoid muscle is in the neck. The inguinal muscle is at the base of the abdomen. (p. 321)

2. **(B)** Expiration is a passive process in which the intercostal (rib) muscles and the diaphragm relax, causing the chest cavity to decrease in size and forcing air from the lungs. (p. 321)

3. **(C)** Although rhythm must be observed, it is not included under the quality of breathing. Quality includes breath sounds (diminished, unequal, or absent?), chest expansion

(inadequate or unequal?), and depth of respirations (labored, increased respiratory effort, use of accessory muscles?). (pp. 322–323).

4. **(C)** An unresponsive patient with shallow, gasping breaths with only a few breaths per minute (agonal respirations) is clearly breathing inadequately. You must provide artificial ventilation with supplemental oxygen preferably via pocket face mask. (pp. 323–324)

5. **(B)** Accessory muscles, such as those in the neck and abdomen, assist in breathing, especially when a patient is having difficulty breathing. Sub-diaphragmatic is a location below the diaphragm. Smooth muscles line blood vessels. Extra muscles is an inventive distracter. (p. 323)

6. **(D)** Blue-colored skin (cyanosis) that feels clammy and cool is usually a sign of inadequate breathing. (p. 323)

7. **(A)** Snoring and gurgling sounds usually indicate a partially obstructed airway. Wheezing can be a sign of anything from airway obstruction to bronchoconstriction. Sniffling is usually from a runny nose. Whistling or grunting is a distracter. (p. 323)

8. **(C)** Respiratory conditions account for a large percentage of deaths in infants and children. Motor-vehicle collisions cause child deaths, but not as high a percentage as respiratory conditions. Heart attacks are more rare in children. Infections are high in infants, but decrease in children. (p. 324)

9. **(D)** The cricoid cartilage of infants and children is less developed and less rigid than is an adult's. (p. 324)

10. **(B)** Infants and children depend more heavily on the diaphragm for breathing because the chest wall is softer. They do not inhale twice the air, and they may grunt only when they are in respiratory distress. (p. 324)

11. **(D)** Signs of inadequate breathing in infants and children include nasal flaring (widening of the nostrils), grunting, seesaw breathing, and retractions. Lip quivering is a distracter. (p. 324)

12. **(C)** It is not enough to simply make sure the patient is breathing. The patient must be breathing adequately. (p. 324)

13. **(B)** The best method involves the BVM with two rescuers and supplemental oxygen. (p. 324)

14. **(D)** If you are unsure about whether a patient needs artificial ventilation, you should provide artificial ventilation. (p. 324)

15. **(B)** Artificially ventilate at a rate of 12 breaths per minute for an adult and 20 breaths per minute for infants and children according to American Heart Association standards. (p. 324)

16. **(C)** See answer #15. (p. 324)

17. **(C)** A low pulse in infants and small children in the setting of a respiratory emergency usually means trouble. In infants and children with respiratory difficulties, you may observe a slight increase in pulse early, but soon the pulse will drop significantly. (p. 325)

18. **(B)** Increase the force of ventilations for any patient—adult, child, or infant—if the chest does not rise and fall with each artificial ventilation, or the pulse does not return to normal. If the chest still does not rise, check that you are maintaining an open airway. (p. 325)

19. **(A)** With certain lower airway respiratory diseases or infections, it is dangerous to probe or place anything in the patient's mouth or pharynx because this may set off spasms along the airway. (p. 325)

20. **(D)** Patients with lower airway obstruction may be wheezing, have increased breathing effort upon exhalation, and have rapid breathing without stridor. Their skin may be pale or blue, but not yellow. Yellow skin is an indication of liver abnormalities. (p. 325)

21. **(C)** A patient with breathing difficulty frequently speaks in short, choppy sentences. The other choices are distracters. (p. 326)

22. **(B)** In a tripod position, the patient is leaning forward with hands resting on the knees or table. The recovery position is lying on the side, which allows fluid to drain from the mouth. Supine with knees flexed is helpful with abdominal pain. (p. 326)

23. **(D)** Headache and vomiting are not commonly associated with breathing difficulties. Crowing, retractions, an increased pulse, and coughing are all common signs associated with breathing difficulty. Restlessness, shortness of breath, and chest tightness are common symptoms of patients with breathing difficulty. (p. 326)

24. **(B)** If a patient is suffering from breathing difficulty and is breathing adequately, administer oxygen via nonrebreather mask. The BVM and pocket mask are for patients in severe distress. (p. 327)

25. **(C)** If a patient is experiencing breathing difficulty and is breathing adequately, it is best to place him in a position of comfort. This is frequently the sitting-up position. Most patients with breathing difficulty feel they can breathe better this way. The tripod position is a position the patient with breathing difficulty assumes. A patient with *inadequate* breathing would need to be supine to receive assisted ventilations. (p. 327)

26. **(C)** An inhaler, also referred to as a puffer, is commonly used for patients with respiratory problems that cause bronchoconstriction. (p. 327)

27. **(C)** When giving a medication by an inhaler, a syringe is not needed. The patient must be alert and cooperative, and the right dose of unexpired medication must be given. (p. 327)

28. **(A)** Prior to coaching the patient in the use of an inhaler, first shake it vigorously. It is not necessary to test the unit by spraying it into the air. (p. 329)

29. **(B)** To ensure that the most medication is absorbed when using an inhaler, encourage the patient to hold the breath as long as possible so the medication can be absorbed by the lungs. Unless the medication is held in the lungs, it will have minimal or no value. (pp. 329–331)

30. **(C)** When documenting a respiratory complaint, ask the patient to describe the difficulty in his own words. Answering history questions is also helpful. It is not necessary to count respirations for two minutes. (p. 329)

COMPLETE THE FOLLOWING

1. Conditions of inadequate breathing include: (p. 323)
   - breathing rate that is out of normal range
   - agonal respirations
   - irregular rhythm (not an absolute indicator)
   - diminished or absent breath sounds
   - inadequate or shallow depth of respirations

- inadequate or unequal chest expansion and increased respiratory effort
- use of accessory muscles in breathing
- pale or cyanotic, cool and clammy skin
- snoring or gurgling (in patients with a diminished level of responsiveness or who are totally unresponsive)

2. Signs of inadequate breathing in infants and children are: (p. 324)
   - nasal flaring (widening of the nostrils)
   - grunting
   - seesaw breathing
   - retractions between the ribs

3. Signs of breathing difficulty include: (any eight) (p. 326)
   - increased pulse rate
   - decreased pulse rate
   - changes in breathing rate
   - changes in breathing rhythm
   - pale, cyanotic, or flushed skin
   - noisy breathing that may be described as: audible wheezing, gurgling, snoring, crowing, stridor
   - inability to speak in full sentences
   - use of accessory muscles to breathe
   - altered mental status
   - coughing
   - flared nostrils
   - pursed lips
   - patient positioning
   - unusual anatomy (barrel chest)

LABEL THE DIAGRAMS (p. 322)

1. Relaxation
2. Contraction (inspiration begins)
3. Inspiration
4. Relaxation (passive expiration begins)

VIRTUAL STREET SCENES

1. Anything related to the patient's respiratory condition is pertinent to the current problem. Document it!
2. Yes.
3. As you learned in Chapter 6, the procedures for airway evaluation, opening the airway, and artificial ventilation are best carried out with the patient lying supine, or flat on the back. However, if the patient must sit, sit her up on the stretcher, lay her head back, and work with her breathing efforts. This takes patience and practice.

Chapter 18: Cardiac Emergencies

MATCH TERMINOLOGY/DEFINITIONS

▶ **Part A**

1. **(I)** Acute myocardial infarction—condition in which a portion of the myocardium dies as a result of oxygen starvation; often called a heart attack by laypersons
2. **(B)** Aneurysm—dilation, or ballooning, of a weakened section of the wall of an artery
3. **(J)** Angina pectoris—pain in the chest that occurs when the blood supply to the heart is reduced and a portion of the heart muscle is not receiving enough oxygen
4. **(G)** Arrhythmia—irregular, or absent, heart rhythm

5. **(D)** Arteriosclerosis—condition in which artery walls become hard and stiff due to calcium deposits
6. **(E)** Asystole—when the heart has ceased generating electrical impulses
7. **(A)** Atherosclerosis—buildup of fatty deposits on the inner walls of arteries
8. **(F)** Cardiac compromise—blanket term for any kind of heart problem
9. **(C)** Congestive heart failure—condition of excessive fluid buildup in the lungs and/or other organs and body parts because of the inadequate pumping of the heart
10. **(H)** Coronary artery disease—diseases that affect the arteries of the heart

▶ **Part B**

1. **(J)** Edema—swelling resulting from a buildup of fluid in tissues
2. **(G)** Embolism—clot of blood and plaque that has broken loose from the wall of an artery and then moves to smaller arteries and blocks blood flow
3. **(B)** Occlusion—blockage
4. **(C)** Pedal edema—accumulation of fluid in the feet or ankles
5. **(E)** Pulmonary edema—accumulation of fluid in the lungs
6. **(I)** Pulseless electrical activity—condition in which the heart's electrical rhythm remains relatively normal, yet the mechanical pumping activity fails to follow the electrical activity, causing cardiac arrest
7. **(D)** Sudden death—cardiac arrest that occurs within two hours of the onset of symptoms
8. **(H)** Thrombus—clot formed of blood and plaque attached to the inner wall of an artery
9. **(A)** Ventricular fibrillation—condition in which the heart's electrical impulses are disorganized, preventing the heart muscle from contracting normally
10. **(F)** Ventricular tachycardia—condition in which the heartbeat is quite rapid; if rapid enough, it will not allow the heart's chambers to fill with enough blood between beats to produce blood flow sufficient to meet the body's needs

MULTIPLE-CHOICE REVIEW

1. **(C)** Cardiac compromise is a term that refers to any kind of problem with the heart. A period of time when the heart stops is cardiac arrest. (p. 337)
2. **(C)** Tearing pain is usually the result of a dissecting aortic aneurysm. Chest pain from the heart is normally described as dull, squeezing, or crushing. (p. 338)
3. **(A)** The pain or discomfort from a heart problem commonly radiates to the arms and jaw. It may also radiate down to the upper abdomen. (p. 339)
4. **(C)** In addition to chest pain or discomfort, the patient with cardiac compromise will also complain of dyspnea. The patient with gastrointestinal distress will complain of diarrhea. Cardiac compromise patients usually have a sudden onset of sweating, <u>not</u> shivering. A headache is a side effect of nitroglycerin. (p. 339)
5. **(C)** Patients with heart problems may complain of pain in the center of the chest, mild chest discomfort, and difficulty breathing. They do not have sudden onset of sharp abdominal pain. (pp. 338–340)

6. **(B)** If the heart is beating too fast or too slow, the patient with cardiac compromise may also lose consciousness. This is due to an inadequate supply of oxygenated blood to the brain. (p. 340)

7. **(C)** The signs and symptoms of cardiac compromise do not include sharp pain in the lower abdomen combined with a fever. (p. 340)

8. **(C)** The patient with cardiac compromise should be administered high-concentration oxygen; the nasal cannula does not provide high-concentration oxygen. (p. 340)

9. **(C)** The "position of comfort" for a patient who is having chest pain is typically sitting up. Patients who are hypotensive (systolic blood pressure less than 90) will usually feel better lying down since this position allows more blood flow to the brain. (p. 340)

10. **(C)** A patient with prescribed nitroglycerin should be given or assisted in taking nitroglycerin (up to three doses). Vital signs and chest pain should be reassessed after each dose. If this patient's blood pressure falls below 100 systolic, then treat for shock and transport promptly. (p. 340)

11. **(B)** You should consider using nitroglycerin when the patient is carrying his own nitro and has crushing chest pain. A side effect of nitro is a headache. Nitro is not given to unconscious patients or to those who are hypotensive, below 100 systolic. (p. 340)

12. **(C)** The role of medical direction in the treatment of a cardiac compromise patient is authorizing the EMT-B to assist the patient in taking his prescribed nitroglycerin. (p. 340)

13. **(C)** In order to give nitroglycerin, the patient's blood pressure must not be lower than 100 systolic. Medical direction should authorize the administration of nitroglycerin, and the patient's physician should have prescribed it. (p. 340)

14. **(C)** The maximum number of doses of nitro routinely given in the field is three. (p. 344)

15. **(C)** If after administering three doses of nitroglycerin, the patient's blood pressure falls below 100 systolic, you should treat for shock and transport promptly. (p. 344)

16. **(A)** Nitroglycerin is contraindicated for a patient who has a head injury. (p. 343)

17. **(D)** Palpitations are not a side effect of nitroglycerin. They are a symptom of cardiac compromise, however. The common side effects of nitro administration include hypotension, headache, and changes in the pulse rate. (p. 343)

18. **(C)** After administering nitro, it is important to reassess the vital signs. It is not necessary to lay the patient down unless his blood pressure drops. Continue the oxygen administration. (p. 343)

19. **(D)** The majority of cardiovascular emergencies are not a result of complications of cardiovascular surgery. Rather, they are a result of changes in the inner walls of arteries or problems with the heart's electrical and mechanical functions. (p. 344)

20. **(A)** When the body is subjected to exertion or stress, the heart rate will normally increase. It would be unusual for the heart to stop with normal exertion. (p. 344)

21. **(C)** Arteriosclerosis is a stiffening or hardening of the artery wall resulting from calcium deposits that cause a vessel to lose its elasticity, which restricts the amount of blood passing through the artery. Atherosclerosis is a buildup of fatty deposits on an artery's inner wall, which also restricts the amount of blood passing through it. (pp. 344–345)

22. **(D)** Risk factors for coronary artery disease include lack of exercise, cigarette smoking, and obesity; other risk factors include heredity, age, hypertension, elevated blood levels of cholesterol and triglycerides. (p. 345)

23. **(C)** Hypertension as well as smoking and diet are risk factors that can be modified to reduce the risk of coronary artery disease. Unfortunately, a patient cannot change his age or heredity factors. (p. 345)

24. **(A)** The reason an emergency occurs in most cardiac-related medical emergencies is due to reduced blood flow to the myocardium. This may in turn cause cardiac arrest, loss of consciousness, or breathing difficulty. (p. 345)

25. **(B)** Angina pectoris means, literally, a pain in the chest. (p. 346)

26. **(B)** Nitroglycerin is administered to the patient with chest pain because it dilates the blood vessels and decreases the work of the heart. A drop in blood pressure is a side effect of nitro. Nitro should not be administered to unconscious patients. (p. 346)

27. **(B)** A condition in which a portion of the myocardium dies as a result of oxygen starvation is known as acute myocardial infarction. A coronary occlusion occurs when the coronary artery is completely blocked. Myocardial starvation is a distracter. (p. 346)

28. **(C)** When a cardiac arrest occurs within two hours of the onset of cardiac symptoms, this is referred to as sudden death. (p. 346)

29. **(B)** Unfortunately, nearly 25% of the patients who experience a cardiac arrest within two hours of the onset of symptoms have no previous history of cardiac problems. (p. 346)

30. **(C)** Changes in the field care of the acute myocardial infarction (AMI) have made thrombolytics and defibrillation two of the most important treatment methods. Defibrillation of a patient with a shockable rhythm offers the best chance for survival. Thrombolytics (clotbusters) break up the clot, saving heart muscle tissue. (p. 346)

31. **(B)** Congestive heart failure is a condition in which excessive fluids build up in the lungs and/or other organs. An infection in the heart is a distracter. A chronic lung condition that requires a low concentration of oxygen administration is COPD. (p. 347)

32. **(B)** When there is damage to the left ventricle and blood backs up into the lungs, this usually presents in the form of pulmonary edema. Pedal edema is the accumulation of fluid in the feet or ankles. Thrombolytics are medications that dissolve blood clots. Diaphoresis is profuse sweating. (p. 347)

33. **(D)** The chain of survival does not include early diagnosis. The elements of the chain of survival include early access, early CPR, early defibrillation, and early advanced care. (p. 348)

34. **(D)** Ways to decrease the EMS access time include installing a 9-1-1 system, placing 9-1-1 stickers on telephones, and providing public information workshops. (p. 348)

35. **(B)** CPR training by heart specialists is unnecessary in order to decrease the time it takes to start CPR on a cardiac arrest victim. (p. 348)

36. **(A)** The typical cardiac arrest victim is a male in his sixties. (p. 349)

37. **(D)** The most common witness to a cardiac arrest is a female in her sixties. (p. 349)

38. (D) Early defibrillation is the single most important factor in determining survival from cardiac arrest. If the time from the call is received to arrival of the defibrillator is longer than 8 minutes, virtually no one survives cardiac arrest. (p. 349)

39. (B) See answer #38. (p. 349)

40. (B) When treating a cardiac arrest patient and there is no ACLS unit in the community, the EMT-B should then package quickly and transport to the closest medical facility. To call for ACLS from another town and wait for their arrival would take too much time. Do not delay on the scene until the patient regains a pulse. Transport! (pp. 349–350)

41. (D) The EMT-B does not need to know how to administer epinephrine via IV or ET tube to manage a patient in cardiac arrest. Epinephrine administration is designed for allergic or anaphylactic patients. (pp. 349–350)

42. (D) When using a fully automated defibrillator, it is unnecessary to press the button to deliver the shock. This is because a <u>fully</u> automated defibrillator delivers the shock automatically once enough energy has been accumulated. (pp. 350–351)

43. (B) The primary electrical disturbance resulting in cardiac arrest is ventricular fibrillation. (p. 351)

44. (A) The shockable rhythms include ventricular fibrillation, ventricular tachycardia, and pulseless ventricular tachycardia. Asystole and PEA are not shockable. (p. 351)

45. (A) A nonshockable rhythm that can be the result of a terminally sick heart or severe blood loss is called pulseless electrical activity. (p. 351)

46. (C) A nonshockable rhythm that is commonly called "flatline" is named asystole. This condition is called "flatline" because the wavy line displayed on an ECG when there is electrical activity goes flat with asystole. (p. 351)

47. (B) When the AED is analyzing the patient's heart rhythm, the EMT-B must avoid touching the patient. If you are touching the patient, there can be interference from the electrical impulses of your heart and from movement of the patient's muscles. This can fool the AED's computer into believing there is a shockable rhythm when there really isn't one or vice versa. Also, it's possible a shock could be delivered to you if you are touching the patient, which could injure you. (p. 352)

48. (D) The AED should routinely be used on patients with shockable rhythms. It is not designed to be used on trauma victims, who usually are in PEA or asystole; patients under 55 pounds, because the power of the shock would be too high; and patients under 8 years of age, for the same reason. (pp. 352, 357)

49. (C) The AED pads are first attached to the cables. Then the pad attached to the red cable is placed over the left lower ribs. The pad attached to the white cable is placed in the angle between the sternum and the right clavicle. (p. 352)

50. (C) After the first set of three stacked shocks, if the patient has a pulse and is breathing adequately, give high-concentration oxygen via nonrebreather mask and then transport. (p. 357)

51. (B) After six shocks, the EMT-B should transport the patient unless local protocol says otherwise. Termination of an arrest can only be done with the approval of medical direction. (p. 358)

52. (A) Defibrillation comes first! Don't hook up oxygen or do anything that delays analysis of the rhythm or defibrillation. (p. 358)

53. (D) A patient with an implanted defibrillator can be defibrillated immediately. Emergency care, CPR, and defibrillation for this patient are the same as for other cardiac patients. A trauma patient with severe blood loss should not be defibrillated. If a patient is soaking wet or is touching anything metallic that another person is touching, you could receive a shock. Move these patients before defibrillating. (p. 361)

54. (A) If it is necessary to remove a nitro patch to defibrillate a patient, you should wear gloves to prevent the nitro from being absorbed into your skin. Do not use alcohol to cleanse the patient's skin; this could burn the patient's skin during defibrillation. (p. 360)

55. (C) If a patient has a cardiac pacemaker and needs to be defibrillated, the EMT-B should place the pad several inches away from the pacemaker battery. If you do not do this, you could damage the pacemaker with the AED shock. You cannot change the AED's power setting. EMT-Bs do not remove pacemakers; this involves surgery. (p. 361)

COMPLETE THE FOLLOWING

1. The chain of survival includes: (p. 348)
   - early access
   - early CPR
   - early defibrillation
   - early advanced care

LABEL THE DIAGRAM (Chapter 4, pp. 57–59)

1. Aorta
2. Pulmonary vein
3. Left lung
4. Left ventricle
5. Artery
6. Arterioles
7. Capillary bed
8. Venules
9. Vein
10. Right ventricle
11. Inferior vena cava
12. Superior vena cava
13. Pulmonary artery

VIRTUAL STREET SCENES

1. Cardiac patients can deteriorate very quickly. This is usually due to fluid in the lungs, intense chest pain, or dysrhythmia. Each of these problems can be monitored and managed by advanced life support (ALS) personnel, so call for them early.

2. Give the patient (or help the patient take) nitroglycerin if *all* of the following conditions are met: she complains of chest pain; she has a history of cardiac problems; her physician has prescribed nitroglycerin (NTG); she has the nitroglycerin with her; her systolic blood pressure is greater that 100; medical direction authorizes administration of the medication.

3. If the AED does not shock a pulseless patient, it means the patient does not have a shockable rhythm.

4. This patient is in critical condition, so she is a high priority. Vital signs should be taken every 5 minutes on a critical patient.

MATCH TERMINOLOGY/DEFINITIONS

1. **(D)** Convulsions—uncontrolled muscular movements

2. **(B)** Diabetes mellitus—condition brought about by decreased insulin production; also called "sugar diabetes" or simply "diabetes"

3. **(G)** Epilepsy—medical condition that sometimes causes seizures

4. **(A)** Glucose—form of sugar that provides the body's basic source of energy

5. **(H)** Hyperglycemia—high blood sugar

6. **(F)** Hypoglycemia—low blood sugar

7. **(C)** Insulin—hormone produced by the pancreas or taken as a medication by many diabetics that aids cells in utilizing glucose

8. **(I)** Seizure—sudden change in sensation, behavior, or movement that can, in its most severe form, produce convulsions

9. **(E)** Status epilepticus—prolonged seizure, or when a person suffers two or more convulsive seizures without regaining full consciousness

10. **(J)** Stroke—blockage or bursting of a major blood vessel supplying the brain; also called a cerebrovascular accident (CVA)

MULTIPLE-CHOICE REVIEW

1. **(C)** The relationship of glucose to insulin is often described as a lock and key mechanism. In order for sugar to enter the body's cells, insulin must be present. The relationship is not oppositional, synergistic, or antagonistic. (p. 371)

2. **(A)** The condition brought about by decreased insulin production is known as diabetes mellitus. Hypotension is low blood pressure resulting from hypoperfusion, or shock, or other causes; hypoglycemia is low blood sugar. A cerebrovascular accident occurs when an artery in the brain is blocked or ruptured. (p. 371)

3. **(C)** The most common medical emergency for the diabetic patient is called hypoglycemia. See also answer #2. (p. 371)

4. **(A)** When a diabetic overexercises or overexerts, a medical condition called hypoglycemia can develop because sugars in the body are used faster than normal. Hyperglycemia (high blood sugar) occurs because the diabetic does not produce enough natural insulin, which is needed to pass sugar from the blood into the cells. Acute pulmonary edema is fluid in the lungs, which is usually the result of left heart failure. (p. 373)

5. **(B)** Potential causes of hypoglycemia: the patient may have taken too much insulin by mistake, the patient has been vomiting, or the patient has been fasting. A person does not lower sugar in the blood by eating a box of candy; this increases the blood sugar level. (p. 371)

6. **(A)** If sugar is not replenished quickly, the hypoglycemic patient may have permanent brain damage. (p. 372)

7. **(C)** The clues that a patient is a diabetic include a medical identification bracelet, the presence of insulin in the refrigerator, and information provided by family members. The fact that the patient eats low fat food would have no effect on the patient's condition. (p. 373)

8. **(B)** Sugunoil is a distracter and is not an oral medication used to treat diabetes. (p. 373)

9. **(D)** An intoxicated appearance and uncharacteristic behavior are typical of diabetic emergency. (pp. 373, 376)

10. **(B)** Diabetics often present the EMT-B with cold, clammy skin, anxiety, and combativeness. It is unusual for them to have a decreased heart rate. (pp. 373, 376)

11. **(A)** In order for the EMT-B to consider administering oral glucose, the patient must have altered mental status and have a history of diabetes and be awake enough to swallow. Oral glucose is not administered to the patient with an absent gag reflex or a patient with a seizure history who is not a diabetic. (p. 376)

12. **(C)** When reassessing a patient to whom you have administered oral glucose, and you note the patient's condition has not improved, you should consult medical direction about whether to administer more glucose. (p. 376)

13. **(C)** The recovery position prevents aspiration of fluids or stomach content into the lungs. The position is utilized for all non-spine injured patients who are unresponsive or have an altered mental status. (p. 376)

14. **(C)** Children are less likely to eat correctly, are more active, and as a result are more likely to exhaust blood sugar levels. As a result, children are more at risk for developing diabetes. (p. 376)

15. **(C)** A sudden onset or a change in mental status may indicate an alteration in the patient's blood sugar level. (p. 376)

16. **(B)** Before and after administering oral glucose, make sure you document the mental status of the patient. Increasing the oxygen flow rate is not necessary since it should remain at 15 liters per minute by nonrebreather mask. The glass of water is not needed. (p. 376)

17. **(D)** One trade name of oral glucose is Insta-glucose. D_5W is an intravenous solution of five percent dextrose in water. Lactose is another form of sugar, and insulin is a hormone produced by the pancreas to help the body break down sugar. (p. 377)

18. **(D)** When a patient is very confused and disoriented, before deciding the patient has a behavioral problem, the EMT-B should consider a potential head injury, a brain tumor, and hypoxia. There is no such thing as an allergy to glucose. (p. 376)

19. **(B)** Diabetics routinely test the level of sugar in their blood using a glucose meter. (pp. 372–373)

20. **(D)** Complications of diabetes include: kidney failure, heart disease, and blindness. (p. 378)

21. **(C)** The reading on the glucose meter is reported in milligrams of glucose per deciliter of blood (p. 372)

22. **(D)** A diabetic with sugar level below 80 is considered hypoglycemic. (p. 373)

23. **(A)** A diabetic with a sugar level above 120 is considered hyperglycemic (p. 373)

24. **(C)** The most common cause of seizures in adults is not taking anti-seizure medication. (p. 379)

25. **(A)** Seizures are commonly caused by high fever, brain tumor, and infection. They are not generally a result of cold exposure. (p. 379)

26. **(A)** Idiopathic seizures occur spontaneously, have an unknown cause, and often start in childhood. Seizures in

children who frequently have them are rarely life-threatening, but you should treat seizures in an infant or child as if they are life-threatening. (p. 379)

27. **(A)** Convulsive seizures may be seen with epilepsy or hypoglycemia. They are not seen with asthma, AMI, pulmonary embolism, or anaphylaxis. (pp. 378–379)

28. **(B)** The best-known condition that results in seizures is epilepsy. (p. 379)

29. **(A)** Not all seizures are alike. The type of seizure that most people associate with epilepsy and seizure disorders is called generalized tonic-clonic seizure. The patient falls to the floor and has severe convulsions. (p. 379)

30. **(D)** The family's reaction to the seizure (e.g., they called 9-1-1 or were frightened by the seizure) is not important to emergency care. When obtaining the medical history of a seizure patient, find out how long the seizure lasted, what the patient did after the seizure, and what the patient was doing prior to the seizure. (pp. 379–380)

31. **(C)** If a seizure patient becomes cyanotic, provide artificial ventilations with supplemental oxygen. (pp. 379–380)

32. **(B)** When you arrive on the scene of a seizure patient, and you notice that a bystander has placed a tongue blade in the corner of the patient's mouth, you should carefully remove the object from his mouth. Any object in the patient's mouth could cause an airway obstruction. Then begin oxygen administration. (pp. 379–380)

33. **(A)** A seizure will normally last about 1 to 3 minutes. (p. 380)

34. **(B)** When a patient has two or more back-to-back seizures without regaining consciousness (or a seizure lasts over 5 to 10 minutes), this is called status epilepticus. Status asthmaticus is a continuous asthmatic attack. Convulsions are uncontrolled muscular movements. (p. 380)

35. **(D)** If you suspect a conscious patient has had a stroke, transport in the semi-sitting position. If a suspected stroke patient was unconscious, you should transport in the recovery position. (pp. 381–382)

36. **(B)** When a stoke patient has difficulty saying what he is thinking even though he clearly understands you, this is called expressive aphasia. (pp. 381–382)

37. **(C)** When the patient can speak clearly but cannot understand what you are saying, this is called receptive aphasia. (pp. 381–382)

38. **(D)** A common sign of a cerebrovascular accident is headache. (pp. 381–382)

39. **(D)** Signs and symptoms of a stoke include: vomiting, seizures, and loss of bladder control. (pp. 381–382)

40. **(B)** When a patient has many of the signs and symptoms of a stroke, which completely resolve in less than 24 hours, this is called a TIA. (pp. 381–382)

COMPLETE THE FOLLOWING

1. The signs and symptoms of a diabetic emergency include: (any six) (p. 376)
   - Rapid onset of altered mental status
   - Intoxicated appearance, staggering, slurred speech, to unconsciousness
   - Elevated heart rate
   - Cold, clammy skin
   - Hunger

   - Seizures
   - Uncharacteristic behavior
   - Anxiety
   - Combativeness

2. Hyperglycemia occurs because the diabetic does not produce enough natural insulin, which is needed to pass sugar out of the blood and into the cells. It usually involves a situation in which the diabetic: (p. 378)
   - has not taken enough insulin to make up for the deficiency in natural insulin.
   - has forgotten to take his insulin.
   - has overeaten.
   - has an infection that has upset his insulin/glucose balance.

VIRTUAL STREET SCENES

1. They should be told how important it is that the patient eats, since the oral glucose will wear off. Tell them not to hesitate to call EMS again if there is any change in the patient's mental status.

2. Too much exercise for the amount of sugar taken in, too much insulin, or vomiting a meal also could cause hypoglycemia.

3. If medical direction permits it, you could have tried giving the patient some orange juice with a teaspoon of sugar in it.

Chapter 20: Allergic Reactions

MATCH TERMINOLOGY/DEFINITIONS

1. **(C)** Allergen—something that causes an allergic reaction

2. **(B)** Anaphylaxis—severe or life-threatening allergic reaction in which the blood vessels dilate, causing a drop in blood pressure, and the tissues lining the respiratory system swell, interfering with the airway

3. **(E)** Auto-injector—syringe (pre-loaded with medication) that has a spring-loaded device that pushes the needle through the skin when the tip of the device is pressed firmly against the body

4. **(D)** Epinephrine—hormone produced by the body; as a medication, it constricts blood vessels and dilates respiratory passages and is used to relieve severe allergic reactions

5. **(A)** Hives—red, itchy, possibly raised blotches on the skin that often result from an allergic reaction

MULTIPLE-CHOICE REVIEW

1. **(C)** An exaggerated response of the body's immune system to any substance is called an allergic reaction. Vasoconstricting is the constriction of the vessels. A syncopal episode is when the patient passes out momentarily. (p. 389)

2. **(D)** Allergic reactions are sometimes treated as a high priority because they can cause airway obstruction. In anaphylaxis (a severe allergic reaction), exposure to the allergen will cause blood vessels to dilate rapidly and cause a drop in blood pressure. Many tissues swell, including those that line the respiratory system. This swelling can obstruct the airway, leading to respiratory failure. Vomiting and hives are not life-threatening. Most patients can tolerate a rapid pulse for a short while. (p. 389)

3. **(C)** The first time a patient is exposed to an allergen, the person's immune system forms antibodies, which are an attempt by the body to "attack" the foreign substances (allergens). (p. 389)

4. **(A)** The second time a patient is exposed to an allergen, the body reactions include dilation of the blood vessels, massive swelling, and difficulty in breathing. (p. 389)

5. **(D)** Red fruits and vegetables are not common causes of allergic reactions. Causes include hornet stings, eggs and milk, poison ivy, and penicillin. (pp. 389–390)

6. **(A)** It is important to find out if a patient is allergic to latex so you do not wear gloves that could cause an allergic reaction. Latex allergy does not cause antitoxins, immediate cardiac arrest, or an allergy to other substances such as milk. (p. 390)

7. **(B)** Hives are not a <u>respiratory</u> sign or symptom but are an effect of an allergic reaction on the skin. The respiratory signs and symptoms of anaphylactic shock include rapid breathing, cough, and stridor, as well as tightness in the throat or chest, labored or noisy breathing, hoarseness or loss of voice, and wheezing. (p. 392)

8. **(D)** The effects of an allergic reaction on the cardiac system could include increased heart rate and decreased blood pressure. (p. 392)

9. **(C)** To be considered a severe allergic reaction, a patient must have signs and symptoms of shock and/or respiratory distress. (p. 392)

10. **(B)** After administering epinephrine, the EMT-B should reassess the patient after 2 minutes. Do not decrease the oxygen and do not allow the patient to remain at home. (p. 393)

11. **(B)** If a patient has no history of allergies and is having her first allergic reaction, you should treat for shock and transport immediately. (p. 393)

12. **(A)** If a patient has an epinephrine auto-injector, besides helping him take the medication you should always ask if the patient has any spare auto-injectors for the trip to the hospital just in case you need to recontact medical direction for permission to administer another dose of epinephrine to the patient. (p. 393)

13. **(B)** The location for injection with the auto-injector is the lateral mid-thigh. Injecting epinephrine in the back could cause a pneumothorax. Injection into the buttocks would require too much medication and take too long to act. (p. 393)

14. **(B)** The adult epinephrine auto-injector contains 0.3 mg and the child's contains 0.15 mg, or $1/2$ the adult dose. The child dose is indicated for children weighing less than 66 pounds. (p. 397)

15. **(B)** Children commonly outgrow allergies as they mature. Infants rarely experience anaphylaxis; anaphylactic reactions are common in <u>older</u> children. Parents frequently can provide useful medical history. (p. 397)

COMPLETE THE FOLLOWING

1. The signs and symptoms of allergic reaction or anaphylactic shock can include: (any ten) (pp. 391–392)
   - itching
   - hives
   - flushing

   - swelling of the face, especially the eyes and lips
   - warm, tingling feeling in the face, mouth, chest, feet, and hands
   - feeling of tightness in the throat or chest
   - cough
   - rapid breathing
   - labored breathing
   - noisy breathing
   - hoarseness
   - muffled voice
   - loss of voice entirely
   - stridor
   - wheezing
   - increased heart rate
   - decreased blood pressure
   - itchy, watery eyes
   - headache
   - runny nose
   - sense of impending doom
   - altered mental status
   - flushed, dry skin or pale, cool, clammy skin
   - nausea or vomiting
   - vital sign changes to: increased pulse, increased respirations and decreased blood pressure

2. The important thing to recognize in any presentation is the presence of either respiratory distress or signs and symptoms of shock. (p. 392)

LABEL THE DIAGRAMS (p. 390)

1. Insect bites or stings
2. Food
3. Plants
4. Medications

VIRTUAL STREET SCENES

1. Yes, it would be appropriate but only with medical direction's permission. It should get injected into the thigh.

2. Yes, it would be appropriate. If ALS will not be on scene momentarily, then you could plan for an intercept en route.

3. Your priorities would be the patient's ABCs and defibrillation.

CASE STUDY—The Lakefront Emergency

1. No, there is only one patient.

2. Yes, to the scene, or at least an intercept en route to the hospital due to the breathing difficulty.

3. Because she has breathing difficulty and cannot inhale deeply enough to speak for normal time periods.

4. She is alert and oriented.

5. The sound is most likely a wheeze, which can be caused by asthma, upper airway obstruction, anaphylaxis, or right heart failure (cor pulmonale).

6. The posture or position of the patient, like an upright tripod position, intercostal separation or retractions, accessory muscle use, cyanosis, and others.

7. This patient should be given oxygen by a nonrebreather mask at 15 liters per minute.

8. This is a high priority patient due to her breathing difficulty, and she should be rapidly transported.

9. The position of comfort is generally best. But if she is able to breathe adequately, lay her down to improve her dizziness.

10. SAMPLE (signs and symptoms, allergies, medications, past medical history, last intake, and events leading up to illness).

11. A) Epinephrine.
    B) It would be appropriate to assist her with her epinephrine auto-injector.

12. A) You must call medical direction for permission to administer epinephrine to the patient.
    B) Make sure the epinephrine auto-injector is prescribed to the patient, is not expired, and is clear.

13. A) Chief complaint is breathing difficulty with chest pain.
    B) OPQRST findings, vital signs, SAMPLE findings.
    C) Treatment given thus far (e.g., oxygen, positioning, epinephrine auto-injector per medical direction).

14. The paramedic would establish an IV, administer saline or Ringer's Lactate, evaluate the need for airway or breathing management, and assess the need for additional epinephrine or other medications such as Benadryl. Some EMS systems may use the PASG (MAST).

Chapter 21: Poisoning and Overdose Emergencies

MATCH TERMINOLOGY/DEFINITIONS

1. (D) Absorbed poisons—poisons that are taken into the body through unbroken skin

2. (H) Activated charcoal—substance that adsorbs many poisons and prevents them from being absorbed by the body

3. (O) Antidote—substance that will neutralize a poison or its effects

4. (J) Delirium tremens—severe reaction that can be part of alcohol withdrawal, characterized by sweating, trembling, anxiety, and hallucinations

5. (I) Dilution—thinning down or weakening by mixing with something else

6. (E) Downers—depressants, such as barbiturates, that depress the central nervous system

7. (L) Hallucinogens—mind-affecting or mind-altering drugs that act on the central nervous system to produce excitement and distortion of perceptions

8. (F) Ingested poisons—poisons that are swallowed

9. (K) Inhaled poisons—poisons that are breathed in

10. (G) Narcotics—class of drugs that affect the nervous system and changes many normal body activities; their legal use is for relief of pain.

11. (A) Poison—any substance that can harm the body by altering cell structure or functions

12. (M) Toxin—poisonous substance secreted by bacteria, plants, or animals

13. (B) Uppers—stimulants, such as amphetamines, that affect the central nervous system to excite the user

14. (N) Volatile chemicals—vaporizing compounds, such as cleaning fluid, that are breathed in by an abuser to produce a "high"

15. (C) Withdrawal—state in which a patient's body reacts severely when deprived of an abused substance

MULTIPLE-CHOICE REVIEW

1. (B) Empty pill bottles or containers are a good environmental clue of poisoning. Just because a patient has vomited, has an altered level of responsiveness, or has a headache does not necessarily indicate poisoning. (p. 403)

2. (A) A poison is any substance that can harm the body, sometimes seriously enough to create a medical emergency. (p. 403)

3. (C) Although some of the over one million cases of poisoning in the United States each year result from murder or suicide attempts, most poisonings are accidental and involve young children. (p. 403)

4. (B) A substance secreted by plants, animals, or bacteria that is poisonous to humans is called a toxin. A narcotic is a drug that relieves pain; a drug is a chemical used to treat illness. (p. 403)

5. (D) Due to the poisons they produce, plants such as mistletoe, mushrooms, and rubber plants can be dangerous to humans or pets. (p. 403)

6. (B) Botulism is a deadly disease caused by a toxin produced by bacteria. HIV is a virus. Steroids and penicillin are medications that, when used properly, are not deadly. (p. 403)

7. (B) Reactions to poisons are most serious in the ill and elderly. (p. 403)

8. (B) Poisons interfere with, but do <u>not</u> enhance, the normal biochemical processes in the body. Poisons damage the body by destroying skin and other tissues, overstimulating (or depressing) the central nervous system, and displacing oxygen on the hemoglobin. (p. 403)

9. (D) Excretion is not a route of entry to the body but rather is a route of exit. Poisons enter the body through inhalation, ingestion, injection, and absorption. (p. 405)

10. (C) Carbon monoxide, chlorine, and ammonia are examples of inhaled poisons. (p. 405)

11. (A) Insecticides and agricultural chemicals can be absorbed through the skin. Carbon monoxide and ammonia are inhaled. Insect stings and snake bites are injected. Aspirin and LSD are ingested. (p. 405)

12. (B) The venom of a snakebite is an injected poison. (p. 405)

13. (A) It is important to determine the time a poison was ingested because different poisons act on the body at different rates. Other answer choices are incorrect statements. (p. 406)

14. (B) If you suspect poisoning by ingestion, after assuring a child has a patent airway, ask the parent for the child's weight because the effects of most chemicals are weight dependent. (p. 406)

15. (B) The most common results of poisoning by ingestion are nausea and vomiting. All the other answers are plausible but not the most common. (p. 406)

16. (C) Activated charcoal is used to prevent poisons from being absorbed by the body. It does not speed up the digestion of most chemicals, rather, it prevents digestion. It does not dilute the poison or act as an antidote. (p. 406)

17. (A) The difference between activated charcoal and regular charcoal is that activated charcoal is manufactured to have many cracks and crevices that increase the amount of surface for the poison to bind to. (p. 406)

18. **(C)** The decision on when to use activated charcoal is best made with medical direction or poison-control center consultation. It is not necessary to wait until the patient gets to the emergency department. The patient's family physician need not be consulted. (p. 406)

19. **(D)** Activated charcoal is not routinely used with ingestion of caustic substances, strong acids, or strong alkalis. (p. 406)

20. **(B)** Venom is an injected poison from a snakebite or other animal. Examples of caustic substances include lye, toilet bowl cleaner, and oven cleaner. (p. 406)

21. **(A)** A patient who continues to cough violently after a gasoline ingestion should not be given activated charcoal as he may aspirate the gasoline into his lungs. (p. 406)

22. **(C)** When a physician orders dilution of an ingested substance, you can use either water or milk. A cola drink will burn the stomach as well as produce gas from the carbonation. Coffee has caffeine in it, which will speed up the heart. (p. 409)

23. **(C)** The most common inhaled poison is carbon monoxide. Carbon dioxide is a colorless gas that we exhale. Nitrogen is a gas that makes up about 79% of the air. Phosgene is a nerve gas. (p. 410)

24. **(A)** As you approach a patient who has passed out while cleaning a large tank, if you smell an unusual odor, you should stand back and attempt to learn more about the chemical involved. This action will also prevent you or your crew from being overcome by the chemical. (p. 410)

25. **(B)** The principal prehospital treatment of a patient who has inhaled poison is administering high-concentration oxygen. (p. 410)

26. **(C)** Besides motor-vehicle exhaust, you might also find carbon monoxide around an improperly vented wood-burning stove. Malfunctioning oil, gas, and coal-burning furnaces and stoves can also be sources of carbon monoxide. (pp. 410, 412)

27. **(B)** Carbon monoxide affects the body by preventing the normal carrying of oxygen by the red blood cells. It does not cause severe respiratory burns or airway swelling, nor does it stimulate the central nervous system to decrease oxygen consumption. (pp. 410, 412)

28. **(D)** Cherry red lips are <u>not</u> typically seen. A conscious patient who you suspect has carbon monoxide poisoning may exhibit cyanosis, altered mental status, and dizziness. (pp. 410, 412)

29. **(A)** If a patient has been contaminated by poisonous powder, you should brush off as much as possible, then irrigate after determining that the powder does not react with water. (p. 413)

30. **(B)** If you smell alcohol on the breath or clothes of a patient, you should not let this sidetrack you from doing a complete assessment. Calling the police is not necessary unless the patient is a threat to your safety. (pp. 414, 416)

31. **(A)** Acetone breath is not seen with alcohol abuse but is with diabetes. Do not confuse the odor of alcohol on the breath with acetone breath. (p. 416)

32. **(C)** Sweating, trembling, anxiety, and hallucinations found in the alcohol withdrawal patient are called delirium tremens. (p. 416)

33. **(B)** The patient who has mixed alcohol and other drugs will exhibit with depressed vital signs. (pp. 416–417)

34. **(B)** When interviewing an intoxicated patient, do not begin by asking if he has taken any drugs because the patient may think you are accusing him of a crime. (pp. 416–417)

35. **(A)** Drugs that stimulate the nervous system to excite the user are called uppers. (p. 417)

36. **(B)** Tranquilizers or sleeping pills are examples of downers. (p. 417)

37. **(B)** Drugs that have a depressant effect on the central nervous system are called downers. (p. 417)

38. **(C)** Drugs capable of producing stupor or sleep that are often used to relieve pain are called narcotics. Narcotics also depress the respiratory system. (p. 417)

39. **(D)** Mind-altering drugs that act on the nervous system to produce an intense state of excitement or distortion of the user's perceptions are called hallucinogens. (p. 417)

40. **(C)** A class of drugs that have few legal uses and are dissolved in the mouth are called hallucinogens. In illegal forms, they usually are found as a colored dot on a piece of paper or in sugar cubes. (p. 417)

41. **(B)** Cleaning fluid, glue, and model cement are examples of volatile chemicals. Diuretics are medications that tend to increase the flow of urine in order to eliminate excess body fluids. (p. 417)

42. **(A)** A patient who has overdosed on an upper may have signs and symptoms such as excitement, increased pulse and breathing rates, dilated pupils, and rapid speech. (p. 419)

43. **(B)** A patient who has overdosed on a downer may have signs and symptoms such as sluggishness, sleepiness, and lack of coordination of body and speech. (p. 419)

44. **(C)** A patient who has overdosed on a hallucinogen may have signs and symptoms such as fast pulse rate, dilated pupils, flushed face, and "see" or "hear" things. (p. 419)

45. **(D)** A patient who has overdosed on a narcotic may have signs and symptoms such as reduced pulse rate and rate and depth of breathing, constricted pupils, and sweating. (p. 419)

COMPLETE THE FOLLOWING

1. If you suspect poisoning, document the following information: (pp. 413–414)
   - Route of poisoning
   - Substance
   - Amount
   - Time
   - Interventions
   - Patient's weight
   - Effects of poisoning
   - Effects of treatment

2. The signs and symptoms of alcohol abuse include: (any six) (p. 416)
   - Odor of alcohol on a patient's breath or clothing.
   - Swaying and unsteadiness of movement.
   - Slurred speech
   - A flushed appearance to the face
   - Nausea or vomiting
   - Poor coordination
   - Slowed reaction time
   - Blurred vision
   - Confusion
   - Hallucinations
   - Lack of memory
   - Altered mental status

1. Inhalation
2. Injection
3. Ingestion
4. Absorption

COMPLETE THE CHART (p. 418)

1. Upper
2. Narcotic
3. Mind-altering
4. Mind-altering
5. Volatile chemical
6. Downer
7. Downer
8. Upper
9. Upper
10. Downer
11. Mind-altering
12. Mind-altering
13. Mind-altering
14. Narcotic
15. Volatile chemical
16. Mind-altering
17. Upper
18. Narcotic
19. Downer
20. Narcotic

VIRTUAL STREET SCENES

1. No. Do not give activated charcoal to any patient with an altered mental status.

2. Your highest priority should be to keep the patient's airway clear and patent.

3. It is necessary to take the oil to the hospital so that hospital chemists can identify the substance that was ingested.

Chapter 22: Environmental Emergencies

MATCH TERMINOLOGY/DEFINITIONS

▶ Part A

1. **(C)** Active rewarming—application of an external heat source to rewarm the body of a hypothermic patient

2. **(B)** AGE—abbreviation that stands for arterial gas embolism

3. **(J)** Air embolism—gas bubble in the bloodstream; more accurately called an arterial gas embolism

4. **(H)** Central rewarming—application of heat to the lateral chest, neck, armpits, and groin of a hypothermic patient

5. **(F)** Conduction—direct transfer of heat from one material to another through direct contact

6. **(D)** Convection—carrying away of heat by currents of air or water or other gases or liquids

7. **(G)** Decompression sickness—condition resulting from nitrogen trapped in the body's tissues caused by coming up too quickly from a deep, prolonged dive

8. **(E)** Drowning—death caused by changes in the lungs resulting from immersion in water

9. **(A)** Evaporation—change from liquid to gas; as perspiration on the skin vaporizes, the body experiences a cooling effect.

10. **(I)** Hyperthermia—increase in body temperature above normal; life-threatening in its extreme

▶ Part B

1. **(F)** Hypothermia—generalized cooling that reduces body temperature below normal; life-threatening in its extreme

2. **(E)** Local cooling—cooling or freezing of particular parts of the body

3. **(A)** Near-drowning—condition of having begun to drown; the patient may be conscious, unconscious with heartbeat and pulse, or with no heartbeat or pulse but still able to be resuscitated.

4. **(B)** Passive rewarming—covering a hypothermic patient and taking other steps to prevent further heat loss and help the body rewarm itself

5. **(C)** Radiation—sending out energy, such as heat, in waves into space

6. **(D)** Respiration—breathing; during this process, the body loses heat as warm air is exhaled from the body.

7. **(G)** Toxins—substances produced by animals or plants that are poisonous to humans

8. **(I)** Venom—toxin produced by certain animals such as snakes, spiders, and some marine life-forms

9. **(H)** Water chill—chilling caused by conduction of heat from the body when the body or clothing is wet

10. **(J)** Wind chill—chilling caused by convection of heat from the body in the presence of air currents.

MULTIPLE-CHOICE REVIEW

1. **(A)** Water conducts heat away from the body 25 times faster than still air. (p. 425)

2. **(C)** The body loses heat from respiration, radiation, conduction, convection, and evaporation. Excretion is the elimination of solid wastes, and induction is to place something into the body. Condensation is the accumulation of moisture on an object. (pp. 425–426)

3. **(C)** When there is more wind, there is greater heat loss. (pp. 425–426)

4. **(C)** Most radiant heat loss occurs from a person's head and neck. This is why one should always cover the head when going outside on a cold day. (p. 425)

5. **(D)** Having a headache does not predispose the patient to hypothermia. Predisposing factors to hypothermia include burns, diabetes, and spinal-cord injuries. Other predisposing factors include shock, head injuries, generalized infection, and hypoglycemia. Also the elderly and infants and young children are at risk. (pp. 426–427)

6. **(D)** Infants and children do not have more body fat than adults. Infants and children are more prone to hypothermia because they have small muscle mass, they have large skin surface in relation to their total body mass, and they are unable to shiver effectively. (p. 427)

7. **(B)** You should consider hypothermia when a patient has been in a cold environment for a considerable length of time. (p. 427)

8. **(B)** When a patient's core body temperature drops below 90°F, the patient may no longer be shivering. (p. 428)

9. **(A)** Hypothermic patients do not have a high blood pressure and low pulse. Signs and symptoms of hypothermia include stiff or rigid posture, cool abdominal skin temperature, and loss of motor coordination. (p. 428)

10. **(B)** Passive rewarming involves simply covering the patient. Administering heated oxygen and applying heat packs are part of active rewarming. Never massage the limbs of any hypothermic patient. (p. 428)

11. **(C)** Never give hot liquids to a hypothermic patient quickly. You can give warm liquids slowly. The treatment of the hypothermic patient includes removal of all of the patient's wet clothing, actively rewarming the patient during transport, providing care for shock, and providing oxygen. (pp. 428–429)

12. **(A)** When actively rewarming a patient, apply heat to the chest, neck, armpits, and groin. Never give the person stimulants to drink. (p. 428)

13. **(A)** The reason why you should rewarm the body's core first is to prevent blood from collecting in the extremities due to vasodilation, which could cause a fatal form of shock. (p. 428)

14. **(C)** When transporting an alert patient with mild hypothermia, it is recommended you keep the patient at rest. Since the blood is the coldest in the extremities, unnecessary movement could quickly circulate the cold blood and lower the core body temperature. The wet clothing must come off so the patient can be dried and warmed. (pp. 428–429)

15. **(B)** In a heat emergency, EMT-B care of a patient with moist, pale, normal-to-cool skin includes placing the patient in an air-conditioned ambulance, elevating the patient's legs (if appropriate), and administering oxygen. It may also include cooling or fanning, but never so far as to cause the patient to shiver. (pp. 428–429)

16. **(C)** If in a heat emergency a patient with moist, pale, normal-to-cool skin is responsive and not nauseated, the EMT-B should have him drink water. (pp. 428–429)

17. **(C)** When treating an unresponsive patient with severe hypothermia, provide high-concentration oxygen that has been passed through a warm humidifier. If necessary, the oxygen that has been kept warm in the ambulance passenger compartment can be used. If there is no other choice, oxygen from a cold cylinder may be used. (pp. 428–429)

18. **(B)** Because patients with extreme hypothermia may not reach biological death for over 30 minutes, the medical philosophy is "they are not dead until they're warm and dead." In other words, a patient is not considered dead until after he is rewarmed and resuscitative measures are applied. (p. 429)

19. **(A)** A cold injury usually occurring to exposed areas of the body that is brought about by direct contact with a cold object or exposure to cold air is called an early local cold injury. This injury is commonly called frostnip. (pp. 429–430)

20. **(A)** The skin color of a patient with a superficial local cold injury will change from red to white. (p. 430)

21. **(C)** If a superficial local cold injury is on an extremity, the EMT-B should not reexpose the injury to cold. Immersion in hot water will burn the injury. The extremity should be splinted, but should be covered. (p. 430)

22. **(C)** When muscles, bones, deep blood vessels, and organ membranes become frozen, this type of injury is called a deep local cold injury. (p. 430)

23. **(B)** In frostbite, the affected area first appears white and waxy. When the condition progresses to actual freezing, the skin turns mottled or blotchy, the color turns from white to grayish yellow and finally grayish blue. (p. 430)

24. **(C)** Do not allow the frostbite patient to drink alcohol or smoke because constriction of blood vessels and decreased circulation to the injured tissues may result. (p. 430)

25. **(A)** Active rewarming of a frozen part is seldom recommended in the field. Very hot water may burn the part; the patient's face should be left uncovered. (p. 431)

26. **(C)** When assessing a patient you suspect is in extreme hypothermia, check the carotid pulse for 30–45 seconds. (p. 429)

27. **(C)** The environment associated with hyperthermia includes heat and high humidity. (p. 431)

28. **(B)** The higher the humidity, the less your perspiration evaporates. (pp. 431–432)

29. **(B)** The medical problems resulting from dry heat are often worse than those from moist heat because moist heat tires people before they can harm themselves through overexertion. Dry heat does not affect the respiratory system more quickly than humid heat. (pp. 431–432)

30. **(D)** Fluid buildup in the lungs is related to <u>too</u> much salt in the body, not too little. When salts are lost by the body through sweating, the patient may have muscle cramps, weakness or exhaustion, and dizziness or periods of faintness. (p. 432)

31. **(B)** A patient with heat exhaustion will present with moist, pale, normal-to-cool skin. A rapid strong pulse and lack of sweating are sometimes found with heat stroke. (p. 432)

32. **(B)** The signs and symptoms of a heat emergency in patients who have hot, dry or moist skin include seizures. Muscle cramps usually only occur in early heat exposure from salt loss. (p. 433)

33. **(C)** Heat emergency patients with hot, dry or moist skin have little or no perspiration. The signs and symptoms of a heat emergency in patients who have hot, dry or moist skin include generalized weakness, loss of consciousness or altered mental status, and a full and rapid pulse. (p. 433)

34. **(B)** Substance abuse is a large contributor to adolescent and adult drownings. Car crash immersions are rare. (p. 434)

35. **(C)** During a drowning incident, water flowing past the epiglottis causes a reflex spasm of the larynx. (p. 434)

36. **(B)** About 10 percent of the drowning victims die from lack of air (suffocation). (p. 434)

37. **(A)** If you are not an experienced swimmer, you should never attempt to go into the water to do a rescue. You should wear a personal floating device on the shore and the appropriate exposure suit if you are going into the water. Get qualified help immediately. (pp. 434, 435)

38. **(B)** If you suspect that a patient still in the pool has a possible spine injury, you should immobilize and spineboard him while still in the water. Expediting the removal from the water could complicate the injury. Do not encourage the patient to swim as this may further injure him. (p. 435)

39. **(C)** Two special medical problems seen in scuba-diving accidents are decompression sickness and air embolism. (p. 439)

40. **(A)** The risk of decompression sickness is increased by air travel within 12 hours of a dive. (p. 439)

41. **(C)** A toxin produced by some animals that is harmful to humans is called venom. (p. 442)

42. **(D)** Typical sources of injected poisons include spider, scorpion, and snakebites and stings. (p. 442)

43. **(B)** While cleaning out the crawl space below the house, you experience blotchy skin, redness in your arm, weakness, and nausea. It is possible that you were bitten by a poisonous spider. (p. 442)

44. **(A)** Lack of sensation on one side of the body is usually due to a head injury or cerebrovascular accident. Signs and symptoms of injected poisoning include puncture marks, muscle cramps, chest tightening, joint pains, excessive saliva formation, and profuse sweating. (pp. 443)

45. (D) Never transport a live snake in the ambulance. Arrange for separate transport of a live specimen. If you suspect that your patient has been bitten by a snake, you should call for medical direction, clean the injection site with soap and water, and remove rings, bracelets, or other constricting items on the bitten limb. (pp. 445–446)

COMPLETE THE FOLLOWING

1. The signs and symptoms of heat exhaustion include: (any six) (p. 432)
   - muscular cramps
   - weakness or exhaustion
   - rapid, shallow breathing
   - weak pulse
   - moist, pale skin that may feel normal to cool
   - heavy perspiration
   - possible loss of consciousness

2. The signs and symptoms of heat stroke include: (any six) (p. 433)
   - rapid, shallow breathing
   - full and rapid pulse
   - generalized weakness
   - hot, dry or possibly moist skin
   - little or no perspiration
   - loss of consciousness or altered mental status
   - dilated pupils
   - seizures may be seen; no muscle cramps

3. The signs and symptoms of an insect bite or sting include: (any ten) (p. 443)
   - altered state of awareness
   - noticeable stings or bites on the skin
   - puncture marks
   - blotchy skin
   - localized pain or itching
   - numbness in a limb or body part
   - burning sensations at the site
   - redness
   - swelling or blistering at the site
   - weakness or collapse
   - difficult breathing and abnormal pulse rate
   - headache and dizziness
   - chills
   - fever
   - nausea and vomiting
   - muscle cramps, chest tightening, joint pains
   - excessive saliva formation, profuse sweating
   - anaphylaxis

VIRTUAL STREET SCENES

1. Active rewarming involves heat packs, hot air, blankets, and warmed humidified oxygen. In the hospital environment, active rewarming may include warm fluids, dialysis, warm enemas, and bypass.

2. Yes, of course, and prepare to apply the AED.

3. In the early stages of hypothermia, the heartbeat may be rapid. In a later stage, it slows. In this patient's situation, it may have been that he was in early stage hypothermia or he may have had another problem, such as shock from internal bleeding.

CASE STUDY—Too Cold for Comfort

1. Mental status, ABCs, and ruling out trauma.

2. No. The parent is on the way, so you can begin to talk to the children and patient.

3. SAMPLE History and OPQRST of the chief complaint, which is altered mental status in this case.

4. Comfortable, lying supine, wrapped in blankets.

5. A mild case of hypothermia.

6. Yes, oxygen would be helpful via nonrebreather mask.

7. A slightly decreased temperature but not as slow at 90°F, which is considered severe hypothermia.

8. She is a child, she is skinny with little fat insulation, and she has been playing in cold water and the wind all afternoon.

9. Children love to swim and will do so all day long. Suggest that they have frequent breaks to warm up out of the water and wind.

Chapter 23: Behavioral Emergencies

MATCH TERMINOLOGY/DEFINITIONS

1. **(D)** Behavioral emergency—when a patient's behavior is not typical for the situation; when the patient's behavior is unacceptable or intolerable to the patient, his family, or the community; or when the patient may harm himself or others

2. **(E)** Behavior—manner in which a person acts

3. **(C)** Positional asphyxia—death of a person due to a body position that restricts breathing for a prolonged time

4. **(A)** Soft restraint—humane device made of leather used to hold a patient still to prevent the patient from injuring himself or others

5. **(B)** Stress reaction—display of emotions, such as fear, grief, or anger, in response to an accident, serious illness, or death

MULTIPLE-CHOICE REVIEW

1. **(D)** Differing lifestyles are not a physical cause of altered behavior. The behaviors of persons from other cultures and with different lifestyles may seem unusual to you but might be quite normal to the person performing them. (pp. 451–452)

2. **(C)** Hypoactivity is a distracter and incorrect response. Altered behavior ranging from irritability to altered mental status can be due to lack of oxygen (hypoxia), head trauma, or hypoglycemia. (pp. 451–452)

3. **(C)** To calm a patient who is experiencing a stress reaction, you should explain things to the patient honestly. Do not lie, since this will lead to mistrust of anything you say or do. Quick movements not only confuse, but will scare the patient, not calm him. You, not the patient, should control the situation. Quickly restraining the patient will not calm him and should only be used as a last resort. (pp. 452–453)

4. **(B)** Rather than having a neat appearance, a patient experiencing a behavioral emergency is more likely to have an unusual appearance, disordered clothing, or poor hygiene. In addition, he may exhibit panic and anxiety; agitated or unusual anxiety, such as repetitive motions; and unusual speech patterns, such as pressure-sounding speech. (p. 453)

5. **(B)** When you are called to care for a patient who has attempted suicide, or is about to attempt suicide, your first concern must be your own safety. Once you ensure your safety, treat the patient as you would other patients. (pp. 454–455)

6. **(A)** High suicide rates occur at ages 15–25 and over age 40. Also, suicides among the elderly are increasing. (p. 454)

7. **(C)** Most suicidal patients will not deny suicidal thoughts, but rather will express them and tell others they are considering suicide. Take all threats of suicide seriously. Examples of a self-destructive activity include a defined lethal plan of action that has been verbalized, giving away personal possessions, and previous suicide threats. (p. 454)

8. **(C)** A patient who has made the decision to commit suicide may actually appear to be coming out of depression, or improving. The fact that the decision has been made and an end is in sight can cause this apparent improvement. (p. 454)

9. **(D)** Stay out of kitchens when dealing with an aggressive patient. Kitchens are filled with dangerous weapons. Stay in a safe area until the police can control the scene. When assessing an aggressive patient for a possible threat to you or your crew, determine the patient's history of aggressive behavior, pay attention to the patient's vocal activity (is he shouting at you), and the patient's posture (watch body language). (p. 455)

10. **(A)** If a patient stands in a corner of the room with fists clenched and screaming obscenities, you should request police backup and keep the doorway in sight. Raising your voice or challenging him could force a confrontation. Explaining that you would respond to the situation in the same way is simply being dishonest. (pp. 455–456)

11. **(B)** The family's ability to pay for services is not a consideration in evaluating whether or not to restrain a patient. Use of reasonable force to restrain a patient should involve an evaluation of the patient's size and strength, the mental state of the patient, and the available methods of restraint. (p. 456)

12. **(A)** The use of force by an EMT-B is allowed in most states in order to defend against an attack by an emotionally disturbed patient. While the police do not need to be present, it is very desirable to involve them. The fact that a patient has been drinking or refuses care does not take away his decision-making rights. (p. 456)

13. **(D)** Four rescuers, not two, should be used to secure a disturbed patient. This allows one rescuer to control each limb. Monitor all restrained patients carefully. (p. 456)

14. **(D)** Apply a surgical mask, but ensure that the patient is not likely to vomit or does not have breathing difficulties before applying. Placing the patient in a prone position may limit, but will not eliminate, the patient's ability to spit. Never place roller gauze or tape over a patient's mouth due to the risk of aspiration. (p. 456)

15. **(C)** When a patient is a danger to himself and others and needs to be transported against his will, the EMT-B should contact the police for assistance. Most states have a legal provision that will allow such a patient to be transported and gives this authority to law enforcement personnel. Know your laws on treating patients without consent. (pp. 458–459)

COMPLETE THE FOLLOWING

1. Risk factors for suicide include the following: (p. 454)
   - depression
   - high current or recent stress levels
   - recent emotional trauma
   - age
   - alcohol and drug abuse
   - threats of suicide
   - suicide plans
   - previous attempts or suicide threats; history of self-destructive behavior
   - sudden improvement from depression

2. When a patient acts as if he may hurt himself or others, take the following precautions: (p. 455)
   - Do not isolate yourself from your partner or other sources of help.
   - Do not take any action that may be considered threatening by the patient.
   - Always be on the watch for weapons.
   - Be alert for sudden changes in the patient's behavior.

VIRTUAL STREET SCENES

1. Restraint is the responsibility of law enforcement. However, while they call and wait for backup, you may offer your assistance, but remember: never assist unless there are sufficient personnel to do the job; you must be able to ensure your own safety and the safety of the patient; and, if you do assist, make certain the restraints used are humane,

2. The most humane form of restraint is a roller bandage or a sheet and tape. Leather restraints are also helpful. Metal and plastic handcuffs cut and rip the skin and should not be carried by EMTs.

3. No. You may need to convince the patient that vital signs are a part your normal routine, but do not skip them. Remember, there could be more than just a behavioral problem.

Chapter 24: Obstetrics and Gynecological Emergencies

▶ **Part A**

1. **(I)** Abortion—spontaneous (miscarriage) or induced termination of pregnancy

2. **(F)** Abruptio placentae—condition in which the placenta separates from the uterine wall

3. **(D)** Afterbirth—placenta, umbilical cord, and some tissues from the lining of the uterus that are delivered after the birth of the baby

4. **(K)** Amniotic sac—thin, membranous "bag of waters" that surrounds the developing fetus

5. **(M)** Breech presentation—when the buttocks or both legs of a baby deliver first during birth

6. **(A)** Cephalic presentation—normal head-first birth

7. **(B)** Cervix—neck of the uterus at the entrance to the birth canal

8. **(O)** Crowning—when the presenting part of the baby first appears through the vaginal opening

9. **(C)** Ectopic pregnancy—implantation of the fertilized egg in an oviduct, the cervix of the uterus, or in the abdominopelvic cavity

10. **(E)** Fetus—baby developing in the womb

11. **(G)** Induced abortion—deliberate actions to stop a pregnancy

12. **(J)** Labor—three stages of the delivery of a baby that begin with the contractions of the uterus and end with the expulsion of the placenta

13. **(L)** Meconium staining—amniotic fluid that is greenish or brownish-yellow rather than clear; an indication of possible maternal or fetal distress during labor

14. **(H)** Multiple birth—when more than one baby is born during a single delivery

15. **(N)** Perineum—skin between the vagina and the anus

▶ **Part B**

1. **(H)** Placenta—organ of pregnancy where exchange of oxygen, foods, and wastes occurs between a mother and fetus

2. **(I)** Placenta previa—condition in which the placenta is formed in an abnormal location (usually low in the uterus and close to or over the cervical opening) that will not allow for a normal delivery of the fetus

3. **(F)** Premature infant—any newborn weighing less than $5\frac{1}{2}$ pounds or one that is born before the 37th week of pregnancy

4. **(A)** Prolapsed umbilical cord—when the umbilical cord presents first and is squeezed between the vaginal wall and the baby's head

5. **(C)** Spontaneous abortion—when the fetus and placenta deliver before the 28th week of pregnancy, commonly called a miscarriage

6. **(E)** Stillborn—born dead

7. **(B)** Supine hypotensive syndrome—dizziness and a drop in blood pressure caused when the mother is in a supine position and the weight of the uterus, infant, placenta, and amniotic fluid compress the inferior vena cava, reducing return of blood to the heart and cardiac output

8. **(G)** Umbilical cord—fetal structure containing the blood vessels that carry blood to and from the placenta

9. **(D)** Uterus—muscular abdominal organ where the fetus develops; also called the womb

10. **(J)** Vagina—birth canal

MULTIPLE-CHOICE REVIEW

1. **(B)** The nine months of pregnancy are divided into three-month trimesters. During the second trimester, the uterus grows very rapidly while the woman's blood volume, cardiac output, and heart rate increase. (p. 464)

2. **(B)** The normal birth position is head first and is called a cephalic birth. Breech is buttocks or feet first birth. (p. 464)

3. **(C)** The first stage of labor starts with regular contractions of the uterus. This can occur earlier or later than nine months. It ends with full dilatation of the cervix. (p. 464)

4. **(D)** The second stage of labor starts with the entry of the baby into the birth canal. (p. 464)

5. **(A)** The third stage of labor begins with the birth of the baby. (p. 464)

6. **(B)** The third stage of labor is complete when the afterbirth is expelled. Expulsion should occur within 20 minutes from the birth of the baby. (p. 464)

7. **(B)** The process by which the cervix gradually widens and thins out is called dilation. (p. 464)

8. **(A)** As the fetus moves downward and the cervix dilates, normally the amniotic sac breaks and fluid leaks out. If this fluid is greenish or brownish-yellow in color, it may indicate fetal or maternal distress. (p. 465)

9. **(C)** The greenish or brownish-yellow fluid expelled from the amniotic sac is called meconium staining. There is no such thing as amniotic bile. Bile is a chemical that helps break down fats during digestion. (p. 465)

10. **(C)** When a mother in labor states she feels the need to move her bowels, this means the birth moment is nearing. This does not indicate that the baby is in distress. (p. 466)

11. **(B)** The contraction duration is timed from the beginning of contraction to when the uterus relaxes. The contraction interval is defined in answer #12. (p. 466)

12. **(A)** The contraction interval, or frequency, is timed from the start of one contraction to the start of the next. The contraction duration is defined in answer #11. (p. 466)

13. **(B)** Delivery is imminent when the contractions last 30 seconds and are 2 to 3 minutes apart. (p. 466)

14. **(B)** The EMT-B's primary roles at a normal childbirth scene are to determine whether the delivery will occur at the scene and, if so, to assist the mother as she delivers the child. If delivery is imminent, do not delay it. There is no need to immobilize the patient during emergency childbirth. (p. 466)

15. **(C)** The sterile obstetrical kit does <u>not</u> contain heavy flat twine to tie the cord. Occasionally, in an off-duty situation, you may be required to improvise using heavy flat twine or new shoelaces to tie the cord. (pp. 466–467)

16. **(B)** When evaluating the mother for a possible home delivery, the EMT-B should ask the frequency and duration of contractions. If the mother feels the need to urinate, this is a normal process, but if she has to move her bowels, this is a signal that the infant is moving down the birth canal. The father's blood type is not important to field care but would be important to hospital care if a transfusion is necessary. (p. 467)

17. **(A)** It is important to ask the mother if you can examine for crowning if the mother is straining during contractions. If she is, birth will probably occur too soon for transport. EMT-Bs do not automatically examine every woman in her ninth month for crowning, and you would need the patient's permission to do so. (pp. 467–468)

18. **(C)** You should ask the mother if her water broke and prepare for a quiet ride to the hospital. Since this is her first pregnancy and only an 8-month term, this may be false labor or just the beginning of labor. (pp. 467–468)

19. **(A)** If you determine that the delivery is imminent based on the presence of crowning and other signs, you should contact medical direction, or follow your local protocol. Do not ask the mother to go to the bathroom first, as the infant may be expelled into the toilet. Do not attempt to hold back a delivery by asking the mother to hold her legs closed. (p. 469)

20. **(B)** When a full-term pregnant woman in a supine position complains of dizziness and you note a drop in blood pressure, this could be due to a condition called supine hypotension syndrome. This is a condition in which the heavy mass created by the weight of the uterus, coupled with the infant's weight, placenta, and amniotic fluid, compresses the inferior vena cava, reducing return of blood to the heart, reducing cardiac output and resulting in low blood pressure. Cushing's reflex occurs in head injuries. (p. 468)

21. (B) To counteract the pressure of the uterus on the inferior vena cava, you should transport the patient on her left side to lessen the pressure. See answer #20. (p. 469)

22. (D) During a delivery, the EMT-B will need infection control gear such as surgical gloves, a mask, and eye protection as well as a gown. A Tyvek suit is not needed for protection against blood spraying. (p. 469)

23. (D) During delivery, encourage the mother to breathe deeply through her mouth. She may feel better if she pants, although she should be discouraged from breathing rapidly and deeply enough to bring on hyperventilation. (p. 469)

24. (A) Do not pull on the baby's shoulders or any other part of the baby. When supporting the baby's head during a delivery, the EMT-B should apply gentle pressure to control the delivery, place one hand below the head, and spread fingers evenly around the baby's head. (p. 469)

25. (B) If the amniotic sac has not broken by the time the baby's head is delivered, use your finger to puncture the membrane. Then pull the membranes away from the baby's mouth and nose. (p. 470)

26. (C) If you cannot loosen or unwrap the umbilical cord from around the infant's neck, you should clamp the cord in two places and cut between the clamps. This way the child will not strangle, the cord will not tear, and the blood supply will not be cut off. (p. 470)

27. (A) Most babies are born face down and then rotate to either side. (p. 470)

28. (B) When suctioning a newborn, compress the syringe before placing it in the baby's mouth to avoid blowing fluids into the baby's airway. (p. 470)

29. (B) Once the baby's feet are delivered, lay the baby on her side with head slightly lower than its torso. This is done to allow blood, fluids, and mucus to drain from the mouth and nose. Remember, newborns are very slippery; never pick up a baby by the feet since you could drop the child. (pp. 470, 472)

30. (D) To assess the newborn, the EMT-B does not check the response to a sternal rub; this could injure the child. A general evaluation usually calls for noting ease of breathing, the heart rate, crying (vigorous crying is a good sign), movement (the more active, the better), skin color (blue coloration at the hands and feet may or may not disappear, but it should not spread to other parts of the body). (p. 472)

31. (C) It is necessary to suction the baby's mouth before the nose because suctioning the nose first may cause the baby to gasp or begin breathing and aspirate any meconium, blood, fluids, or mucus from the mouth into the lungs. (p. 472)

32. (C) If assessment of the infant's breathing reveals shallow, slow, or absent respirations, the EMT-B should provide artificial ventilations at 40 to 60 per minute. Do not use an oxygen mask. (pp. 472–473)

33. (A) In a normal birth, the infant must be breathing on his own before you clamp and cut the cord. (p. 473)

34. (D) The first umbilical cord clamp should be placed about 10 inches from the baby. (p. 473)

35. (C) The second umbilical cord clamp should be placed about 7 inches from the baby. (p. 473)

36. (D) If the placenta does not deliver within 20 minutes of the baby's birth, transport the mother and baby to a medical facility without delay. (p. 475)

37. (B) It is not uncommon for the mother to tear part of the perineum during a delivery. If this occurs, apply a sanitary napkin and apply gentle pressure. Let the mother know that torn tissue is normal and that the problem will be quickly cared for at the medical facility. (pp. 475–476)

38. (D) Initiate rapid transport on recognition of a breech presentation. Never pull on the baby's legs. Provide high-concentration oxygen. Place the mother in a head down position with the pelvis elevated. (p. 477)

39. (A) If you see the umbilical cord presenting first, gently push up on the baby's head or buttocks to take pressure off of the cord. This may be the only chance that the baby has for survival, so continue to push up on the baby until you are relieved by a physician. All patients with prolapsed cords require rapid transport! (pp. 477–478)

40. (D) When a baby's limb presents first, the EMT-B should begin rapid transport of the patient immediately. Do not try to replace the limb into the vagina. (p. 478)

41. (B) When assisting with the delivery of twins, clamp the cord of the first baby before the second baby is born. Labor contractions will continue after the first baby is born. (p. 480)

42. (C) Premature infants are at high risk for hypothermia because they lack fat deposits that would normally keep them warm. (pp. 480–481)

43. (B) When oxygen is administered to an infant, it should be given by flowing it past the baby's face. Use humidified oxygen, if available, so it doesn't dry out the baby's respiratory tract. (p. 481)

44. (B) If you suspect meconium staining when the infant is born, avoid stimulating the infant before suctioning the oropharynx. This reduces the risk of aspiration. (p. 481)

45. (D) A condition in which the placenta is formed low in the uterus and close to the cervical opening preventing the normal delivery of the fetus is called placenta previa. (p. 481)

46. (D) Seizures in pregnancy are usually associated with extreme swelling of the extremities. In addition, the patient will have <u>elevated</u> blood pressure. Seizures tend to occur <u>late</u> in pregnancy and pose a threat to <u>both</u> the mother and unborn baby. (p. 482)

47. (C) Massive bleeding and shock are the gravest dangers associated with blunt trauma to the pregnant woman's abdomen or pelvis. Perform a patient assessment and treat her injuries as you would those of any trauma patient. (pp. 483–484)

48. (A) Because of the physiology of a pregnant woman, the vital signs of a pregnant woman may be interpreted as suggestive of shock when they are actually normal. The pregnant woman has a pulse rate 10–15 beats per minutes <u>faster</u> than her nonpregnant counterpart and a blood volume as much as 48% <u>higher</u> than her nonpregnant state. Shock is <u>more</u> difficult to assess in the pregnant patient, and it is the most likely cause of prehospital death from injury to the uterus. (p. 483)

49. (B) Unless a back or neck injury is suspected, all pregnant women who have suffered blunt trauma injury should be transported in the left lateral recumbent position. If you suspect neck or back injury, first secure the mother to a spine board, then tip board and patient as a unit to the left, relieving pressure on the abdominal organs and vena cava. (p. 484)

50. (C) If vaginal bleeding is associated with abdominal pain, treat the patient as if she has a potentially life-threatening condition. The most serious complication of vaginal bleeding is hypovolemic shock due to blood loss. (p. 485)

COMPLETE THE FOLLOWING

1. When evaluating the expectant mother, the EMT-B should: (pp. 467–468)
   - Ask her name and age and expected due date.
   - Ask if this is her first pregnancy.
   - Ask her how long she has been having labor pains and how often, and if the "bag of waters" has broken.
   - Ask if she is straining or feels the need to move her bowels.
   - With patient's permission, examine for crowning.
   - Feel for uterine contractions.
   - Take vital signs.

2. Take the following steps when providing care for the premature infant: (pp. 480–481)
   - Keep the baby warm.
   - Keep the airway clear.
   - Provide ventilations and/or chest compressions.
   - Watch the umbilical cord for bleeding.
   - Provide oxygen.
   - Avoid contamination.
   - Transport the infant in a warm ambulance.
   - Call ahead to the emergency department.

LABEL THE DIAGRAMS (p. 465)

1. Amniotic sac
2. Umbilical cord
3. Placenta
4. Uterus
5. Pubic bone
6. Cervix
7. Vagina

VIRTUAL STREET SCENES

1. If the amniotic sac has not broken by the time the baby's head is delivered, use your finger to puncture the membrane. Then pull the membranes away from the baby's mouth and nose.

2. This is called *meconium staining*. Meconium-stained amniotic fluid is caused by fetal feces (wastes) released during labor, usually because of maternal or fetal stress. If meconium is present, suction the infant immediately—first the mouth and then the nose. Maintain an open airway and be prepared to provide artificial ventilation or CPR if needed. Transport as soon as possible.

3. Be sure to put the mother on high-concentration oxygen via nonrebreather mask, keep her warm, elevate her legs, and massage her abdomen above the uterus. It also may be helpful to encourage the mother to nurse the infant, since sucking stimulates the uterus to contract.

Chapter 25: Putting It All Together for the Medical Patient

MATCH TERMINOLOGY/DEFINITIONS

1. **(E)** Action taken to correct a patient's problem.
2. **(C)** Movement of blood throughout the body.
3. **(A)** Passageway by which air enters and leaves the body.
4. **(H)** Decision on the seriousness of the patient's condition.

5. **(G)** Orders from the on-duty physician given directly to an EMT-B in the field by radio or telephone.
6. **(B)** Respiration, or the process by which a person inhales and exhales air.
7. **(F)** Pain in the chest, occurring when blood supply to the heart is reduced and a portion of the heart muscle is not receiving enough oxygen.
8. **(D)** Form of sugar, the body's basic source of energy.

MULTIPLE-CHOICE REVIEW

1. **(A)** EMT-Bs do not normally administer intravenous fluids to patients unless they have received special training. (p. 491)
2. **(C)** When a patient presents with more than one condition or a familiar condition but under unusual circumstances, the EMT-B should assess the patient as usual and then seek advice if necessary. (p. 491)
3. **(A)** When a patient tells you that he has a disease with which you are unfamiliar, it is best to respond by saying "I'm not familiar with that disease. Could you tell me more about it?" (p. 495)
4. **(C)** When a patient has two or more medical conditions that are presenting symptoms at the same time, it is good to consult with medical direction for advice. (pp. 491–492)
5. **(D)** The patient with slurred speech may have had a cardiovascular accident, an overdose, or a seizure. (p. 492)
6. **(C)** Patients who have had a seizure generally do not have chest pain. (p. 491)
7. **(A)** A patient who is vomiting coffee ground colored material probably has internal bleeding (such as a gastrointestinal bleed). (p. 493)
8. **(D)** A wheeze is a common breathing sound found in patients having an asthma attack, an allergic reaction, or bronchospasm. (p. 494)
9. **(B)** There is no specific EMT-B intervention for the patient with abdominal pain. (p. 495)
10. **(C)** The EMT-B has been trained to cool down and apply oxygen to the patient suspected of having hyperthermia. (p. 494)

COMPLETE THE FOLLOWING

Examples of EMT-B interventions for medical patients include the following: (p. 494)
- Assisting a patient in using his own inhaler (respiratory difficulty)
- Assisting a patient in taking his own nitroglycerin (cardiac compromise)
- Application of an automated defibrillator (cardiac arrest)
- Administration of oral glucose (diabetics with altered mental status)
- Assisting a patient in using his own epinephrine auto-injector (allergic reaction)
- Administration of activated charcoal (overdose or poisoning)
- Talking down and restraining (behavioral emergencies)
- Assisting in delivery of an infant (patient in labor)
- Cooling or warming (environmental emergency)

Chapter 25 (continued)

VIRTUAL STREET SCENES

1. BSI precautions should include gloves, mask, and eye-shield if you suspect an infectious disease.

2. Patients with dizziness should be encouraged to go to the hospital for evaluation, since there are many serious problems associated with the symptom.

3. If the patient is a diabetic, he might be having a "silent MI." Be very careful to encourage sick diabetics to seek medical attention.

Interim Exam 2

1. **(D)** The initial assessment includes assessing the airway, mental status, and circulation, as well as breathing. Blood pressure is a vital sign taken during the focused history and physical exam. (p. 163)

2. **(B)** Evaluating extremity mobility is not part of the initial assessment. Determining patient priority, forming a general impression, and assessing breathing are all part of the initial assessment. (p. 163)

3. **(B)** Environmental clues during the general impression of a child would include recognizing that the child is holding pieces of a toy (perhaps he/she swallowed one of the pieces). Vital signs and associated signs or symptoms like nausea are not part of the general impression. (pp. 163–164)

4. **(C)** The patient's position, age, sex, sounds he/she is making, and smells from the environment are part of the general impression. Vital signs are not. (pp. 163–164)

5. **(B)** Assessing mental status is the step of the initial assessment that comes after the general impression. (p. 164)

6. **(C)** AVPU stands for alert, response to verbal stimulus, response to painful stimulus, unresponsive. (p. 164)

7. **(B)** See answer #6. (p. 164)

8. **(D)** The lowest and most serious mental status is U, or unresponsive. (pp. 163–164)

9. **(B)** If a patient's level of responsiveness is lower than Alert, you should at least administer high-concentration oxygen by nonrebreather mask. Consider this patient a high priority transport. (pp. 164–165)

10. **(C)** If a patient is talking or crying, assume an open airway. However, this condition may change, so you need to monitor the patient. (p. 169)

11. **(C)** If the patient is not alert and breathing rate is slower than 8 breaths per minute, use a bag-valve mask to assist the ventilations. (p. 169)

12. **(B)** Pale and clammy skin indicates poor circulation, or hypoperfusion. (p. 169)

13. **(A)** A patient who gives a poor general impression is a high priority. (p. 169)

14. **(B)** The patient whose only complaint is nausea and vomiting is not generally considered a high priority. (p. 169)

15. **(A)** The initial assessment varies depending on the age of the patient and whether there is a medical or trauma problem. The medical history does not change the initial assessment. (p. 169)

16. **(C)** The capillary refill is used to evaluate the circulation of infants and children but is no longer advocated as an effective, reliable test for adults. (p. 172)

17. **(B)** Check the mental status of an unconscious infant by talking to the infant and flicking the infant's feet. The sternal rub would be too aggressive and could cause injury. (p. 172)

18. **(B)** A fever and a rash are not generally considered high priority. However, don't forget to take BSI precautions and consider the need for a mask when treating such conditions. (p. 169)

19. **(A)** The difference between the general impression steps for a medical patient and that of a trauma patient is the need to provide manual stabilization of the head if you suspect spine injury in the trauma patient. (p. 173)

20. **(C)** Documenting examination findings that are negative (things that are not true) is called documenting a pertinent negative. (p. 297)

21. **(D)** When writing the PCR narrative section, do not state your personal opinion of the patient's condition. Only relevant facts, not subjective statements, should be documented. (pp. 296–297)

22. **(B)** An important concept of EMS documentation is "if it is not written down, you did not do it." (The presumption is that at the time of the incident you had the opportunity to document everything that you observed and treated.) (p. 298)

23. **(A)** If a patient does not wish to go to the hospital, document with a refusal-of-care form. Be sure to consult medical direction whenever there is a patient refusal. (p. 298)

24. **(B)** Failure to perform an important part of patient assessment or care is an error of omission. Errors of commission are performing actions that are wrong or improper. (p. 301)

25. **(C)** "Making up vitals" is falsification and could endanger the patient's care. (p. 301)

26. **(C)** An objective statement describes something that is measurable, observable, or verifiable, such as vital signs. (p. 296)

27. **(A)** Stating that "the patient is alert and oriented" is an example of objective information that you observe but the patient does not tell you. (p. 296)

28. **(D)** Statements from patients, bystanders, or family should be put in quotes on the PCR. (p. 297)

29. **(A)** Statements about the rudeness of the family members are usually not relevant or needed on the PCR. (p. 297)

30. **(A)** After establishing unresponsiveness in the initial assessment, proceed to open the airway. (p. 163)

31. **(A)** The EMT-B's "sixth sense" refers to clinical judgment, which is developed with experience. (p. 164)

32. **(B)** The vital signs are pulse, respirations, blood pressure, pupils, and skin condition, color and temperature. (p. 179)

33. **(B)** The normal adult pulse rate at rest is between 60 and 100. (p. 181)

34. **(D)** The initial pulse rate for patients 1 year and older is normally taken at the radial pulse. (p. 181)

35. **(D)** When the pulse force is weak and thin, it is described as thready. (p. 182)

36. **(B)** Normal adult at-rest respiration rates vary from 12 to 20 breaths per minute. (p. 183)

37. **(D)** Crowing is a noisy, harsh sound heard during inhalation that indicates a partial airway obstruction. A gurgling sound is caused by fluid in the airway, which requires suctioning. (p. 184)

38. (C) The systolic blood pressure is the arterial pressure created when the left ventricle of the heart contracts. (p. 186)

39. (B) Diastolic blood pressure is the arterial pressure created by relaxation and refilling of the left ventricle of the heart. (p. 186)

40. (B) When a stethoscope is used along with a sphygmomanometer to take the blood pressure, this technique is called auscultation. (p. 188)

41. (A) Determining blood pressure by palpation is not as accurate as the auscultation method. This procedure is used when there is lots of noise around a patient. It is documented as the systolic reading/P. (p. 189)

42. (A) Information that you see, hear, feel, and smell are called signs and can be measured. Information the patient tells you are symptoms. (p. 190)

43. (B) When asking the patient "Have you recently had any surgery or injuries?", you are inquiring about the patient's pertinent past history. (p. 191)

44. (A) When you ask the patient "Are you on birth control pills?" you are inquiring about the patient's medications. This may give some clues about the patient's present problem. (p. 191)

45. (C) An acronym used to remember what questions to ask about the patient's present problem and past history is SAMPLE. AVPU is the level of responsiveness, PEARL is the status of the pupils, and CUPS is a way of categorizing the patient status. (p. 191)

46. (D) When conducting a patient interview on an adult patient, the EMT-B should position oneself close to the patient, identify oneself and reassure the patient, and gently touch the patient's shoulder or rest a hand over the patient's. It is necessary to ask the patient's age. (p. 191)

47. (D) Normal diastolic pressures range from 60 to 90 mm Hg. See Table 9-6. (p. 187)

48. (C) Using the formula presented in the text, a 36-year-old man would have an estimated systolic blood pressure of 136 mmHg (100 + age). See Table 9-6. (p. 187)

49. (B) Using the formula presented in the text, a 26-year-old woman would have an estimated systolic blood pressure of 116 mmHg (90 + age). See Table 9-6. (p. 187)

50. (A) The stethoscope should not be placed under the cuff and then inflated when evaluating the blood pressure because it may give a false reading. (p. 188)

51. (C) When taking a patient's blood pressure, the stethoscope is placed over the brachial artery. The femoral artery is in the leg. (p. 188)

52. (C) The mechanism of injury is the best indication of potential injury. (p. 151)

53. (B) When there are no apparent hazards at the scene of a collision, the danger zone should extend 50 feet in all directions from the wreckage. (pp. 146, 149)

54. (C) In the up-and-over head-on injury pattern, the patient is most likely to sustain head injuries. Chest and neck injuries are also common. Leg, knee, and hip injuries are usually the result of a down-and-under injury pattern. (p. 153)

55. (C) A keen awareness that there may be injuries based on the mechanism of injury is called index of suspicion. (p. 156)

56. (C) The purpose of the initial assessment is to discover and treat life-threatening conditions. (p. 163)

57. (C) The first step in the focused history and physical exam of any trauma patient is to reconsider the mechanism of injury. (p. 198)

58. (C) The "A" in DCAP-BTLS stands for abrasions. (p. 199)

59. (D) Clues to determining the patient's need for a cervical collar include mechanism of injury, level of responsiveness, and location of injuries. The breathing rate will not assist in determining the need for a cervical collar. (p. 202)

60. (B) The rapid assessment evaluates areas of the body where the greatest threats to the patient may be. (pp. 211–212)

61. (A) The detailed physical exam is most often performed on the trauma patient with a significant mechanism of injury. (p. 219)

62. (A) To obtain a history of a patient's present illness, ask the OPQRST questions. These will focus on the chief complaint and potential causes. (p. 237)

63. (C) The "P" in OPQRST stands for provokes, which refers to questions such as "Can you think of anything that might have triggered this pain?" (p. 237)

64. (A) The correct order in the focused history and physical exam of the unresponsive medical patient is conduct a rapid physical exam, obtain baseline vital signs, gather the history of the present illness (OPQRST) from bystanders and family, and gather a SAMPLE history from bystanders and family. (p. 238)

65. (C) For a stable patient, the EMT-B should perform the ongoing assessment every 15 minutes. For an unstable patient, perform the ongoing assessment every 5 minutes. (p. 250)

66. (A) During the ongoing assessment, whenever you believe there may have been a change in the patient's condition, you should repeat the initial assessment. (p. 250)

67. (D) Cool, clammy skin most likely indicates hypoperfusion (shock). Exposure to cold causes dry, cold skin. Fever results in clammy and warm or hot skin. (p. 185)

68. (D) As an EMT-B, your overriding concern at all times is your own safety. Certainly your crew's safety is a priority, but your personal safety MUST come first. (p. 145)

69. (A) During the detailed physical exam of the head of a trauma patient, inspect the ears and nose for blood or clear fluids. (p. 220)

70. (B) Meningitis and head trauma can cause the fontanelle to bulge in an infant. (p. 266)

71. (C) Infants and young children under the age of 8 are abdominal breathers. (p. 266)

72. (C) Adolescents generally feel that they are indestructible but may have fears of permanent injury or disfigurement. (p. 267)

73. (C) Geriatric patients have decreased elasticity of the lungs and decreased activity of cilia that results in decreased ability to clear foreign substances from the lungs. (p. 268)

74. (D) As a normal process of aging, geriatric patients lose skin elasticity and sweat glands shrink. This results in thin, dry, wrinkled skin. (p. 268)

75. (B) Geriatric patients usually have diminished function of the thyroid gland that results in decreased energy and tolerance of heat and cold. (p. 268)

76. (C) When an elderly patient falls, this may indicate a more serious problem such as abnormal heart rhythm, which may cause a diminished cardiac output. (p. 268)

77. (B) Repeaters are devices used when radio transmissions must be carried over long distances. (p. 276)

78. **(C)** If possible, position yourself at or below the patient's eye level. This will be less threatening to the patient. (pp. 284–285)

79. **(B)** The first item given to the hospital in your medical radio report to the receiving facility is your unit identification/level of provider. (p. 283)

80. **(D)** The patient's attitude is not an essential component of the verbal report to the receiving hospital. (p. 284)

81. **(C)** Medical radio reports should paint a picture of the patient's problem in words. (p. 283)

82. **(D)** Always question orders from medical direction that you do not understand. (pp. 283–284)

83. **(A)** Medications that are carried on the ambulance and that EMT-Bs can administer include activated charcoal, oxygen, and oral glucose. Nitroglycerin, epinephrine, and the prescribed inhaler are medications that the EMT-B may assist the patient with administration. (p. 309)

84. **(D)** Any action of a drug other than the desired action is called a side effect. (p. 312)

85. **(D)** When a drug is administered subcutaneously, this means the drug is injected under the skin. (p. 313)

86. **(D)** Infants and children depend more on the diaphragm for respiration than adults do. (p. 324)

87. **(B)** The best method involves a BVM, two rescuers, and supplemental oxygen. (p. 324)

88. **(B)** The adequate rate of artificial ventilation for a non-breathing adult patient is 12 breaths per minute. (p. 324)

89. **(C)** The adequate rate of artificial ventilation for a non-breathing infant or child patient is 20 breaths per minute. (p. 324)

90. **(A)** If an unresponsive adult makes snoring or gurgling sounds, he most likely has a serious airway problem requiring immediate intervention. (p. 323)

91. **(D)** The skin of a patient with inadequate breathing may be blue (or pale) in color and will feel cool and clammy. (p. 323)

92. **(C)** If a patient is experiencing breathing difficulty, but is breathing adequately, it is usually best to place him in a position of comfort. This is generally a sitting-up position. (p. 327)

93. **(D)** The cause of adult chest pain due to a decreased blood supply to the heart is angina pectoris. Arrhythmia is an irregular heart rhythm. (p. 346)

94. **(C)** Most heart attacks are caused by narrowing or occlusion of a coronary artery. The coronary arteries supply the heart muscle with blood. (p. 346)

95. **(D)** Acute myocardial infarction is the condition in which a portion of the heart muscle dies because of oxygen starvation. (p. 346)

96. **(B)** An irregular or absent heart rhythm is called arrhythmia. (p. 346)

97. **(A)** A pulse slower than 60 beats per minute is called bradycardia. (p. 340)

98. **(C)** An at-rest heart beat faster than 100 beats per minute is referred to as tachycardia. (p. 340)

99. **(A)** Congestive heart failure is the condition caused by excessive fluid buildup in the lungs and/or other organs and body parts because of the inadequate pumping of the heart. (p. 347)

100. **(D)** A conscious patient with a possible heart attack is best placed in the position of comfort. For ease of breathing, this is usually a sitting position. (p. 340)

101. **(A)** A diabetic found with a weak, rapid pulse and cold, clammy skin who complains of hunger pangs is probably suffering from hypoglycemia. Hyperglycemic patients often have warm, red, dry skin and an acetone breath. (pp. 375–376)

102. **(B)** In hyperglycemia, the patient will have acetone smelling breath. (p. 378)

103. **(A)** A conscious hypoglycemic patient who is able to swallow is frequently administered oral glucose, with permission given by medical direction or standing orders. (p. 376)

104. **(C)** If you cannot administer glucose to the diabetic patient because she is not awake enough to swallow, you should treat her like any other patient with altered mental status. Secure the airway, provide artificial ventilations if necessary, and be prepared to perform CPR if needed. (p. 376)

105. **(C)** The first time a person is exposed to an allergen, the person's immune system forms antibodies. (p. 389)

106. **(C)** To be considered a severe allergic reaction, a patient must have signs and symptoms of shock or respiratory distress. (p. 392)

107. **(B)** If a patient has no history of allergies and is having his first allergic reaction, you should treat for shock and transport immediately. (p. 393)

108. **(C)** Carbon monoxide, chlorine, and ammonia are examples of inhaled poisons. (p. 405)

109. **(A)** It is important for the EMT-B to determine when the ingestion of a poison occurred because different poisons act on the body at different rates. (p. 406)

110. **(B)** The principal prehospital treatment of a patient who has inhaled poison is administering high-concentration oxygen. (p. 410)

111. **(B)** If mixing alcohol and other drugs, the patient will exhibit with depressed vital signs. (p. 416)

112. **(D)** Activated charcoal is contraindicated for patients who have ingested alkalis, gasoline, or acids. (p. 406)

113. **(C)** Most cases of poisoning involve young children. (p. 403)

114. **(C)** Poisons that are swallowed are ingested poisons. (p. 405)

115. **(B)** A patient with hot and dry or hot and moist skin is experiencing a true emergency that requires rapid cooling and immediate transport. (pp. 432–433)

116. **(A)** As frostbite progresses and exposure continues, the skin will turn from white and waxy to blotchy and grayish yellow and finally to grayish blue. (p. 430)

117. **(C)** To treat a patient with deep frostbite, cover the frostbitten area, handle it as gently as possible, and transport patient. Do not rub the area or apply cold. Do not rewarm the area unless you can ensure it will not refreeze. (p. 430)

118. **(D)** With frostbite, the affected area feels frozen, but only on the surface. (p. 430)

119. **(A)** The initial sign of hypothermia is shivering. (p. 426)

120. **(A)** Extreme hypothermia is characterized by unconsciousness and absence of discernible vital signs. If there is shivering, numbness, and drowsiness, the patient is not yet in severe hypothermia. (p. 429)

121. **(D)** The emergency care steps for a hypothermic patient include keeping the patient still and dry and applying heat to raise the patient's core body temperature. Do not encourage the patient to walk. (p. 428)

122. **(C)** After calming a snakebite victim and treating for shock, you locate the fang marks. Next, you should cleanse the wound site with soap and water. (p. 445)

123. **(A)** When a patient who was working in a hot environment complains of severe muscle cramps in the legs and feels faint, you should move the patient to a cool place and begin care by administering oxygen by nonrebreather. (p. 432)

124. **(C)** The first step in caring for a rescued near-drowning victim is to establish an airway and evaluate the need for CPR. (p. 435)

125. **(D)** Your first step when called to care for any attempted suicide victim is to ensure your own safety. This may mean waiting for police assistance, depending on the circumstances of the suicide attempt. (p. 455)

126. **(C)** If you are unable to perform normal assessment and care procedures because the patient is aggressive and hostile, you should seek advice from medical direction. (p. 456)

127. **(B)** The EMT-B is allowed to use reasonable force to defend against attack by an emotionally disturbed patient. (p. 456)

128. **(B)** The developing unborn baby is called a fetus. (p. 463)

129. **(C)** The muscular organ in which the fetus develops is the uterus. (p. 463)

130. **(A)** The organ of pregnancy in which exchange of oxygen, nutrients, and wastes occurs between mother and fetus is the placenta. (p. 463)

131. **(C)** While developing, the fetus is protected by a thin, membranous "bag of waters" called the amniotic sac. (p. 463)

132. **(A)** When the presenting part of the baby first bulges from the vaginal opening, this is called crowning. (p. 464)

133. **(C)** The first stage of labor begins with uterine contractions. (p. 464)

134. **(B)** The second stage of labor ends with infant delivery. (p. 464)

135. **(C)** The third stage of labor ends with delivery of the placenta. (p. 464)

136. **(D)** If a woman is having her first baby, the first stage of labor will usually last 16 hours on the average. (p. 465)

137. **(B)** During the most active stage of labor, the uterus usually contracts every 2 to 3 minutes (with contractions commonly lasting 30 seconds to 1 minute). (p. 466)

138. **(C)** If the amniotic sac does not break during delivery, the EMT-B should puncture it with a finger; then remove the membranes from the baby's nose and mouth. (p. 470)

139. **(B)** To assist the mother in delivering the baby's upper shoulder, gently support the baby's head. Do not pull on the infant. (p. 470)

140. **(B)** After delivery, first position the newborn on his side, then suction the baby's nose and mouth before clamping

the cord. We do not slap infants on their buttocks as this may injure them, or worse, you may drop the slippery child. (p. 472)

141. **(C)** If spontaneous respiration does not begin after suctioning the baby's mouth and nose, the EMT-B should vigorously rub the baby's back; then consider mechanical ventilatory assistance. (pp. 472–473)

142. **(C)** The first clamp placed on the umbilical cord should be about 10 inches from the baby. (p. 473)

143. **(A)** If bleeding continues from the umbilical cord after clamping and cutting, the EMT-B should clamp the cord again, close to the original clamp. (pp. 473–474)

144. **(A)** The maximum amount of time to wait for the placenta to be delivered before transporting is 20 minutes. (p. 475)

145. **(A)** Delivery of the placenta is usually accompanied by the loss of no more than 500 cc of blood. (p. 475)

146. **(B)** The first step to control vaginal bleeding after birth is to place a sanitary napkin over the vaginal opening. Do not pack the vagina. Consider massaging the uterus if bleeding persists. Allow the mother to nurse the baby, which will control bleeding by stimulating contraction of the uterus. (pp. 475–476)

147. **(B)** The presenting part of the baby in a breech birth is the buttocks or legs. (p. 476)

148. **(B)** If upon viewing the vaginal area, you see the umbilical cord presenting first (a prolapsed cord delivery), you should gently push up on the baby's head or buttocks to keep pressure off the cord. Do not cut the cord since it is the infant's blood supply. Never attempt to push the cord back into the vagina. (pp. 477–478)

149. **(C)** If an arm presentation without a prolapsed cord is noted, the EMT-B should transport immediately, providing high-concentration oxygen. (p. 478)

150. **(C)** A baby is considered premature if the baby weighs less than 5 pounds or is born before the 37th week. (p. 480)

CHAPTER 26: Bleeding and Shock

MATCH TERMINOLOGY/DEFINITIONS

▶ **Part A**

1. **(J)** Artery—blood vessel with thick, muscular walls that carries oxygen-rich blood away from the heart

2. **(A)** Brachial artery—major artery of the upper arm

3. **(C)** Capillary bleeding—bleeding that is characterized by a slow, oozing flow of blood.

4. **(H)** Cardiogenic shock—lack of perfusion brought on by inadequate pumping action of the heart

5. **(B)** Compensated shock—when the patient is developing shock, but the body is still able to maintain perfusion

6. **(E)** Decompensated shock—condition that occurs when the body can no longer compensate for low blood volume or lack of perfusion; late signs, such as falling blood pressure, develop.

7. **(F)** Femoral artery—major artery supplying the thigh

8. **(I)** Golden hour—optimum time limit between time of injury and surgery at the hospital; survival rates are best if surgery takes place within this time period.

9. (G) Hemorrhage—severe bleeding; a major cause of shock

10. (D) Hemorrhagic shock—shock resulting from blood loss

▶ **Part B**

1. (J) Hypoperfusion—inadequate circulation of the blood in which the body's cells and organs do not receive adequate supplies of oxygen and nutrients and dangerous waste products build up

2. (H) Hypovolemic shock—shock resulting from uncontrolled bleeding or plasma loss

3. (E) Irreversible shock—when the body has lost the battle to maintain perfusion to the organ systems; cell damage occurs, especially to the liver and kidneys.

4. (I) Neurogenic shock—shock resulting from uncontrolled dilation of blood vessels due to nerve paralysis (sometimes caused by spinal-cord injuries)

5. (C) Perfusion—adequate circulation of blood throughout the body, filling the capillaries and supplying cells and tissues with oxygen and nutrients

6. (G) Pressure dressing—bulky dressing held in position with a tightly wrapped bandage to help control bleeding

7. (D) Pressure point—site where a large artery lies near the surface of the body and directly over a bone; pressure on such a location can control profuse bleeding in the extremities.

8. (F) Shock—another name for hypoperfusion

9. (A) Tourniquet—device that closes off all blood flow to and from an extremity

10. (B) Vein—blood vessel that has one-way valves and carries blood back to the heart

MULTIPLE-CHOICE REVIEW

1. (B) Blood that has been depleted of oxygen and loaded with carbon dioxide empties into the veins, which carry it back to the heart. (p. 501)

2. (A) Cells and tissues of the brain, spinal cord, and kidneys are the most sensitive to inadequate perfusion. (p. 502)

3. (B) The use of BSI (body substance isolation) precautions is essential whenever bleeding is discovered or anticipated. (p. 503)

4. (C) Bleeding is classified as arterial, venous, and capillary. There is no category called cellular bleeding. (p. 503)

5. (B) Arterial bleeding is often rapid and profuse. Blood in arteries is maintained under high pressure by thick, muscular walls. For this reason, arterial hemorrhage is more difficult to control. Clot formation is also difficult because of this pressure. (p. 503)

6. (B) A steady flow of dark red or maroon blood is a result of venous bleeding. Deoxygenated blood travels back to the heart through veins. (p. 503)

7. (C) Bleeding described as oozing is usually a result of capillary bleeding. (p. 504)

8. (B) When a large bleeding vein in the neck sucks in debris or an air bubble (embolism), this can cause heart stoppage or damage the brain or lungs. An evisceration occurs when an organ or part of an organ protrudes through a wound opening. (pp. 503–504)

9. (D) Sudden blood loss of 1,000 cc in an adult is considered serious. This is double the amount that a blood donor gives. (p. 504)

10. (D) Sudden blood loss of 500 cc in a child is considered serious. (p. 504)

11. (D) Sudden blood loss of 150 cc in a 1-year-old infant is considered serious. (p. 504)

12. (D) The body's natural responses to bleeding is constriction of the injured blood vessel(s) and clotting. However, a serious injury may prevent effective clotting, allowing continued bleeding. (p. 504)

13. (B) Do not wait for signs and symptoms of shock to appear before beginning treatment. Any patient with a significant amount of blood loss should be treated to prevent the development of shock. Many signs and symptoms of shock appear late in the process. (p. 504)

14. (D) The major methods used to control external bleeding include direct pressure, elevation, and pressure points. Vessel clamps are used in surgery. (p. 505)

15. (B) Administering supplemental oxygen improves oxygenation of the tissues. Blood loss decreases perfusion, which means that less oxygen is delivered to the tissues. Supplemental oxygen increases the oxygen saturation of the blood still present in the circulatory system. (p. 505)

16. (D) The most common and effective way to control external bleeding is direct pressure. This can be done with your gloved hand, a dressing and your gloved hand, or by a pressure dressing and a bandage. (p. 507)

17. (C) The initial, or first, dressing should not be removed from a bleeding wound because it is a necessary part of clot formation. Removing it may destroy developing clots or cause further injury. (p. 507)

18. (B) After controlling bleeding from an extremity using a pressure bandage, be sure to check the distal pulse to make sure the bandage is not too tight. If administering oxygen, use a nonrebreather mask at 15 liters per minute. (p. 507)

19. (D) Elevation is used to assist in bleeding control for the following reasons: it slows bleeding, raises the limb above the heart, and helps to reduce blood pressure in the limb. Actually, shock speeds up the pulse. (pp. 507–508)

20. (C) It is inappropriate to use elevation to assist in bleeding control if you suspect musculoskeletal injuries because you could further injure the patient. (pp. 507–508)

21. (A) A pressure point is a site where a main artery lies near the surface of the body directly over the bone. Any site where a pulse can be felt is a pressure point. (p. 508)

22. (C) Use of a pressure point may not be effective if the wound is at the distal end of a limb. Blood is being sent to this area of the limb from many other smaller arteries. (p. 508)

23. (A) An air splint is most effective for controlling venous and capillary bleeding. It is not usually effective for arterial bleeding, at least not until the arterial pressure has decreased below that of the pressure in the splint. An air splint may be used to maintain pressure on a bleeding wound after other manual methods have already controlled the bleeding. (pp. 508–509)

24. (D) Do not insert the ice directly into the wound. When applying cold to a bleeding area, wrap the ice pack/cold pack in a cloth or towel, do not apply directly onto the skin, and do not leave the ice pack/cold pack in place for more than 20 minutes. (p. 509)

25. **(B)** Many experts agree that the pneumatic anti-shock garment is useful for controlling bleeding from areas the garment covers. It is contraindicated for penetrating chest trauma and the patient in cardiogenic shock. (p. 509)

26. **(A)** Bleeding from a clean-edged amputation is usually initially cared for with a pressure dressing. This is because injured blood vessels seal themselves shut as a result of spasms produced by the muscular walls of the vessels. (p. 510)

27. **(C)** Rough-edged amputations, usually produced by crushing or tearing injuries, often bleed heavily because the nature of the injury does not allow for vasoconstriction. Bleeding from these wounds are difficult to control and in some isolated cases require a tourniquet as a last resort. (p. 510)

28. **(A)** Once a tourniquet is in place, it must not be removed or loosened unless ordered by medical direction. Do not loosen, as toxins will flow into the bloodstream. Never cover the extremity because you must visually monitor the wound site and the effectiveness of the tourniquet. (p. 510)

29. **(C)** A blood pressure cuff can be used as a tourniquet if inflated to 150 mmHg or more. (p. 511)

30. **(D)** Allow the drainage to flow freely. The head injury has resulted in increased pressure within the skull, which is forcing fluid out of the cranial cavity. Do not attempt to stop this bleeding or fluid loss; this may increase the pressure in the skull. (p. 511)

31. **(B)** The medical term for a nosebleed is epistaxis. (p. 511)

32. **(D)** A cold pack applied to the bridge of the nose, by itself, will not control bleeding. To stop a nosebleed, place the patient in a sitting position, leaning forward; apply direct pressure by pinching the nostrils; and keep the patient calm. (p. 511)

33. **(A)** The leading cause of internal injuries and bleeding is blunt trauma. (pp. 511–512)

34. **(A)** A blast injury is not usually considered penetrating trauma, unless the blast propels sharp flying objects that penetrate the patient. (p. 512)

35. **(B)** Bradycardia and a flushed face are not commonly associated with internal bleeding. Signs of internal bleeding include vomiting a coffee ground-like substance; dark, tarry stools; and a tender, rigid, or distended abdomen. (p. 512)

36. **(D)** A laceration to the forearm would be considered external, not internal, bleeding. A patient who has internal bleeding may have painful, swollen, or deformed extremities (from bleeding within the limb); signs and symptoms of shock; or bright red blood in the stool. (p. 512)

37. **(C)** Inadequate perfusion is referred to as shock or hypoperfusion. (p. 513)

38. **(D)** An isolated injury to the head does not commonly produce shock because there is not enough room within the adult skull to permit enough bleeding to cause shock. Shock may develop from pump failure, lost blood volume, or dilated blood vessels. (p. 513)

39. **(D)** Hypovolemic (hemorrhagic) shock caused by uncontrolled bleeding is the type of shock most often seen by EMT-Bs. (p. 514)

40. **(C)** The heart attack patient is in shock as a result of pump failure, not the other mechanisms described. (p. 514)

41. **(C)** Neurogenic shock may result from the uncontrolled dilation of blood vessels due to nerve paralysis caused by spinal-cord injuries. Septic shock may also result in the massive dilation of blood vessels. (p. 514)

42. **(A)** When a patient is in shock but the body is still able to maintain perfusion to the vital organs, this is called compensated shock. (pp. 513–514)

43. **(D)** Early signs of shock that are the body's compensating mechanisms are increased heart rate; increased respirations; pale, cool skin; and increased capillary refill time in infants and children. (pp. 513–514)

44. **(D)** When the body has lost the battle to maintain perfusion to the organ systems, this is called irreversible shock. (p. 514)

45. **(A)** The patient in shock feels nauseated because blood flow is diverted from the digestive systems to the vital organs. Digestion of food is not a priority for the patient in shock. (p. 514)

46. **(C)** The pulse of a patient in shock will increase in an attempt to pump more blood. (pp. 514–515)

47. **(D)** A drop in blood pressure is a late sign of shock. The falling blood pressure signifies that the patient has entered the decompensated stage of the shock process. (p. 515)

48. **(D)** Additional signs of shock may include thirst, dilated pupils, and cyanosis around the lips and nail beds. The shock patient will present with pale, cool, clammy skin, not flushed, warm skin, because blood is quickly directed away from the skin and sent to organs such as the heart and brain. (p. 515)

49. **(B)** The EMT-B should be especially careful when evaluating pediatric shock patients because they may have very few signs until a large percentage of their blood volume (approximately 50%) is lost. There is no problem giving them high-concentration oxygen. (p. 515)

50. **(A)** "Platinum ten minutes" is the optimum on-scene time limit when treating a trauma patient. The golden hour is the time from injury to surgical treatment (p. 515)

COMPLETE THE FOLLOWING

1. The major types of shock include: (p. 514)
   - hypovolemic
   - cardiogenic
   - neurogenic

2. The signs and symptoms of shock include: (pp. 514–515)
   - altered mental status
   - pale, cool, clammy skin
   - nausea and vomiting
   - vital sign changes such as increased pulse, decreased blood pressure, and increased respirations
   - thirst
   - dilated pupils
   - cyanosis
   - delayed capillary refill in children

VIRTUAL STREET SCENES

1. The rib cage protects the stomach, spleen, liver, gall bladder, pancreas, and parts of the intestine.

2. Yes. If it is available, ALS should be requested to intercept if they are not on scene when you are ready to transport.

3. Changes to mental status due to hypoperfusion or internal bleeding are indicators that the patient may be decompensating and needs surgery right away to stop the blood loss.

Chapter 26 (continued)

CASE STUDY—Convenience Store Shooting

1. It ensures that the shooter is no longer on the scene.

2. Safety issues, number of patients, the need for additional resources

3. Internal and external bleeding is present. He is going into decompensated shock. This is recognized by the fast, weak radial pulse. Estimate his blood pressure at less than 90 systolic.

4. He is in hypovolemic, or hemorrhagic, shock from blood loss.

5. His brain interprets his blood loss (fluid) as "low fluid volume." Therefore, he asks for fluids. In this case, it is too late to restore his fluid volume by asking him to drink fluids. He needs IV fluids and whole blood in the trauma center.

6. Bullet fragments can easily ricochet into the chest. (Always listen to the lung sounds on a trauma patient to prevent missing potential injuries to the lungs.)

7. Use a nonrebreather mask at 15 liters per minute. Monitor his ventilations closely in case you need to switch to a BVM.

8. Call for ALS immediately. If they have not arrived when you are ready to transport, then arrange an intercept en route to the hospital.

9. A "platinum ten minutes" on the scene

10. A "golden hour" from the time of the injury to the surgery

11. Insert an oral airway if he has no gag reflex. Switch to assisted ventilations if required. When the paramedics arrive, he should be tubed (unless your EMT-B training included endotracheal intubation).

12. That's controversial and dependent on your local protocols. However, since he has internal bleeding and no penetrating chest wound or pulmonary edema, some protocols would allow PASG use.

13. Because this patient is being ventilated (at this time), he is considered critical. And in fact, he is in decompensated shock and moving to irreversible shock.

14. Two large-bore IVs of Normal Saline or Ringer's Lactate, endotracheal intubation, monitor ECG, consider PASG, and assisted ventilations.

15. Review your sample radio report with your instructor.

Chapter 27: Soft-Tissue Injuries

MATCH TERMINOLOGY/DEFINITIONS

▶ Part A

1. (N) Abrasion—scrape or scratch in which the outer layer of the skin is damaged but all layers are not penetrated

2. (K) Air embolus—air bubble in the bloodstream

3. (O) Amputation—surgical removal or traumatic severing of a body part, usually an extremity

4. (H) Avulsion—flap of skin or other soft tissue torn loose or pulled off completely

5. (C) Bandage—any material used to hold a dressing in place

6. (F) Closed wound—internal injury in which there is no open pathway from the outside to the injured site

7. (M) Contusion—bruise

8. (J) Crush injury—injury caused when force is transmitted from the body's exterior to its internal structures

9. (L) Dermis—layer of the skin below the epidermis; it is rich in blood vessels, nerves, and specialized structures such as sweat glands, sebaceous (oil) glands, and hair follicles.

10. (I) Dressing—any material used to cover a wound in an effort to control bleeding and help prevent further contamination

11. (B) Epidermis—outer layer of the skin

12. (E) Evisceration—intestine or other internal organ protruding through a wound in the abdomen

13. (G) Full-thickness burn—burn in which all the layers of the skin are damaged; also called a third-degree-burn

14. (A) Hematoma—swelling caused by the collection of blood under the skin or in damaged tissues as a result of an injured or broken blood vessel

15. (D) Laceration—cut that can be smooth or jagged

▶ Part B

1. (H) Occlusive dressing—any dressing that forms an airtight seal

2. (F) Open wound—injury in which the skin is interrupted, or broken, exposing the tissue underneath

3. (D) Partial-thickness burn—burn in which the epidermis is burned through and the dermis is damaged; also called a second-degree burn

4. (J) Puncture wound—open wound caused by a sharp, pointed object that tears through the skin and destroys underlying tissues

5. (B) Rule of nines—method for estimating the extent of a burn area in which areas on the body are assigned certain percentages of the body's total surface area

6. (I) Rule of palm—method for estimating the extent of a burn area; the palm of the patient's hand, which equals about 1% of the body's surface area, is compared with the patient's burn to estimate its size.

7. (G) Subcutaneous layers—layers of fat and soft tissues below the dermis

8. (C) Sucking chest wound—open chest wound in which air is "sucked" into the chest cavity

9. (E) Superficial burn—burn that involves only the epidermis, the outer layer of the skin; also called a first-degree burn

10. (A) Universal dressing—large bulky dressing

MULTIPLE-CHOICE REVIEW

1. (C) The teeth, bones, and cartilage are not considered soft tissue. The soft tissues of the body include skin, blood vessels, fatty tissues, muscles, fibrous tissues, nerves, glands, and membranes. (p. 525)

2. (D) Blood insulation is a distracter. The functions of the skin include protecting the body by providing a barrier to germs, debris, and unwanted chemicals; shock (impact) absorption; and temperature regulation. (pp. 525–526)

3. (D) Epithelial cells comprise the tissue that covers the respiratory tract. The layers of the skin are the epidermis, dermis, and subcutaneous layers. (pp. 525–526)

4. (A) The layer of the skin called the epidermis is composed of dead cells, which are rubbed off or sloughed off and are replaced continuously. See answers #3, #5, #6. (p. 525)

5. (B) Specialized nerve endings in the skin layer called the dermis are involved with the senses of touch, cold, heat, and pain. (pp. 525–526)

6. **(C)** Shock absorption and insulation are major functions of the subcutaneous layers of the skin. See answers #3, #4, #5. (p. 526)

7. **(C)** Wounds that usually result from the impact of a blunt object are called closed. Wounds resulting from stabbings, lacerations, and perforations are open wounds. (p. 526)

8. **(B)** A closed wound that involves a large amount of tissue damage and a collection of blood at the injury site is called a hematoma. See answer #9 for crush injury. A penetration is a puncture wound. (p. 528)

9. **(C)** A soft-tissue injury caused by a force that can cause rupture or bleeding of internal organs is called a crush injury. (p. 528)

10. **(C)** An open wound is an injury in which the skin is interrupted, exposing the tissues underneath. See answer #9 for crush injury. See answer #8 for hematoma. (pp. 529–530)

11. **(B)** A minor ooze of blood from capillary beds is from an injury called an abrasion. An amputation occurs when an extremity or digit is cut or torn completely off. A laceration is a cut, and a puncture is a penetration or hole made with a sharp object. (p. 530)

12. **(C)** A wound caused by a sharp-edged object such as a razor blade or broken glass is called a laceration. See answer #11 for abrasion. See answer #13 for puncture. See answer #14 for avulsion. (p. 530)

13. **(B)** When a sharp, pointed object passes through the skin or other tissue, a puncture wound has occurred. (p. 530)

14. **(A)** When the tip of the nose is cut or torn off, this is an avulsion. Attempt to preserve any avulsed part, since it may be possible to surgically restore the part or to use it for skin grafts. (p. 531)

15. **(A)** The priority when treating severe open wounds is to control bleeding. While cleaning the wound, preventing contamination, and bandaging are important, it is necessary to first control bleeding by direct pressure (with elevation if necessary). (pp. 533–534)

16. **(D)** Care for a laceration includes checking the pulse distal to the injury. Also check sensory and motor function. The patient may need stitches, plastic surgery, or a tetanus shot at the hospital, so do not put on butterfly bandages and release the patient. Never pull apart the edges of a laceration. (pp. 533–534)

17. **(C)** Various types of guns fired at close range can cause burns around the entry wound, injection of air into the tissues (causing severe damage), and damage underlying tissue. Generally the patient would not present with a contusion unless he/she had on a bulletproof vest, which spreads the energy of the impact. (p. 534)

18. **(D)** Never remove an impaled object. Care in the field for a patient with an impaled object includes stabilizing the object, using direct pressure, and leaving the object in place (unless it is impaled in the cheek). See answer #16. (p. 535)

19. **(C)** Never apply pressure to the object, rather, stabilize it with a bulky dressing. An impaled object may be plugging bleeding from a major artery while it is in place. To remove it may cause severe bleeding. Removal could also cause further injury to nerves, muscles, and other soft tissue. (pp. 535–536)

20. **(A)** To control profuse bleeding resulting from an impaled object, position your gloved hands on either side of the object and exert downward pressure. Be careful not to push the actual object in any further. (pp. 535–536)

21. **(A)** If you can see both ends of the object impaled in the cheek, pull it out in the direction it entered the cheek. However, never twist the object. If it is impaled into a deeper structure, stabilize it. The object may go into the oral cavity and create an airway obstruction or bleeding into the mouth may interfere with breathing or cause nausea or induce vomiting. (p. 536)

22. **(C)** If a patient has an impaled object in the eye, your care should include use of 4 × 4s to stabilize the object and a paper cup to cover the impaled object. Make sure to cover the uninjured eye. Never use plastic foam cups as the particles may flake into the eye. (pp. 536–537)

23. **(D)** In cases where an avulsed flap of tissue has been torn loose but not off, the EMT-B should fold the skin back to its normal position, clean the wound surface, control bleeding, and dress the wound. Do not tear off the remainder of the flap. (p. 537)

24. **(C)** Avulsed parts should be treated by placing in a plastic bag and then placing on top of a sealed bag of ice. Do not put the part directly on ice or in dry ice. Follow local protocols with regard to use of saline. (p. 537)

25. **(C)** When treating an amputation, be sure to place a snug pressure dressing over the stump. A tourniquet should only be used if other methods fail. The amputated part should not be placed directly on ice nor should ice be used on the stump. (p. 538)

26. **(B)** When treating an amputation, whenever possible transport the patient and the amputated body part in the same ambulance. This will avoid delays and possibly save the person's limb. (p. 538)

27. **(A)** An air bubble sucked into a large vein in the neck is called an air embolus. The "bends," or decompression sickness, involves nitrogen bubbles in the joints that do not enter the body through an external opening. (p. 538)

28. **(A)** The treatment of neck vein injury is aimed at preventing an embolus, preventing shock, and stopping bleeding. Do not compress the neck as you can injure the trachea or compress the arteries. (p. 538)

29. **(D)** To treat a neck laceration, the EMT-B should use an occlusive dressing to ensure material is not sucked into the wound. Do not use an ACE bandage as it could restrict breathing and arterial flow in the neck. (p. 538)

30. **(B)** When applying pressure to a neck wound, be sure you do not compress both carotids at the same time. This could cut off the blood supply to the brain and cause a stroke or other brain injury. (p. 538)

31. **(D)** The chest can be injured in a number of ways, including blunt trauma, penetrating objects, and compression. (p. 538)

32. **(C)** When the driver of a motor vehicle pitches forward after a head-on collision and strikes the chest on the steering column, this is called a compression injury. The heart can be severely squeezed, the lungs can be ruptured, and the sternum and ribs fractured. (p. 538)

33. **(B)** All open wounds to the chest should be considered life-threatening. Such open wounds impede the patient's breathing ability. (p. 540)

34. **(C)** An injury that has both an entrance and an exit is called a perforating puncture wound. (p. 540)

35. **(B)** When the delicate pressure balance within the chest cavity is compromised, initially the lung on the injured side will collapse. The patient will limit chest expansion due to the pain involved in breathing. (p. 540)

36. **(C)** When the chest cavity is open to the atmosphere, this is referred to as a sucking chest wound. A hemothorax is a condition in which the chest cavity fills with blood. (p. 540)

37. **(B)** Binding the chest will make it even harder for the patient to breathe. The treatment for an open chest wound includes maintaining an open airway, administering high-concentration oxygen, and sealing the open wound. (p. 540)

38. **(D)** When air becomes trapped in the chest cavity, it will <u>not</u> increase the ventilatory volume of the chest because this would increase pain when breathing. Trapped air in the chest can put pressure on the unaffected lung and heart, reduce cardiac output, and affect oxygenation of the blood. (p. 542)

39. **(D)** The signs and symptoms of a pneumothorax or tension pneumothorax include tracheal deviation to the uninjured side, distended neck veins, and uneven chest wall movement. The depth of respiration is <u>not</u> increased. (pp. 540–541)

40. **(B)** Coughed-up frothy blood is <u>not</u> a sign of traumatic asphyxia. The signs and symptoms include distended neck veins; head, neck, and shoulders that appear dark blue; and bloodshot and bulging eyes. (p. 541)

41. **(B)** When taping an occlusive dressing in place, have the patient forcefully exhale as you tape. (pp. 542–543)

42. **(B)** When an open wound to the abdomen is so large and deep that organs protrude, this is called an evisceration. (p. 544)

43. **(D)** Contusions over the upper ribs are signs of chest injury but not abdominal injuries. The signs of an abdominal injury include lacerations and puncture wounds to the lower back, large bruises on the abdomen, and indications of developing shock. (p. 544)

44. **(B)** Partially digested blood that is vomited looks like coffee grounds. (p. 544)

45. **(C)** Headache is not normally a symptom of an abdominal injury. The symptoms of an abdominal injury include cramps, nausea, and thirst. Patients may also experience pain that is initially mild and then rapidly becomes intolerable. (p. 544)

46. **(B)** Consider positioning the patient with an abdominal injury supine, with legs flexed at knees. This position relaxes the abdominal muscles and reduces pain. (p. 544)

47. **(C)** The treatment of an evisceration should <u>never</u> include replacing or touching the exposed organ. This could cause serious damage to the part and increase the chance of infection. (pp. 544–545)

48. **(C)** When covering an exposed abdominal organ, apply a saline-moistened dressing directly over the wound site. Do not use aluminum foil since it can cut eviscerated organs. (p. 545)

49. **(D)** Burn injuries often involve structures below the skin, such as muscles, nerves, bones, and blood vessels. (p. 545)

50. **(B)** In addition to physical damage caused by burns, patients often suffer emotional and psychological problems due to the lengthy recovery process and possibility of permanent disfigurement. (p. 545)

51. **(A)** When caring for a burn patient, think beyond the burn. Was there a possible medical emergency that caused the burn or did the burn aggravate an existing injury? (p. 545)

52. **(A)** When caring for burn patients, do not neglect assessment in order to begin burn care. A decision to transport immediately would be based on other injuries found. (p. 545)

53. **(D)** At normal temperature, distilled water is not a chemical that can burn a patient. Examples of agents causing burns are AC current, hydrochloric acid, and dry lime. (p. 545)

54. **(A)** A burn that involves only the epidermis is called a superficial burn. Epi-thickness is a distracter. (p. 545)

55. **(B)** A burn that results in deep intense pain, blisters, and mottled skin is called a partial-thickness burn. (pp. 545, 547)

56. **(C)** To distinguish between a partial-thickness burn and a full-thickness burn, look for dry and white areas, which indicate a full-thickness burn. Charred black or brown areas are also indicative of full-thickness burns. (pp. 545, 547)

57. **(B)** Electrical burns are of special concern since they pose a great risk of severe internal injuries. Chemical burns may remain on the skin and continue to burn for hours. Radiation burns may cause the patient to lose his hair over time. (p. 547)

58. **(C)** Chemical burns are of special concern since they may remain on the skin and continue to burn for hours. Superheated gases are usually present in a room with a fire in which the ceiling temperature is very hot. Electrical burns may travel from one extremity to the other and pose a great potential for internal injury. (p. 547)

59. **(D)** Burns to the face are of special concern because they may involve airway injury. They may also involve eye injury. (p. 548)

60. **(C)** Burns that can interrupt circulation to distal tissues are called circumferential burns. The resulting encircling scarring tends to limit normal functions. (p. 548)

61. **(B)** You are treating an adult patient who has partial-thickness burns to the entire left arm (9), chest (9), face, and neck (4 1/2). The size of the burn area is 22.5%. (pp. 548–549)

62. **(D)** You are treating an adult patient who has partial-thickness burns totally covering the legs (18 + 18), chest (9), and abdomen (9). The size of the burn area is 54%. (pp. 548–549)

63. **(A)** A burn the size of five palms would cover approximately 5% of the body surface area. (p. 549)

64. **(B)** The age of the patient is an important factor in burns. Patients under 5 and over 55 years of age have the most severe responses to burns. They also have a greater risk of death from burns. (p. 549)

65. **(A)** A partial-thickness burn that involve less than 15% of the body surface is classified as a minor burn per Table 27-3 in the text. (p. 550)

66. **(B)** A partial-thickness burn that involves between 15% and 30% of the body surface area is classified as a moderate burn per Table 27-3 in the text. (p. 550)

67. **(C)** A partial-thickness burn that involves more than 30% of the body surface area is classified as a critical burn per Table 27-3 in the text. (p. 550)

68. **(D)** Partial-thickness burns on the wrist would not be considered critical unless the hand was involved. Critical burns include circumferential burns, moderate burns in an infant or elderly patient, and burns complicated by musculoskeletal injuries. (p. 550)

69. **(B)** A partial-thickness burn that involves between 10% and 20% of the body surface area of a child under 5 years of ages is classified as a moderate burn per Table 27-4 in the text. (p. 550)

70. **(C)** A full-thickness burn to the front of the right forearm would not be considered a critical burn since it is only a small percentage of the body surface area. (p. 550)

71. **(A)** If a patient has a partial-thickness burn to the entire back, the patient should be wrapped in a dry, sterile burn sheet. (p. 551)

72. **(B)** The primary care for a patient with a chemical burn is to wash away the chemical with flowing water. (p. 552)

73. **(C)** You are treating a patient who was burned. The patient is having visual difficulties, is restless and irritable, has an irregular pulse rate, and muscle tenderness. This patient probably has an electrical burn. (p. 554)

74. If dry lime is the burn agent, brush it from the patient's skin and then flush with water. (p. 553)

75. **(A)** An occlusive dressing is used to form an airtight seal. (p. 556)

COMPLETE THE FOLLOWING

1. The signs of abdominal injury include: (any eight) (p. 544)
   - pain, cramps, nausea, weakness, thirst
   - obvious lacerations and puncture wounds
   - lacerations and puncture wounds to the pelvis and middle or lower back or chest wounds near the diaphragm
   - indications of blunt trauma
   - indications of developing shock
   - coughing up or vomiting blood
   - rigid and/or tender abdomen
   - distended abdomen
   - the patient tries to lie very still with legs drawn up

2. The parts of the body that account for 9% each in the rule of nines are: (pp. 548–549)
   - head and neck
   - each upper extremity
   - chest
   - abdomen
   - upper back
   - lower back and buttocks
   - front of each lower extremity
   - back of each lower extremity

3. The signs and symptoms of an electrical injury include: (any five) (p. 554)
   - burns where energy enters and exits
   - disrupted nerve pathways displayed as paralysis
   - respiratory difficulties or respiratory arrest
   - irregular heartbeat or cardiac arrest
   - muscle tenderness with or without muscular twitching
   - elevated blood pressure or low blood pressure with signs and symptoms of shock
   - restlessness or irritability if conscious, or loss of consciousness
   - visual difficulties
   - fractured bones and dislocations from severe muscle contractions or from falling
   - seizures

LABEL THE DIAGRAM (p. 547)

1. Superficial
2. Partial-thickness
3. Full-thickness
4. Skin reddened
5. Blisters
6. Charring

VIRTUAL STREET SCENES

1. Apply direct pressure as you elevate the arm. If that doesn't control the bleeding, hold a pressure point until the bleeding stops. Then firmly wrap the wound with a pressure bandage.

2. If the patient has an impaled object, do not attempt to remove it. Instead, stabilize the object in place with bulky dressings, applying pressure as each layer is positioned. Then secure the dressings in place with adhesive strips or tape. Be careful not to move the piece of glass.

3. If the patient already has low blood pressure, she is in very serious condition and needs rapid transport. Administer high-concentration oxygen, place her in a Trendelenburg position, keep her warm, and arrange for an ALS intercept en route to the hospital if possible.

Chapter 28: Musculoskeletal Injuries

MATCH TERMINOLOGY/DEFINITIONS

1. **(A)** Bones—hard but flexible living structures that provide support for the body and protection for vital organs

2. **(I)** Cartilage—connective tissue that covers the outside of the bone ends and acts as a surface for articulation allowing for smooth movements at joints

3. **(N)** Closed extremity injury—injury to an extremity in which the skin is not broken

4. **(E)** Crepitus—grating sensation or sound caused when broken bone ends rub together

5. **(B)** Dislocation—disruption or "coming apart" of a joint

6. **(H)** Extremities—portion of the skeleton that includes the clavicles, scapulae, arms, wrists, hands, pelvis, thighs, legs, ankles, and feet

7. **(G)** Fracture—any break in a bone

8. **(L)** Joints—places where bones articulate, or meet

9. **(O)** Ligaments—connective tissue that supports joints by attaching the bone ends and allowing for a stable range of motion

10. **(K)** Manual traction—process of applying tension to straighten and realign a fractured limb before splinting

11. **(C)** Open extremity injury—extremity injury in which the skin has been broken or torn through from the inside by an injured bone or from the outside by something that has caused a penetrating wound with associated injury to the bone

12. **(M)** Sprain—stretching and tearing of ligaments

13. **(J)** Strain—muscle injury caused by overstretching or overexertion of the muscle

14. **(F)** Tendons—bands of connective tissue that bind muscles to bones

15. **(D)** Traction splint—special splint that applies constant pull along the length of the leg to help stabilize the fractured bone and reduce muscle spasms

MULTIPLE-CHOICE REVIEW

1. **(B)** As we age, our bones become deficient in calcium. (p. 565)

2. **(C)** The strong white fibrous material covering the bones is called the periosteum. (p. 565)

3. **(B)** In children, the majority of the long bone growth occurs in the growth plate (located at the ends of bones). Fractures in this area can be very serious and can lead to a shortening of a limb. (p. 567)

4. **(D)** Musculoskeletal injuries are caused by indirect, direct, and twisting forces. (p. 569)

5. **(B)** Fractures of the femur typically cause a 2-pint blood loss over the first two hours. If there are additional complications, such as an artery laceration, blood loss could be more severe. Blood loss from a fracture of tibia/fibula would be about 1 pint; and a pelvis fracture would cause a 3 to 4 pint loss. (p. 571)

6. **(C)** The death rate from closed fracture of the femur dropped from 80% to 20% in the post WWI period due to the invention of the traction splint. The PASG was extensively used in the Vietnam conflict. (p. 572)

7. **(A)** The coming apart of a joint is referred to as a dislocation. A fracture is a break in a bone. See answer #8 for definitions of sprain and strain. (p. 572)

8. **(C)** The stretching or tearing of ligaments is called a sprain. A strain is caused by overstretching or overexertion of the muscle. (p. 572)

9. **(B)** A break in the continuity of the skin of a painful, swollen, deformed extremity is considered an open bone or joint injury. A simple fracture and a closed fracture have no break in the skin. Grating is not a type of fracture. (p. 572)

10. **(C)** Proper splinting of a possible closed fracture is designed to prevent closed injuries from becoming open ones. (p. 574)

11. **(C)** The signs and symptoms of a bone or joint injury include grating, swelling, and bruising. If shock develops, vomiting may occur. (p. 573)

12. **(A)** When a joint is locked into position, the EMT-B should splint the joint in the position found. Do not disregard splinting and transport immediately unless the patient is a high priority for some other reason. If this is the case, then a long backboard would be used as a splint. (p. 574)

13. **(C)** The procedure, which is done at least twice whenever a splint is applied, is assessment for pulses, motor function, and sensation (PMS) distal to the injury. Once traction is applied, it is not reapplied. (p. 575)

14. **(B)** The treatment of a painful, swollen extremity includes these steps: take BSI precautions, splint the injury, elevate the extremity, and apply a cold pack. Do not elevate the extremity until it is splinted. (p. 576)

15. **(C)** Multiple fractures, especially of the femur, can cause life-threatening external and internal bleeding. (p. 576)

16. **(A)** Applying a cold pack to a possible fracture will help to reduce the swelling. It does not stop bleeding from the bone, nor does it stop all pain and discomfort. Do not use a pressure bandage at the site of a fracture since it may damage the bone ends. (p. 574)

17. **(D)** If the initial assessment of a patient with a musculoskeletal injury reveals the patient is unstable, do not take time to splint each individual injury. It is not in the patient's best interest to waste the "Golden Hour" treating minor injuries. (p. 574)

18. **(D)** A splint properly applied to a closed bone injury should help prevent damage to muscles, nerves, or blood vessels caused by broken bones, as well as prevent an open bone injury and motion of bone fragments. The splint should not prevent circulation to the extremity. (p. 574)

19. **(D)** Complications of bone injuries include excessive bleeding, increased pain from movement, and paralysis of the extremity. Distal circulation usually decreases. (p. 574)

20. **(C)** The objective of realignment is to assist in restoring circulation and to fit the extremity into a splint. (p. 574)

21. **(A)** If there is a severe deformity of the distal extremity or it is cyanotic or pulseless, the EMT-B should align with gentle traction before splinting. The PASG should not be used for alignment. If you delay splinting until en route to the hospital, the circulation to the extremity could be hindered. (p. 574)

22. **(A)** The types of splints generally carried by EMT-Bs include rigid, formable, and traction. Other listings are examples of the three types of splints. (p. 575)

23. **(D)** Rigid splints are not used to immobilize joint injuries in the position found. Formable splints are used for this purpose. (p. 575)

24. **(C)** Traction splints are used specifically for fractures of the femur. (p. 575)

25. **(D)** When splinting, the EMT-B should immobilize the injury site and joints above and below. Do not leave open wounds exposed as they may get infected. Sometimes protruding bone ends fall back into place when the limb is placed in a splintable position. However, it is not the EMT-B's responsibility to reduce a fracture in the field. (p. 575)

26. **(C)** To ensure proper immobilization and increase patient comfort when using a rigid splint, pad the spaces between the body part and the splint. (p. 575)

27. **(B)** The method of splinting is always dictated by the severity of the patient's condition and the priority decision. If the patient is a high priority for "load and go" transport, choose a fast method of splinting. If the patient is a low priority for transport, choose a slower-but-better splinting method. (p. 575)

28. **(D)** If the patient with a musculoskeletal injury is unstable, the EMT-B should care for life-threatening problems first, consider aligning the injuries to an anatomical position, and immobilize the entire body to a long spine board. In the case of a critical patient, consider using a long backboard as a total body splint and lifting/spinal immobilization device. (p. 576)

29. **(D)** Hazards of improper splinting include aggravation of a bone or joint injury, reduced distal circulation, and delay in transport of patient with life-threatening injury. (p. 576)

30. **(C)** If the lower leg is cyanotic or lacks a pulse when a knee joint injury is assessed, the EMT-B should realign with gentle traction if no resistance is met. Call medical direction if you need some encouragement. An attempt at restoring a pulse must be made, otherwise the patient could lose the lower leg. (p. 576)

31. **(B)** Examples of a bipolar traction splint include Hare, Fernotrac, and half-ring. (p. 576)

32. **(B)** The amount of traction the EMT-B should pull when applying a Sager traction splint is about 10% of the body weight up to 15 pounds. (p. 582)

33. **(B)** The indications for a traction splint are a painful, swollen, deformed mid-thigh with no joint or lower leg injury. (p. 582)

34. **(B)** Whenever possible, three rescuers should be used to apply a traction splint. This allows one rescuer to support the injury site when the limb is lifted to position the traction splint. (p. 582)

35. (C) If the patient has multiple leg fractures and exhibits signs of shock (hypoperfusion), the EMT-B should apply the PASG as a splint. The patient will most likely be in shock so the PASG will serve a dual purpose. (p. 585)

36. (D) Signs and symptoms of a knee injury include pain and tenderness, swelling, and deformity. (p. 585)

37. (A) Elderly patients are more susceptible to hip fractures because of brittle bones or bone weakened by disease. (p. 584)

38. (B) When a patient has a fractured hip, the injured limb may appear shorter. (p. 584)

39. (C) When a patient who was involved in a serious fall has an unexplained sensation of having to empty his or her bladder, the patient may have a pelvic fracture. (p. 583)

40. (D) When immobilizing a patient who has a pelvic injury, you should not raise the lower legs. (p. 583)

COMPLETE THE FOLLOWING

1. Signs and symptoms of a musculoskeletal injury include: (p. 573)
   - pain and tenderness
   - deformity or angulation
   - grating, or crepitus
   - swelling
   - bruising
   - exposed bone ends
   - joints locked into position
   - nerve and blood vessel compromise

2. Signs and symptoms of a hip fracture include: (p. 584)
   - localized pain
   - sensitive to pressure on the lateral prominence of the hip
   - surrounding tissues discolored (delayed sign)
   - swelling
   - unable to move the limb while on the back
   - unable to stand
   - foot on the injured side is turned outward
   - injured limb may appear shorter

LABEL THE DIAGRAM (p. 566)

1. Skull
2. Cervical spine
3. Manubrium
4. Sternum
5. Xiphoid process
6. Thoracic spine
7. Costal cartilage
8. Lumbar spine
9. Iliac crest
10. Pelvis
11. Femur head
12. Acetabulum
13. Pubis
14. Medial malleolus
15. Lateral malleolus
16. Clavicle
17. Scapula
18. Ribs
19. Humerus
20. Elbow
21. Ulna
22. Radius
23. Sacral spine
24. Femur
25. Patella
26. Tibia
27. Fibula
28. Tarsals
29. Metatarsals
30. Phalanges

VIRTUAL STREET SCENES

1. You would have observed an open cut or laceration with bleeding where the bone exited the skin.

2. Yes. In order to apply a splint to a grossly deformed long bone, it will be necessary to move the bone into a splintable (straight) position with gentle traction on the extremity.

3. If the patient does not have a distal pulse, contact medical direction, who may allow you to gently manipulate the extremity once to try to restore the pulse.

4. If the patient's vital signs are stable and there is no evidence of multiple fractures, as ALS unit is probably not needed.

Chapter 29: Injuries to the Head and Spine

MATCH TERMINOLOGY/DEFINITIONS

1. **(O)** Autonomic nervous system—nervous system that consists of nerves that control involuntary functions such as the heartbeat and breathing

2. **(K)** Central nervous system—brain and spinal cord

3. **(I)** Cerebrospinal fluid (CSF)—fluid that surrounds the brain and spinal cord

4. **(B)** Concussion—mild closed head injury without detectable damage to the brain.

5. **(J)** Contusion—bruised brain caused when the force of a blow is great enough to rupture blood vessels

6. **(H)** Cranium—bony structure making up the forehead, top, back, and upper sides of the skull

7. **(D)** Malar—cheek bone; also called the zygomatic bone

8. **(M)** Nasal bone—bones that form the upper third, or bridge, of the nose

9. **(C)** Nervous system—body system that is divided into two subsystems and that provides overall control of thought, sensation, and the voluntary and involuntary motor functions of the body. (The major components of the nervous system are the brain and the spinal cord.)

10. **(N)** Orbits—bony structures, or sockets, around the eyes

11. **(A)** Peripheral nervous system—pairs of nerves that enter and exit the spinal cord between the vertebrae, twelve pairs of cranial nerves that travel between the brain and organs without passing through the spinal cord, and all of the body's other motor and sensory nerves

12. **(E)** Spinous process—bony bump on the vertebra that you can feel on a person's back

13. **(L)** Temporal bones—bones that form part of the side of the skull and floor of the cranial cavity

14. **(G)** Temporomandibular joint—movable joint formed between the mandible and the temporal bones; also called the TM joint

15. **(F)** Vertebrae—bones of the spinal column

MULTIPLE-CHOICE REVIEW

1. **(B)** The function of the spinal column is to protect the spinal cord. (p. 613)

2. **(C)** The spine is made up of 33 vertebrae. (p. 613)

3. **(C)** When a patient has a scalp injury, expect profuse bleeding since the scalp is very vascular. Do not try to determine the wound depth or palpate the site with fingertips. (p. 615)

4. **(C)** A bruise behind the ear is called Battle's sign. (p. 617)

5. **(B)** Discoloration of the soft tissues under both eyes is called raccoon's eyes. (p. 617)

6. **(A)** The signs and symptoms of a skull or brain injury include blood or fluid leakage from the ears and/or nose. (p. 617)

7. **(B)** Skull or brain injury may result in altered mental status and unequal pupils. Difficulty moving below the waist is a sign of a spine injury. (p. 617)

8. **(A)** Temperature increase is a late sign of brain or skull injury. It is due to inflammation, infection, or damage to temperature-regulating centers. (p. 618)

9. **(C)** Shock (hypoperfusion) from blood loss is generally <u>not</u> a sign of head injury, except in infants. There simply is not enough room within the adult skull to permit enough bleeding to cause shock. If there is a head injury with shock, evaluate for blood loss occurring elsewhere. (p. 618)

10. **(B)** The significance of an increase in carbon dioxide in the injured brain is that it causes brain tissue swelling. Hyperventilating the patient with supplemental oxygen at a rate of at least 25 ventilations per minute will reduce brain tissue swelling. (p. 618)

11. **(A)** A patient with a GCS of less than 8 should be taken to a trauma center. (p. 621)

12. **(D)** If an object has penetrated a patient's skull, stabilize the object with bulky dressings. This will minimize accidental movement of the object. (p. 622)

13. **(B)** The primary concern for emergency care of facial fractures or jaw injuries is the patient's airway. Such fractures create the potential for bleeding into the airway and difficulty maintaining a patent airway. (p. 622)

14. **(D)** The cervical and lumbar vertebrae are most frequently injured because they are not supported by other bony structures. (p. 623)

15. **(C)** When the spine is excessively pulled, which commonly occurs during a hanging, this is called a distraction injury. (p. 623)

16. **(C)** On your size-up of an automobile collision, you notice that both sides of the windshield have a spider-web crack. It is wise to call for a backup ambulance because both the driver and the passenger will need to be treated for spinal injury. (pp. 623–624)

17. **(D)** A fall from <u>three</u> times the patient's height is considered a high index of suspicion for a spinal injury. The EMT-B should also maintain a high degree of suspicion for a spinal injury when the patient has been involved in a motor-vehicle collision, motorcycle crash, or has open fractures to the ankles that resulted from a fall. (p. 624)

18. **(D)** Lateral bending injuries are caused by using improper lifting techniques. Diving accidents commonly cause flexion, extension, or compression injuries of the cervical spine. (p. 624)

19. **(A)** The unconscious trauma patient should be treated as if he has a potential spine injury. (p. 624)

20. **(D)** The most reliable source of spinal-cord injury in the conscious patient is paralysis of the extremities. (p. 624)

21. **(B)** A lack of spinal pain does not rule out the possibility of spinal-cord injury because other painful injuries may mask it. (pp. 624–625)

22. **(A)** When assessing a suspected spine-injured patient and you note a reversal of the normal breathing pattern, this is likely a result of damage to the nerves that control the rib cage. (p. 625)

23. **(D)** If a patient is found on her back with arms extended above the head, this may indicate a cervical-spine injury. (p. 625)

24. **(A)** If a patient is up and walking around at the scene of a high-speed collision, the EMT-B should assess for a potential spinal injury. (p. 625)

25. **(A)** If a patient has the mechanism of injury for a spinal injury, do not assess for spinal pain by asking the patient to move. Keep the patient as still as possible, and assess for equality of strength and tingling in the extremities. (p. 625)

26. **(A)** After performing the initial assessment and rapid trauma exam on a spine-injured patient, your next step is to determine the patient's priority, since this will be important in deciding how to immobilize him. (p. 626)

27. **(B)** If a patient complains of pain when you are attempting to place the head in a neutral in-line position, steady the head in the position found. (p. 626)

28. **(B)** When treating a patient with a spine injury, one EMT-B should maintain constant manual in-line stabilization until the patient is secured to a backboard. (p. 626)

29. **(C)** The cervical collar does not completely eliminate neck movement. All other answer choices are true. (p. 626)

30. **(C)** If a stable patient is found in a sitting position on the ground and is complaining about back pain, the EMT-B should immobilize with a short spine board or an extrication vest. This will immobilize the head, neck, and torso until he can be transferred to a long spine board. (pp. 626, 630)

31. **(B)** The rapid extrication procedure is <u>not</u> used for stable, low-priority patients. All other answer choices are true. (p. 630)

32. **(A)** When immobilizing a 6-year-old-or-younger child on a long backboard, provide padding beneath the shoulder blades. This eliminates the void behind the shoulders caused by the child's large head. (p. 634)

33. **(B)** If a helmet has a snug fit that allows little or no movement of the patient's head within the helmet, the helmet may be left in place. (p. 638)

34. **(B)** The correct order of steps for applying a short spine immobilization device: position device behind the patient; secure the device to patient's torso; evaluate torso fixation and pad behind the neck as necessary; secure the patient's head to the device. (pp. 628–629, 630)

35. **(D)** Prior to and after immobilization, the EMT-B should assess distal pulses, motor function, and sensation (PMS) in all extremities. (pp. 636, 637)

COMPLETE THE FOLLOWING

1. Signs of skull fracture or brain injury include: (any six) (pp. 617–618)
   - visible bone fragments
   - altered mental status
   - deep laceration or severe bruise or hematoma
   - depressions or deformity of the skull
   - any severe head pain
   - Battle's sign
   - raccoon's eyes
   - unequal pupils
   - one "sunken" eye
   - clear fluid from ears and/or nose
   - increase in blood pressure
   - equilibrium problems
   - paralysis or disability on one side of body
   - bleeding from the ears or nose
   - personality changes
   - temperature increase

- blurred or multiple image vision
- impaired hearing
- projectile vomiting
- seizures
- deteriorating vital signs
- posturing
- irregular breathing patterns

2. Types of brain injuries include: (p. 619)
   - concussion
   - contusion
   - hematoma (subdural, epidural)

LABEL THE DIAGRAM (p. 617)

1. cervical
2. thoracic
3. lumbar
4. sacral
5. coccyx

VIRTUAL STREET SCENES

1. The airway is always the highest priority for assessment and treatment.

2. The decision to immobilize him is based on the mechanism of injury, not on whether or not he has neck pain.

3. Serious head injuries are associated with irregular breathing patterns, high blood pressure, and a pulse rate under 60.

CASE STUDY—Deep Dive in a Shallow Pool

1. You would want to know if the patient struck his head, where he entered the pool, if there was any loss of consciousness, exactly how he flipped over, and did the patient at any point have any movement or sensation in his arms or legs.

2. As long as the patient is floating with assistance and manual stabilization of his head and neck is being maintained, you can float him to the shallow end of the pool where it will be easier to apply a long backboard.

3. Equipment needed includes a long backboard that floats, a rigid cervical collar, a head immobilizer, some padding, and straps or cravats.

4. Ask him if he remembers what happened, if he is having trouble breathing, and if he has feeling or sensation in his arms and legs. You should ask the OPQRST questions about his chief complaint.

5. Tell the patient that you are going to do everything you can to properly immobilize his spine and get him to the most appropriate hospital as quickly as possible.

6. Your partner should complete the initial assessment, take baseline vital signs, make sure the patient is securely immobilized, and reassess distal pulses, motor function, and sensation.

7. Many spine injury calls go to court, so make sure the prehospital care report is very accurate. Be sure to document the actions of the bystander who was in the pool when you arrived and how the injury was reported to have occurred (MOI). Be very specific that the patient stated that he had no sensation or movement in his arms and legs prior to your arrival and that distal pulses, motor function, and sensation were checked and rechecked before and after immobilization.

Chapter 30: Putting It All Together for the Trauma Patient

1. **(D)** Multiple-trauma patient—a patient with more than one serious injury

2. **(C)** Teamwork—cooperation of crew members, each knowing their role and working together to manage the serious patient

3. **(B)** Rapid trauma assessment—quick assessment of the head, neck, chest, abdomen, pelvis, extremities, and posterior of the body to detect signs and symptoms of injury

4. **(G)** Hypoperfusion—inability of the body to adequately circulate blood to the body's cells to supply them with oxygen and nutrients

5. **(A)** Golden hour—the optimum limit of time between the moment of injury and surgery at the hospital

6. **(H)** Emergency move—procedure designed to move a patient quickly when the situation of safety warrants it

7. **(F)** Hematoma—swelling caused by a collection of blood under the skin or in damaged tissues as a result of an injured or a broken blood vessel

8. **(E)** Mechanism of injury—action or forces that may have caused or contributed to the injury

MULTIPLE-CHOICE REVIEW

1. **(B)** The patient with a fractured right leg and a crushed pelvis is called a multiple-trauma patient. (p. 653)

2. **(C)** When a patient has an obvious angulated forearm and is unresponsive, your assessment and treatment priority is the airway. (p. 653)

3. **(C)** The multiple-trauma patient most likely will be stabilized in the surgical suite. (p. 653)

4. **(A)** The three "Ts" involved in the management of a multiple-trauma patient are timing, transport, and teamwork. (p. 653)

5. **(C)** A reasonable goal for scene time when dealing with a critical trauma patient is 10 minutes. (p. 653)

6. **(B)** When a trauma patient is making gurgling sounds as he breathes, you should suction his airway. (p. 654)

7. **(D)** Sometimes a long backboard can act as a full body splint when the critical patient must be immobilized quickly. (p. 658)

8. **(D)** When a patient has two fractured femurs, a crushed pelvis, and a possible abdominal injury, you should not apply a traction splint. Do consider applying a PASG (if local protocol allows), and request an ALS intercept en route to the hospital. (p. 658)

9. **(C)** When trying to minimize the on-scene care of a multiple-trauma patient, do not take the time to bandage all lacerations. (p. 653)

10. **(C)** Even when you are trying to cut scene time for a multiple-trauma patient, the one thing you do not cut out is scene safety—no matter how serious the patient is. (p. 658)

COMPLETE THE FOLLOWING

Treatments that would be appropriate on the scene of a critical trauma patient include: (p. 658)
- Suctioning the airway
- Inserting an oral or nasal airway

- Restoring a patent airway by sealing a sucking chest wound
- Ventilating with a bag-valve mask
- Administering high-concentration oxygen
- Controlling bleeding
- Immobilizing the patient with a cervical collar and a long backboard
- Inflating a pneumatic anti-shock garment

VIRTUAL STREET SCENES

1. Yes, if you suspect supine hypotensive syndrome due to compression of the vena cava by the uterus.

2. You should consider turning the patient and backboard on the side to help clear the airway.

3. No, not with her other problems. Application of a traction splint would take too long.

4. Make sure additional units are responding and that all other patients are assessed and treated.

Chapter 31: Infants and Children

MATCH TERMINOLOGY/DEFINITIONS

1. **(A)** Adolescent—child from 12 to 18 years of age

2. **(C)** Blow-by oxygen—flowing oxygen over the face of a small child so it will be inhaled

3. **(N)** Central line—intravenous line that is placed close to the heart

4. **(L)** Croup—group of viral illnesses that cause inflammation of the larynx, trachea, and bronchi

5. **(I)** Epiglottitis—bacterial infection that produces swelling of the epiglottis and partial airway obstruction

6. **(K)** Febrile seizure—complication of a rapidly rising temperature

7. **(B)** Fontanelle—"soft spot" at the front of an infant's skull where bones have not yet fused together

8. **(F)** Gastrostomy tube—feeding tube placed through the abdominal wall directly into the stomach

9. **(G)** Newborn or infant—child between birth and 1 year of age

10. **(H)** Preschooler—child from 3 to 6 years of age

11. **(D)** School-aged child—child from 6 to 12 years of age

12. **(O)** Shunt—drainage device that runs from the brain to the abdomen to relieve excess cerebrospinal fluid

13. **(J)** SIDS—sudden unexplained death during sleep of an apparently healthy baby in the first year of life

14. **(E)** Toddler—child from 1 to 3 years of age

15. **(M)** Tracheostomy tube—tube placed through the neck into the trachea to create an open airway

MULTIPLE-CHOICE REVIEW

1. **(B)** A toddler is between 1 and 3 years old. (p. 662)

2. **(C)** A school-aged child is between 6 and 12 years old. (p. 662)

3. **(D)** When assessing the toddler, examine the head last, not first. Toddlers fear having their head or face touched by strangers; to build confidence, examine heart and lungs first, then the head. (p. 663)

4. **(C)** Until about age 4, a child's head is proportionately larger and heavier than the adult's. This is why padding needs to be placed behind the shoulders when the child is immobilized. It is also the reason why children fly head first when involved in auto collisions or fall out of a window. (p. 664)

5. **(B)** The soft spot on an infant's skull is called a fontanelle. (p. 664)

6. **(A)** A sunken fontanelle may indicate dehydration. See answer #7. (p. 664)

7. **(B)** A bulging fontanelle may indicate elevated intracranial pressure. It is also a sign of meningitis. It may also bulge when the infant cries. (p. 664)

8. **(D)** Newborns usually breathe through their noses. This is why secretions in and obstruction of the nasal passageways can cause breathing problems. (p. 664)

9. **(B)** In an infant, hyperextension of the neck may result in airway obstruction because hyperextension can close off the flexible trachea. (p. 661)

10. **(D)** If the EMT-B suctions a child's airway for longer than a few seconds at a time, this could lead to cardiac arrest. Suctioning temporarily cuts off the body's oxygen supply; if it is prolonged, it is especially dangerous to infants and children. (p. 661)

11. **(A)** The tongues of infants and children are more likely than an adult's to fall back into and block the airway because their tongues are proportionately larger than the adult's. (p. 661)

12. **(B)** The insertion procedure for an oropharyngeal airway in an infant or child is done with the tip pointing toward the tongue and throat, which is the same position it will be in after insertion. Flipping it over the tongue may cause a tear in the soft palate. (pp. 661–662)

13. **(A)** When assessing the capillary refill of a child 5 years old or younger, peripheral perfusion is considered satisfactory if the color returns in less than 2 seconds. (p. 665)

14. **(D)** Loss of consciousness is not a sign of a partial airway obstruction in an infant or child. (p. 665)

15. **(C)** A child with a complete airway obstruction, or severe partial one, cannot cry and the cough becomes ineffective. (p. 665)

16. **(C)** The effects of hypoxia on an infant and a child is slowed heart rate and altered mental status. Hypoxia is the underlying reason for many of the most serious medical problems with children. (p. 666)

17. **(D)** Always use infection control barriers even when ventilating infants and children. Guidelines to use when ventilating the infant or child include: avoid breathing too hard through the pocket face mask or using excessive bag pressure and volume; use properly sized face masks to assure a good mask seal. Also remember if ventilation is not successful in raising the patient's chest, perform procedures for clearing an obstructed airway, then try to ventilate again. (p. 666)

18. **(B)** The flow-restricted, oxygen-powered ventilation device is contraindicated in infants and children. There are special units that are designed for pediatric patients, which require additional training, but they are not used in the field by EMT-Bs. (p. 666)

19. **(C)** Common causes of shock in a child include infection, trauma, blood loss, and dehydration. (p. 667)

20. **(D)** Croup is not a cause of shock. Less common causes of shock in a child include allergic reactions, poisoning, and cardiac events (rare). (p. 667)

21. **(B)** The blood volume of infants and children is approximately 8% of the total body weight. (p. 667)

22. **(D)** Children decompensate very rapidly, not very slowly! When children are in shock, they compensate very well, appear better than they actually are, and "go sour quickly" once they decompensate. (p. 668)

23. **(C)** When a child is bleeding internally, the EMT-B should avoid waiting for signs of decompensated shock before treating for shock. At this point, the child has approximately 30% blood loss. (p. 668)

24. **(B)** Decreased urine output and absence of tears are signs of shock in infants and children. (p. 668)

25. **(B)** When treating a child in shock, unless there are injuries that would contraindicate it, the EMT-B should elevate the patient's legs. (p. 668)

26. **(A)** Because children have a large skin surface area in proportion to their body mass, they can easily become victims of hypothermia. (p. 669)

27. **(B)** If a child has an airway respiratory disease, it is very important that the EMT-B <u>avoid</u> inserting a tongue blade into the mouth, which could stimulate laryngospasms. Administering blow-by oxygen is an appropriate action. (p. 669)

28. **(A)** Stridor on inspiration is an upper airway problem. The signs of an airway disease in a child include breathing effort on exhalation, rapid breathing, and wheezing. (pp. 670–671)

29. **(C)** A viral illness that causes inflammation of the upper airway and bronchi, which is often accompanied by a "seal bark" cough, is called croup. Epiglottitis is a bacterial infection that produces swelling of the epiglottis that usually develops in an older child; the patient exhibits with drooling due to the inability to swallow. (p. 670)

30. **(C)** About one-third of all pediatric trauma deaths are related to airway mismanagement. (p. 671)

31. **(B)** Hypothermia does <u>not</u> cause fever. Causes of fever in children include upper respiratory infection, pneumonia, and infection. (p. 672)

32. **(B)** Rectal or oral thermometers generally are <u>not</u> used in the prehospital setting unless permitted by local medical direction. (p. 672)

33. **(C)** When treating an infant or child with a high fever, monitor for shivering while cooling with tepid water. Do not use alcohol as it is a fire hazard and can be absorbed by the skin. Do not cover with a towel soaked in ice water, which can rapidly cause hypothermia. (p. 672)

34. **(B)** Infants are more susceptible to dehydration because, compared to adults, a greater percentage of their body is water. (p. 672)

35. **(C)** Fevers are the <u>most</u> <u>common</u> cause of seizures in infants and children. While they are rarely life-threatening in children who have them, they should be considered life-threatening by the EMT-B. (p. 673)

36. **(B)** Severe aspirin poisoning does not cause dehydration. It can cause seizures, shock, and coma. (p. 673)

37. **(A)** A common cause of lead poisoning in children is ingesting chips of lead-based paint. Eating fish from fresh water lakes is generally not a problem unless the lake is polluted. (p. 674)

38. **(C)** If you are treating a child who accidentally ingested a handful of her mother's vitamin tablets, you should be concerned because many vitamin pills contain iron, which can be fatal to a child. (p. 674)

39. **(D)** The majority of meningitis cases occur between the ages of 1 month and 5 years. (p. 675)

40. **(D)** In cases of sudden infant death syndrome, the EMT-B should provide resuscitation and transport to the hospital. You should avoid accusatory actions such as looking for evidence of neglect. Instead, be supportive, since parents who lose a child to SIDS often suffer intense guilt feelings. (p. 676)

41. **(B)** The number one cause of death in infants and children is trauma. Much trauma to infants and children occurs because they are curious and learning about their environment. (p. 676)

42. **(C)** The child who has been struck by a vehicle may present with a triad of injuries that include head injury, lower extremity injury (possibly a fractured femur), and abdominal injury (with possible internal bleeding). (pp. 676–677)

43. **(D)** The most frequent signs of head injury is altered mental status. Respiratory arrest is a common secondary effect. Head injury itself is seldom a cause of shock except in infants. Suspect internal injuries whenever a head-injury child presents with shock. (p. 677)

44. **(D)** Because the musculoskeletal structures of the chest are less developed in infants and children, they are more likely to incur injury to structures beneath the ribs. (p. 677)

45. **(C)** Because the abdominal muscles of infants and small children are immature, there is less protection for underlying organs. (p. 677)

46. **(B)** When using PASG on a pediatric patient, the EMT-B should remember the abdominal section is not generally used on children. (p. 677)

47. **(D)** You must keep the infant or child covered to prevent a drop in body temperature. Burned patients who become hypothermic have a higher death rate. (pp. 677–678)

48. **(D)** A parent's concern about the child's injuries is normal and to be expected. Indications that child abuse may be occurring include repeated responses to provide care for the same child or family, poorly healing wounds or improperly healed fractures, and indications of past injuries. (pp. 678–680)

49. **(C)** Torn clothing on the child is not necessarily an indication of child abuse. When you respond to the home of a person that you think may be a child abuser, observe for a family member who has trouble controlling anger, indications of alcohol and drug abuse, and any adult who appears in a state of depression. (p. 680)

50. **(C)** While you should talk with the child separately about how an injury occurred, it is not your role to ask the child if he/she has been abused. Always report your suspicions to the emergency department staff and in accordance with local policies. (p. 680)

COMPLETE THE FOLLOWING

1. Signs of respiratory distress in a child include: (any ten) (pp. 670–671)
   - nasal flaring
   - retraction of the muscles above, below, and between the sternum and ribs
   - use of abdominal muscles

- stridor
- audible wheezing
- grunting
- breathing rate greater than 60
- cyanosis
- decreased muscle tone
- poor peripheral perfusion
- delayed capillary refill
- altered mental status
- decreased heart rate

2. Potential problems that can occur when caring for a special needs child with a tracheostomy are: (pp. 681–682)
   - obstruction
   - bleeding from the tube or around the tube
   - an air leak around the tube
   - an infection
   - a dislodged tube

3. Four possible complications of central venous lines include: (p. 683)
   - infection
   - bleeding
   - cracked line
   - clotting off the line

COMPLETE THE CHART (p. 667)

1. $1^1/_2$ to 2 sec
2. 1 to $1^1/_2$ sec
3. 1 to $1^1/_2$ sec
4. 10–12 breaths/min
5. 20 breaths/min
6. 20 breaths/min

VIRTUAL STREET SCENES

1. The child may have had a seizure.

2. If the mental status did not improve and you suspected the child had a temperature as well as a rash, there may be an infectious disease involved. Be sure to use a face mask, eye shield, and disposable gloves.

3. Follow up in case there is an infectious disease to which you may have been exposed.

CASE STUDY—The Case of the Poisoned Juice

1. Use gloves, eye shields, and mask.

2. Find out exactly who drank the juice. Separate the healthy children from the juice drinkers to limit the "sympathy" sickness.

3. Dehydration

4. A shunt is a tube to drain excess cerebrospinal fluid in the head into the abdomen. Shunts are used for children who are hydrocephalic.

5. Pulse of 90 to 140, respirations of 25 to 40; BP is usually not taken on a child under 3.

6. Pulse of 80 to 130, respirations of 20 to 30; BP is usually not taken on a child under 3.

7. Pulse of 80 to 120, respirations of 20 to 30, and BP of 99 systolic

8. Have the caretaker hold the child. Be sure to keep the infant warm; warm your stethoscope and hands prior to touching the child. Observe the breathing from a distance.

9. Have the caretaker hold the child. Assure the child that he was not bad. Remove an article of clothing, examine, and then replace the clothing. Examine in a trunk-to-head approach to build confidence.

10. Use a toy, let them help you, and approach from toes to head.

11. In a child safety car seat

12. Ask the parent if this is how the infant normally reacts to this stimuli.

13. They can analyze the contents to determine what organism caused the problem.

Chapter 32: Ambulance Operations

MATCH TERMINOLOGY/DEFINITIONS

1. **(G)** AED—automated external defibrillator

2. **(I)** ATV—automatic transport ventilator

3. **(H)** CID—cervical immobilization device

4. **(A)** Due regard—legal term, which appears in most states' driving laws, referring to the responsibility of the emergency vehicle operator to drive safely and keep the safety of all others in mind at all times

5. **(B)** EMD—Emergency Medical Dispatcher

6. **(E)** Hypothermia thermometer—special thermometer that is designed to go down to 82°F.

7. **(D)** Landing zone (LZ)—large, flat area without aerial obstruction in which a helicopter can land to pick up a patient

8. **(F)** Sager—traction splint for the immobilization of a painful, swollen, deformed thigh

9. **(J)** Thumper—mechanical compressor for performing CPR that is especially helpful to services with transport time to the hospital over 15 minutes

10. **(C)** True emergency—call in which the driver of the emergency vehicle responds with lights and siren because he is of the understanding that loss of life or limb may be possible

MULTIPLE-CHOICE REVIEW

1. **(C)** The federal agency that develops specifications for ambulance vehicle designs is the U.S. Department of Transportation. (p. 687)

2. **(B)** The purpose for carrying an EPA-registered, intermediate-level disinfectant on the ambulance is to destroy mycobacterium tuberculosis. (p. 687)

3. **(D)** The telemetry repeater is used in the ambulance to boost the radio signal. Equipment that should be in the portable first-in kit to be taken directly to a patient's side would include the suction unit, rigid cervical collar, and a blood pressure cuff. (p. 689)

4. **(D)** The suction unit is used in the "A" (airway) step of the initial assessment of a trauma patient. Supplies used for the "C" (circulation) step would include disposable gloves, occlusive dressings, and the AED. (p. 689)

5. **(A)** The rubber bulb syringe is a supply used for childbirth. Equipment used to obtain vital signs includes an adult and a pediatric stethoscope, sphygmomanometer kit, and a penlight. (p. 689)

6. **(A)** A device used to carry patients over a long distance is called a Stokes basket. The scoop stretcher is used to lift and move patients without a spine injury through tight places. See answer #7. (p. 689)

7. **(C)** A Reeves stretcher is used for carrying a patient who must lie supine down stairs when a cot is too heavy or wide. The Stokes, or basket stretcher, is used to carry patients in high-angle rescue. (p. 689)

8. **(D)** A typical fixed oxygen delivery system consists of a 3,000-liter reservoir, a two-stage regulator, and the necessary reducing valve and yokes. (p. 689)

9. **(C)** The automatic transport ventilator is not an essential item to carry on the ambulance for prehospital respiratory care. (pp. 689–690)

10. **(D)** The fixed suction unit in the ambulance should reach a vacuum of at least 300 mmHg within 4 seconds. It should provide an air flow of 30 liters per minute and should be usable by a person at the head of the patient. Oxygen tanks require periodic hydrostatic testing. (pp. 689–690)

11. **(B)** The mechanical CPR compressor is a helpful device but is not essential for assisting with cardiopulmonary resuscitation. (p. 690)

12. **(D)** Burn sheets are not used for immobilization. Equipment carried on an ambulance that is used for immobilization includes a Hare traction splint, triangular bandages, and padded aluminum splints. (pp. 690–691)

13. **(A)** Chemical cold packs are carried on an ambulance for use with musculoskeletal injuries. (pp. 690–691)

14. **(D)** The Hare traction device is for splinting. Supplies used for wound care should include sterile burn sheets, 5 × 9-inch combine dressings, and self-adhering roller bandages. (pp. 690–691)

15. **(B)** Sterilized aluminum foil is used to maintain body heat or as an occlusive dressing. Body parts should be wrapped in a plastic bag and kept cool. Use a paper cup over an avulsed eye. Never use aluminum foil to directly cover an injury since it can cut the patient. (p. 690)

16. **(C)** Large safety pins are used with a sling. Supplies for childbirth include a rubber bulb syringe, sanitary napkins, and sterile surgical gloves. (p. 691)

17. **(C)** Every shift, both you and your partner should complete the equipment checklist. Preventative maintenance, oil changes, and waxing the ambulance are done routinely but not on each shift. (p. 692)

18. **(B)** The battery is checked with the engine off. (p. 692)

19. **(D)** It is not the EMD's job to advise the caller that an ambulance is not needed. The responsibilities of the Emergency Medical Dispatcher (EMD) include dispatching and coordinating EMS resources, interrogating the caller, prioritizing the call, and coordinating with other public safety agencies. (pp. 694–695)

20. **(C)** When an EMD questions a patient or caller, he/she does not routinely ask if the patient has been in the hospital recently. This is part of the EMT-B's SAMPLE history taken at the scene. (pp. 694–695)

21. **(B)** The brand of vehicle is not important to EMS, but would be for the police report. When speaking with a caller who is at the scene of a traffic collision, the EMD should ask if traffic is moving, how many lanes of traffic are open, and if any of the vehicles are on fire. (pp. 694–695)

22. **(D)** To be a safe ambulance operator, the EMT-B should be tolerant of other drivers, always wear glasses or contact lenses if required, and have a positive attitude about his ability as a driver. (pp. 695–696)

23. **(D)** Most state statutes prohibit passing of a school bus that has its red lights blinking. Stop and wait for the bus driver to shut off the red lights, which signals that all the children are in a safe position. Then proceed with caution. State statutes do allow emergency vehicle operators to do all of the following under certain conditions: park the vehicle anywhere so long as it does not damage personal property; proceed past red stop signals, flashing red stop signals, and stop signs; and exceed the posted speed limit as long as life and property are not endangered. (p. 696)

24. **(A)** At the scene of a collision, you examine a patient and find that he is stable. This situation is no longer considered a true emergency; further use of lights and siren would be inappropriate. (pp. 696–697)

25. **(D)** Do not use the siren throughout the call. Use the siren sparingly. Never assume that all motorists will hear your signal, and be prepared for erratic movements of motorists. (pp. 696–697)

26. **(B)** The decision about the use of lights and sirens should always be made with the medical condition of the patient in mind. The continuous sound of a siren may cause a sick or an injured person to suffer increased fear and anxiety, and his condition may deteriorate as stress increases. (pp. 696–697)

27. **(B)** Escorts or multi-vehicle response are a very dangerous means of response. Motorists often do not expect to see the second emergency vehicle and may collide with it. (pp. 697–698)

28. **(D)** The type of emergency does not affect ambulance response; factors that do include time of the day, weather, and road maintenance and construction. See also Complete the Following answer #2. (p. 698)

29. **(B)** Park in front of the wreckage if you are the first emergency vehicle on the scene so your flashing lights can warn approaching motorists before flares and other signals can be placed. Park 100 feet and uphill from a wreckage that involves fire. (pp. 698–700)

30. **(B)** Packaging is the sequence of operations required to ready the patient to be moved and to combine the patient and the patient-carrying device into a unit ready for transfer. (p. 700)

31. **(A)** An unconscious patient who has no potential spine injury should be positioned in the ambulance in the recovery position, which promotes maintenance of an open airway and the drainage of fluids. (p. 701)

32. **(B)** Forming a general impression of the patient is done when you first see the patient, not en route to the hospital. En route, the EMT-B rechecks bandages and splints, performs ongoing assessment, continues to monitor vital signs, and notifies the receiving facility of estimated time of arrival. (pp. 702–703)

33. **(D)** If a patient develops cardiac arrest en route to the hospital, the EMT-B's first action should be to tell the operator to stop the vehicle. (p. 703)

34. **(B)** When delivering the patient to the hospital, the EMT-B should never move a patient onto the hospital stretcher and leave. This is considered abandonment. (pp. 703, 705)

35. **(C)** When approaching a helicopter, first wait for the pilot or medic to wave you in. Then approach from the front or side of the craft. All other approach directions could cause injury or death. Remember to always follow the directions of the flight crew. (p. 712)

COMPLETE THE FOLLOWING

1. List the seven questions an EMD should ask a caller reporting a medical emergency. (p. 694)
   - What is the exact location of the patient?
   - What is your call-back number?
   - What's the problem?
   - How old is the patient?
   - What's the patient's sex?
   - Is the patient conscious?
   - Is the patient breathing?

2. List seven factors that can affect ambulance response. (p. 698)
   - day of the week
   - time of the day
   - weather
   - road maintenance and construction
   - railroads
   - bridges and tunnels
   - schools and school buses

3. List the four major ways the EMT-B on the scene of a collision should describe the landing zone to the air rescue service. (p. 712)
   - terrain
   - major landmarks
   - estimated distance to nearest town
   - other pertinent information

LABEL THE PHOTOGRAPHS (p. 710)

1. Low-level
2. Intermediate
3. High-level
4. Sterilization

VIRTUAL STREET SCENES

1. Notify the dispatcher, call the police, and assure that there are no injuries caused by the collision. While waiting for the police to respond, ask the dispatcher to reassign the initial call to another unit.

2. Because you cannot stop the ambulance fast enough if an unsuspecting motorist drives in front of you. Even with emergency lights and sirens on, you cannot assume that other drivers will see you or hear you approach.

3. The driver of the emergency vehicle would be at fault.

CASE STUDY—The Ambulance Collision

1. Yes, by stopping before proceeding through the intersection.

2. Yes, by wearing a shoulder harness.

3. It was necessary to assign yet another ambulance to handle that call.

4. Do no harm.

5. The service may lose business. The EMS personnel may be ridiculed, and some patients may actually be afraid to get into your ambulance!

6. Because he is allowed to look into incidents of this nature with close scrutiny. This is especially true in the public sector, when injury has occurred.

7. Absolutely. Civilian motorists are not required to drive with "due regard for the safety of all others."

8. He does, unless his service is willing to assist him or unless he has some insurance or legal aid.

9. Yes, he could.

10. Proper driver screening and qualification, driver training, driving SOPs (which include always wearing shoulder harness in the front of the vehicle, how to negotiate an intersection, and proper use of emergency lights and siren), retraining, keeping the vehicles in good shape, and a good quality improvement program.

Chapter 33: Gaining Access and Rescue Operations

MATCH TERMINOLOGY/DEFINITIONS

1. **(H)** A Post—post in front of the driver's compartment that supports the roof and windshield

2. **(A)** B Post—when moving toward the rear of the vehicle, the second post you see, which supports the roof

3. **(L)** Complex—access that requires tools or special equipment to reach the patient

4. **(J)** Cribbing—blocks of hardwood, usually $4 \times 4 \times 18$-inch or $2 \times 4 \times 18$-inch, used to stabilize a vehicle

5. **(M)** Disentanglement—three-part procedure used by rescue personnel to free a patient trapped in a vehicle

6. **(E)** Entrapment—when a patient is pinned and requires assistance, sometimes mechanical, to free him

7. **(N)** Extrication—process by which entrapped patients are rescued from vehicles, buildings, tunnels, or other places

8. **(O)** Glas-Master—saw that is designed to cut laminated windshield glass

9. **(D)** Ground gradient—decreasing circles of voltage on the ground surrounding a point where a charged wire is down

10. **(K)** Inner circle—area immediately around and including the wrecked vehicle

11. **(I)** Laminated glass—safety glass used in automobile windshields made of two sheets of plate glass bonded to a sheet of tough plastic

12. **(C)** Nader Pin—named after a well-known consumer advocate, this case-hardened pin is held by the cams of an automobile's door locking system

13. **(G)** Protective gear—gear designed to prevent the rescuer from being injured while working in the inner circle

14. **(F)** Stabilization—to crib or block a vehicle or structure to prevent further unintended, uncontrolled movement

15. **(B)** Tempered glass—glass used in an automobile's side and rear windows designed to break into small rounded pieces rather than sharp fragments

MULTIPLE-CHOICE REVIEW

1. **(B)** The correct term is specialty rescue teams. Such teams may be provided by a variety of agencies such as EMS, fire, police, industrial or commercial services. (p. 719)

2. **(B)** Defining patient care is not a phase of extrication. The phases of extrication encompass ten steps that include gaining access to the patient, disentangling the patient, and sizing up the situation. See also Complete the Following answer #1. (p. 719)

3. **(A)** An important part of a rescue scene size-up is determining the extent of entrapment. Starting IVs on the patient is not a part of the size-up and is a paramedic skill. Removing shattered glass, if needed, should be done from as far away from the patient as is possible. Informing the patient about the extent of vehicle damage will make him more anxious. Don't lie if asked, but focus on treating the patient. (p. 720)

4. **(C)** During size-up of a collision, you must be able to read a collision and develop an action plan based on your knowledge of rescue operations and estimate of the patient's condition and priority. Knowledge includes previous experience; remember you were called to rescue the patient, not the vehicle! (p. 720)

5. **(B)** When developing an action plan for patient extrication, always keep in mind the "golden hour." The cost of vehicle damage or the type of vehicle is irrelevant to the extrication as is the presence of bystanders, although they should not interfere with your operations. (p. 720)

6. **(C)** If a vehicle has an air bag that deployed, the manufacturer recommends lifting the bag and examining at the steering wheel and dash. If either is damaged, it is likely that patient's chest is damaged, which would mean great potential for internal injury. The use of a HEPA mask is not required; gloves and eye protection are recommended. (p. 720)

7. **(B)** The unsafe act that contributes most to collision scene injuries is failure to wear protective gear during rescue operations. (p. 721)

8. **(D)** By limiting the inner circle to rescuers who are in protective gear, you help to <u>decrease</u> potential injuries. Factors that may contribute to injuries of rescuers at a collision include a careless attitude toward personal safety, a lack of skill in tool use, and physical problems that impede strenuous effort. (p. 721)

9. **(D)** Plastic "bump hats" do not provide adequate protection; use quality headgear. Good protective gear at the scene of a collision includes fire-resistant trousers or turnout pants; steel toe, high-top work shoes; and firefighter or leather gloves. (pp. 721–722)

10. **(A)** To ensure eye protection at the collision scene, the EMT-B should wear safety goggles with a soft vinyl frame. Safety glasses can be worn, but they must have <u>large</u> lenses and side shields. Thermal masks are cold-weather gear. A hinged plastic helmet shield will allow particles to enter from under the shield. (p. 722)

11. **(C)** An aluminized rescue blanket may be used to protect your patient from poor weather and flying particles. The rescuer should be properly attired for cold weather conditions. (p. 722)

12. **(A)** When using flares, the EMT-B should watch for spilled fuel or other combustibles prior to igniting. Do not throw flares out of the moving vehicle or use a traffic wand. Never turn your back on traffic; walk towards the traffic so you can observe oncoming vehicles. (pp. 722, 724)

13. **(C)** When there is an electrical hazard, the safe zone should be far enough away to assure an arcing wire does not cause injury. If you feel a ground gradient, you are already too close to the electricity. (p. 724)

14. **(D)** A material or an object that will carry electricity is called a conductor. (p. 724)

15. **(B)** If a vehicle collides with a broken utility pole with utility wires down, you should tell the vehicle's occupants to stay in the vehicle until the power company arrives. (pp. 724–725)

16. **(B)** In wet weather, a phenomenon known as a ground gradient may provide your first clue that a wire is down. (p. 725)

17. **(A)** If you feel a tingling sensation in your legs and lower torso, you should turn 180 degrees and shuffle with both feet together (or hop on one foot) to safety. Either technique helps prevent your body from completing a circuit with the energized ground, which can cause electrocution. (p. 725)

18. **(D)** Do <u>not</u> apply a short spine board to the driver as this is the time for a quick removal. If there is a fire in the car's engine compartment and people are trapped within the vehicle, you should quickly and carefully remove the patient, assure that the fire department has been called, and don protective gear and use your fire extinguisher. (pp. 725, 727)

19. **(C)** When a vehicle's hood is closed and there is an engine fire, you should <u>not</u> attempt to open the hood as this will fuel the fire with oxygen and the fire will flare up. (p. 725)

20. **(A)** When a vehicle rolls off the roadway into dried grass in a field, it is possible that a fire may occur from the catalytic converter, which is under the car, and its temperature can reach over 1,200 degrees. (pp. 725, 727)

21. **(C)** "Try Before You Pry" is the foundation for the simple access procedure. Disentanglement is removing the vehicle from around the patient who is entrapped. Stabilization is ensuring the vehicle is less likely to roll or move during extrication efforts. (p. 731)

22. **(D)** Once a vehicle is stabilized and an entry point is gained, do <u>not</u> pull a patient out of an access hole prior to spinal immobilization. (p. 731)

23. **(C)** If an unconscious patient is in a sitting position behind the wheel with legs pinned by the vehicle, the best approach to disentanglement would be to cut the roof, displace the doors, then displace the dash. This allows for plenty of room to work and for vertical rapid extrication if the patient's condition deteriorates. (pp. 731, 732)

24. **(D)** Removing the roof of a vehicle does <u>not</u> stabilize a vehicle. (p. 732)

25. **(C)** When an extrication involves displacing the dash or steering wheel but the air bag has not yet deployed, disconnect the battery cable. (p. 732)

COMPLETE THE FOLLOWING

1. The ten phases of the rescue process are: (p. 719)
   - preparing for the rescue
   - sizing up the situation
   - recognizing and managing hazards
   - stabilizing the vehicle prior to entering
   - gaining access to the patient
   - providing initial patient assessment and rapid trauma exam
   - disentangling the patient
   - immobilizing and extricating the patient from the vehicle
   - providing a detailed physical exam, ongoing assessment, treatment, and transporting to the most appropriate hospital
   - terminating the rescue

2. The factors that can increase the potential for an injury at a collision site are: (any six) (p. 721)
   - a careless attitude toward personal safety
   - lack of skill in tool use
   - physical problems that impede strenuous effort

- failure to eliminate or control hazards
- using unsafe tools
- failure to select the proper tool for the task
- failure to recognize mechanisms of injury and unsafe surroundings
- lifting heavy objects improperly
- deactivating safety devices designed to prevent injury
- failure to wear highly visible outer clothing, especially when exposed to highway traffic

LABEL THE PHOTOGRAPHS (pp. 726, 728, 733)

1. Extinguishing fire under vehicle
2. Extinguishing fire under the dash
3. Stabilizing car on wheels
4. Stabilizing car on its side
5. Stabilizing car on its roof
6. Car roof folded back

VIRTUAL STREET SCENES

1. The strategy depends on the abilities, training, and equipment available to the rescuers. However, taking the roof off first has an advantage; if the patient takes a turn for the worse, the patient could be removed through the roof on a long backboard.

2. This is a serious mechanism of injury. The patient should be transported to a trauma center.

3. ALS should be requested right away, due to the mechanism of injury and the patient's unresponsiveness.

Chapter 34: Special Operations

MATCH TERMINOLOGY/DEFINITIONS

1. **(O)** Cold zone—area in which the command post and support functions that are necessary to control the incident are located

2. **(L)** EMS Command—senior EMS person on the scene who establishes an EMS command post and oversees the medical aspects of a multiple-casualty incident

3. **(M)** Hazardous material—any substance or material in a form that poses an unreasonable risk to health, safety, and property when transported in commerce

4. **(N)** Hot zone—area immediately surrounding a dangerous goods incident that extends far enough to prevent adverse effects from released dangerous goods to personnel outside the zone

5. **(K)** Incident Management System (IMS)—system used for the management of a large-scale multiple-casualty incident, involving assumption of responsibility for command and designation and coordination of such elements as triage, treatment, transport, and staging

6. **(J)** Multiple-casualty incident (MCI)—any medical or trauma incident involving three or more patients that places a great demand on EMS equipment and personnel

7. **(I)** Staging officer—person responsible for overseeing and keeping track of ambulances and ambulance personnel at a

multiple-casualty incident and who directs ambulances to treatment areas at the request of the transportation officer

8. **(H)** Staging sector—area in which ambulances are parked and other resources are held until needed

9. **(G)** Transportation officer—person responsible for communicating with sector officers and hospitals to manage transportation of patients to hospitals from the scene of a multiple-casualty incident

10. **(F)** Treatment officer—person responsible for overseeing treatment of patients who have been triaged at a multiple-casualty incident

11. **(E)** Treatment sector—area in which patient care is delivered at a multiple-casualty incident

12. **(C)** Triage—process of quickly assessing patients in a multiple-casualty incident and assigning each a priority for receiving emergency care or transportation to definitive care

13. **(D)** Triage officer—person responsible for overseeing triage at a multiple-casualty incident

14. **(B)** Triage sector—area in which secondary triage takes place at a multiple-casualty incident

15. **(A)** Triage tag—color-coded tag indicating the priority group to which a patient has been assigned

MULTIPLE-CHOICE REVIEW

1. **(A)** Using the *North American Emergency Response Guidebook*, the EMT-B would find that ethyl acetate is a chemical that irritates the eyes and respiratory tract. See Table 34-1. (p. 743)

2. **(B)** Using the *North American Emergency Response Guidebook*, the EMT-B would find that Benzene (benzol) is a chemical that has toxic vapors that can be absorbed through the skin. See Table 34-1. (p. 743)

3. **(D)** The regulations that require training in hazardous materials for responders to hazmat incidents are OSHA 1910.120. (p. 741)

4. **(B)** The level of training for those who initially respond to releases or potential releases of hazardous materials in order to protect people, property, and the environment is called First Responder Operations. (p. 742)

5. **(A)** The level of training for those who are likely to witness or discover a hazardous substance release is called First Responder Awareness. (p. 742)

6. **(C)** The standard that deals with competencies for EMS personnel at a hazardous materials incident is called NFPA 473. (p. 742)

7. **(D)** Pet stores generally are not hazmat locations. Examples of potential hazardous materials locations would include garden centers, chemical plants, and trucking terminals. (p. 742)

8. **(C)** Unless EMS personnel are trained to the level of Hazardous Materials Technician, they must remain in the cold zone. (p. 744)

9. **(C)** All victims leaving the hot zone should be considered contaminated until proven otherwise. (p. 744)

10. **(A)** The primary concern at the scene of a hazardous materials incident is the safety of the EMT-B and crew, patients, and the public. Stabilizing the incident often takes a long time. Exposed patients need to be removed but this, too, does not happen quickly, due to the need to identify the hazmat material and decontaminate the patients. (p. 743)

11. **(B)** Upon arrival at a tanker truck crash where the vehicle has overturned and is rapidly leaking its contents onto the street, the EMT-B should isolate the area and call for the appropriate backup assistance. Do not try to stop or seal the leak since this would expose many rescuers to the chemical. Sending in the least senior EMT-B to assess the patient is not an appropriate move as it could sacrifice a rescuer. (pp. 742–744)

12. **(B)** The "safe zone" of a hazardous materials incident should be established in an upwind/same level location. If it was established downwind, you would increase the chance of being exposed to the chemicals. Zones established downhill may be contaminated by hazardous runoff. (pp. 743–744)

13. **(C)** Initiating rescue attempts inside the hot zone are delayed until the product and proper protection needs are determined. The role of the incident commander at a hazardous materials incident is to delegate responsibility for directing bystanders to a safe area, establishing a perimeter, and evacuating people if necessary. (pp. 742–744)

14. **(A)** When a contaminated victim of a hazardous materials incident comes in contact with other people who are not contaminated, this is referred to as secondary contamination. (p. 744)

15. **(C)** The designations on the sides of tanker trucks are called hazardous material placards. (pp. 744–745)

16. **(B)** The commonly used placard system for fixed facilities is called the NFPA 704 system. (p. 744)

17. **(B)** All employers are required to post in an obvious spot the information about all the chemicals in the workplace on a form called a MSDS (Material Safety Data Sheet). (p. 745)

18. **(A)** The NFPA rules are really only guidelines and do not detail how to manage an incident. Resources that the EMT-B should use at a hazardous materials incident include the local hazmat team, the *North American Emergency Response Guidebook,* and CHEM-TEL. (pp. 745–746)

19. **(A)** CHEMTREC is a 24-hour service for identifying hazardous materials that also provides instructions for handling spills. (pp. 745–746)

20. **(B)** The responsibilities of EMS personnel at a hazardous materials incident are taking care of the injured and monitoring and rehabilitating hazmat team members. (p. 748)

21. **(A)** The rehab sector at a hazardous materials incident should be located in the cold zone, not the warm zone. It should also be protected from the weather, easily accessible to EMS, and free from exhaust fumes. (p. 748)

22. **(D)** As soon as possible after a hazmat team member exits the hot zone, the EMT-B should reassess his vital signs. Remember that hazmat team members should have their baseline vitals taken while suiting up and both pre-entry and exit vitals should be tracked on a flow sheet. (p. 748)

23. **(C)** Always try to contain the runoff water when it is necessary to decontaminate a patient before hazmat specialists arrive. Flushing water down the nearest drain could decontaminate the area's entire water supply. (p. 750)

24. **(D)** A good local disaster plan is not generic, but rather should be written to address the events that are conceivable for a particular location (e.g., Florida needs to plan for hurricanes, Kansas for tornadoes). (p. 751)

25. **(D)** Upon arrival of the first EMS unit at the scene of an MCI, the crew leader should assume EMS command, conduct a scene walk through, and call for backup. Do not begin

patient treatment since even though this might save one or two lives, it would be at the expense of the majority of the patients because response would be delayed and disorganized. (pp. 751, 753)

26. **(C)** Once units arrive at an MCI, as much face-to-face communication as possible should be used, especially between Command and sector officers and between sector officers and subordinates. This will help to reduce radio channel crowding. (p. 753)

27. **(C)** If an MCI involves hazardous materials, a rehabilitation sector would be needed. (p. 755)

28. **(A)** The individual at an MCI who is responsible for the sorting and prioritizing of the patients is the triage officer. (p. 755)

29. **(A)** Patients who are assessed to have decreased mental status at an MCI are considered Priority 1. Other examples of Priority 1 patients are those with airway and breathing difficulties, uncontrolled or severe bleeding, severe medical problems, shock, and severe burns. (pp. 755–756)

30. **(A)** Patients who are assessed to have shock (hypoperfusion) at an MCI are considered Priority 1. See answer #29. (pp. 755–756)

31. **(B)** Patients who are assessed to have multiple-bone or joint injuries at an MCI are considered Priority 2. Other examples of Priority 2 patients are those with burns without airway problems and back injuries with or without spinal-cord damage. (pp. 755–756)

32. **(D)** Patients who are assessed to have died at the MCI scene are considered Priority 4 (or zero). (pp. 755–756)

33. **(C)** The individual at an MCI who is responsible for maintaining a supply of vehicles and personnel at a location away from the incident site is the staging officer. (p. 759)

34. **(C)** The individual at an MCI who is responsible for determining patient destinations and notifying the hospitals of the incoming patients is the transportation officer. (p. 760)

35. **(D)** Patient transport decisions at an MCI are based upon prioritization, destination facilities, and transportation resources. The patient's family preferences are not a consideration in a disaster situation. (pp. 760–761)

COMPLETE THE FOLLOWING

1. The information you should be prepared to give when you call for assistance from CHEMTREC includes:
   (pp. 745–746, 748)
   * Give your name, your call-back number, and your FAX number.
   * Explain the nature and location of the problem.
   * Report the identification number(s) of the material(s) involved if there is a safe way for you to obtain this information.
   * Give the name of the carrier, shipper, manufacturer, consignee, and point of origin.
   * Describe the container type and size.
   * Report if the container is on rail car, truck, open storage, or housed storage.
   * Estimate the quantity of material transported and released.
   * Report local conditions (e.g., the weather, terrain, proximity to schools and/or hospitals).
   * Report injuries and exposures.
   * Report local emergency services that have been notified.
   * Keep the line of communication open at all times.

Chapter 34 (continued)

2. The characteristics of the rehab sector must include the following: (any four) (p. 748)
   - located in the cold zone
   - protected from weather
   - large enough to accommodate multiple rescue crews
   - easily accessible to EMS units
   - free from exhaust fumes
   - allows for rapid re-entry into the emergency operation

COMPLETE THE CHART (p. 756)

1. EMS Staging Officer
2. EMS Safety Officer
3. Transportation Officer
4. Triage Officer
5. Rehab Officer
6. P-2 Tx Leader

VIRTUAL STREET SCENES

1. Yes, a helicopter would be appropriate provided there is a nearby landing zone that will not keep ambulances from transporting patients.

2. With a short transport time, you could have the ambulances turn around and return to the scene to pick up additional patients.

3. Some EMS providers have used a school bus to transport low-priority patients to a hospital. If you ever do so, medically clear each patient on the bus to assure they are low priority and arrange for medical personnel to travel with them on the bus to the hospital.

CASE STUDY—The School Bus MCI

1. Size up the situation, establish EMS command, make contact with the fire and police command officers.

2. You should don the EMS Command or Medical Command vest. Your responsibilities are the overall management of the medical aspects of the incident, working directly with the chief officers of the police and fire departments, assuring the safety of all your personnel, and designating triage, treatment, transport, and staging sector officers.

3. Triage officer

4. Set up the Triage Sector and begin tagging patients and classifying into priority for removal from the scene to the treatment area.

5. Respond three to the scene and seven to a staging area about a mile away with easy access to the scene. The ambulances responding to the scene will help fill out the complement of command officers and provide personnel to triage patients.

6. The first crew leader at the staging sector should be designated as the staging officer and be responsible for the release of ambulances and personnel to the scene as directed by command. If this is a lengthy operation, he should also attend to the human needs of the staging personnel by locating restrooms and food. He will need to be able to communicate with arriving mutual aid units, providing them with maps and directions to the scene and hospital as it becomes necessary.

7. Yes, but only upon direction of Command and/or the staging officer.

8. Transportation and Treatment Sector Officers would be helpful in managing the flow of patients.

9. On long backboards with rigid extrication collars applied

10. Take the patients to the respective section of the treatment area depending on their triage tag priority.

11. P-2

12. P-1

13. P-4 (or zero)

14. P-1

15. Allow one parent per child to assist and stay with the child in the treatment area if space permits.

16. Transportation sector officer

17. Do a roll call of the hospitals for bed availability and the number of patients of each priority they can handle.

18. Consider the use of a medivac helicopter.

19. P-3 patients with minor injuries who are medically cleared. There will still need to be medical personnel on the bus just in case a patient's status changes.

20. Appoint a Public Information Officer, plan for rehab and a light meal after the incident, and consider setting up a Critical Incident Stress Debriefing for all personnel who were at the scene who are interested in talking about what they saw and did.

Interim Exam 3

1. (B) The circulation of blood throughout the body, filling the capillaries and supplying the cells and tissues with oxygen and nutrients is called perfusion. Physiology is the study of how the body functions. Metabolism is the process of all the physical and chemical changes within the body that are necessary for life. (p. 502)

2. (D) With one exception (the pulmonary artery), arteries carry oxygenated blood away from the heart. (p. 501)

3. (A) With one exception (the pulmonary vein), veins carry deoxygenated blood back to the heart. (p. 501)

4. (D) Once an adult loses approximately a liter of blood, his/her condition is considered serious. This is one-sixth of the total blood volume in a 150-pound patient. (p. 504)

5. (C) Once a child loses approximately 500 ml of blood, his condition is considered serious. (p. 504)

6. (B) Once an infant loses approximately 150 cc of blood volume, his condition is considered serious. Note that a cc and a ml are equal measurements. (p. 504)

7. (A) Since internal bleeding is not visible, the EMT-B must base severity of blood loss on signs and symptoms exhibited. Mechanism of injury may also be a good clue to internal injury. What the patient tells you will not reveal how much blood has been lost. (p. 512)

8. (D) The patient's history of diabetes is not significant in determining bleeding severity. The factors on which severity of bleeding depends are the rate of bleeding and the amount of blood loss, the patient's age and weight, and the ability of the patient's body to respond and defend against blood loss. (p. 504)

9. (B) Blood that oozes and is dark red is most likely from a capillary. Venous bleeding will be a steady flow of dark red or maroon blood. Arteries spurt and blood is usually bright red. (pp. 503–504)

10. **(C)** You are treating a patient who has a slashed wrist, which is spurting bright red blood. After trying direct pressure and elevation to control the bleeding, the next step would be to press on the brachial artery. See answer #11. (p. 505)

11. **(D)** When all other methods have failed to control bleeding, the EMT-B should apply a tourniquet as the last resort. (p. 505)

12. **(C)** Vomiting bile is usually not a sign of internal bleeding. Signs of internal bleeding include painful, swollen, or deformed extremities; a tender, rigid abdomen; and bruising. (p. 512)

13. **(C)** A fall from a height will usually produce a blunt injury, unless the patient falls onto something that penetrates, such as a fence. Examples of penetrating trauma include handgun bullet wounds, carving-knife wounds, and screwdriver stab wounds. (p. 512)

14. **(C)** Gunshot wounds are considered penetrating trauma. Examples of blunt trauma include blast injuries, auto-pedestrian collisions, and falls. (p. 512)

15. **(A)** The signs and symptoms of internal bleeding are the same as those of shock (hypoperfusion). Patients with these signs are difficult to stabilize in the field. (p. 512)

16. **(B)** Hypovolemic, cardiogenic, and neurogenic are all types of shock. Hydrophobia is another name for rabies. (p. 514)

17. **(C)** At a point when the body can no longer compensate for the low blood volume, decompensated shock begins. Anaphylactic shock is a severe allergic reaction with respiratory distress and hypotension. (pp. 513–514)

18. **(C)** The brain and spinal cord are the major components of the central nervous system. The peripheral nerves branch out from the spinal cord. (p. 613)

19. **(D)** The nervous system is divided into the central, peripheral, and autonomic nervous systems. Voluntary is a type of skeletal muscle that allows movement. (p. 613)

20. **(D)** The cranium consists of the forehead, top, back, and upper sides of the skull. The maxilla is the upper jaw, and the mandible is the lower jaw. (pp. 614–615)

21. **(A)** The bones forming the face include the zygomatic, mandible, and maxillae. Vertebrae are bones of the spine. (p. 615)

22. **(A)** The brain and spinal cord are bathed in cerebrospinal fluid. Lymphatic fluid is responsible for maintaining our immune system. Synovial fluid lubricates the joints. (p. 615)

23. **(B)** The spine is divided into sections called vertebrae. Coccygeal is the name of one section of the vertebrae. (p. 615)

24. **(B)** The lumbar area of the spine includes 5 vertebrae. (p. 615)

25. **(C)** The cervical area of the spine includes 7 vertebrae. (p. 615)

26. **(B)** When a patient strikes her head and states she feels groggy and has a headache, she most likely has a concussion. (p. 619)

27. **(D)** While the patient most likely has a concussion, any altered mental status after striking the head, such as "just sitting there staring off into space for a few minutes," can be an early indication of a contusion, a concussion, or a coup injury. An attention deficit is not usually injury induced. (p. 619)

28. **(B)** When a patient has some memory loss after a head injury, this is referred to as amnesia. (p. 619)

29. **(C)** When a bruising of the brain occurs on the side of the injury, this is referred to as a coup injury. When bruising occurs on the opposite side, this is called contrecoup. A hematoma is a collection of blood within tissue. A hematoma in the cranium is usually named by its location such as epidural (outside the dura), subdural (below the dura), or intracerebral (within the brain). (p. 619)

30. **(D)** A collection of blood within the skull or the brain is called a subdural, epidural, and intracerebral hematoma depending on the specific location. See answer #29. (p. 619)

31. **(D)** Decreased respiration does not lead to increased cellular perfusion, rather, it decreases perfusion. Head injury is made worse by limited room for expansion inside the skull. As pressure in the skull increases, it becomes more difficult for blood to flow into the head. This leads to carbon dioxide level increases in the brain. (p. 619)

32. **(B)** An assessment strategy used to check an extremity for injury or paralysis in the conscious patient is assessing equality of strength by checking hand grip or pushing against the patient's hands and feet. (pp. 625–626)

33. **(A)** The type of immobilization device used for a patient depends on patient priority. (p. 626)

34. **(D)** If a patient has a brain injury with skull fracture, the patient's pupils will tend to be unequal. (p. 617)

35. **(D)** The vitals of a patient with a brain injury are increased blood pressure, decreased pulse. (pp. 617–618)

36. **(A)** Consider the possibility of a cranial fracture whenever you note deep lacerations or severe bruises to the scalp or forehead. (p. 618)

37. **(B)** The spinal column is made up of 33 irregularly shaped bones. (p. 615)

38. **(B)** Any blunt trauma above the clavicles may damage the cervical vertebrae. (p. 623)

39. **(A)** Priapism is a persistent erection of the penis. (p. 625)

40. **(B)** Often with a cervical-spine injury, the patient in a supine position may have his arms stretched out above his head. (p. 625)

41. **(A)** The first step in the care of a scalp injury is to control bleeding. (p. 615)

42. **(C)** An unstable object impaled in the cheek wall should be pulled out if easily done. This minimizes the potential for bleeding into the airway. (p. 536)

43. **(A)** If possible, a patient with facial fractures should be transported on a long spine board in the supine position. Then the patient and board can be rotated to the side to ensure drainage from the patient's mouth. (p. 622)

44. **(D)** The pressure point for controlling bleeding from the leg is the femoral artery. (p. 508)

45. **(A)** Do not pick embedded particles out of the cut. Care for an open wound includes controlling bleeding, bandaging the dressing in place, and cleaning the wound surface. (pp. 533–534)

46. **(B)** The best method for control of nasal bleeding is pinching the nostrils together. (p. 511)

47. **(C)** The first step in caring for possible internal bleeding after ensuring respiration and circulation and controlling life-threatening external bleeding is treating for shock. Do not place the patient in a sitting position if you suspect shock. (p. 513)

48. (D) A razor blade cut is an example of a laceration. The term "incision" was used in the old curriculum. (p. 530)

49. (D) The condition in which flaps of skin are torn loose or pulled off completely is called avulsion. (p. 531)

50. (C) If a patient has an object impaled in the forearm, after the control of profuse bleeding, you should stabilize the object. Do not remove the object. (p. 535)

51. (D) Pale, cool, clammy skin is a sign of shock. (p. 514)

52. (A) An object impaled in the eye should be stabilized with gauze and protected with a disposable cup. It is also important to cover the other eye to limit movement of the eyes. (pp. 536–537)

53. (C) A lacerated eyelid or injury to the eyeball should be covered with folded 4 × 4s to carefully hold it in place. (pp. 536–537)

54. (A) All open wounds to the chest should be considered life-threatening. (pp. 539–540)

55. (C) Before moving a supine patient with possible spinal injuries onto a long spine board, you should always apply a rigid collar. A KED is not needed for a supine patient. (p. 626)

56. (A) The initial effort to control bleeding from a severed neck artery should be direct pressure or pinching. Then apply the occlusive dressing. Remember BSI precautions. (p. 538)

57. (B) The most reliable sign of spinal-cord injury in conscious patients is paralysis of extremities. Tenderness along the spine may indicate injury to the bones or muscles. (p. 624)

58. (D) When caring for an open abdominal wound with evisceration, do not replace the organ but cover with a moistened dressing. (p. 544)

59. (C) A patient in acute abdominal distress without vomiting should be transported face up with the knees bent to relieve the pressure on the abdominal muscles. (pp. 544–545)

60. (C) When a joint is locked into position, the EMT-B should splint it in the position found. Do not apply force to move a joint. (pp. 575–576)

61. (A) A splint properly applied to an extremity should prevent an open bone injury, motion of bone fragments, and damage to muscles and blood vessels. It should not impede circulation. (p. 574)

62. (B) A fractured clavicle is best cared for with a sling and swathe. Do not tie the sling over the injured clavicle. (p. 582)

63. (B) A fracture to the humerus shaft is best cared for by immobilizing with a rigid splint or sling and swathe, which limits movement in all directions. (p. 590)

64. (D) A fracture to the proximal end of the humerus is best cared for by immobilizing with a sling and swathe. (p. 590)

65. (B) The best way to immobilize a fractured elbow when the arm is found in the bent position and there is a distal pulse is to keep the arm in its found position and apply a short paddled splint. Do not straighten fractured joints that have pulses. (p. 591)

66. (B) When splinting, if a severe deformity exists or distal circulation is compromised, you should align to the anatomical position with gentle traction. (p. 574)

67. (C) The first step in immobilizing a fractured wrist with distal pulse is to place the broken hand in its position of function. (p. 593)

68. (A) A patient with a fractured pelvis should be immobilized on an orthopedic stretcher or long spine board with legs bound together with wide cravats. An antishock garment could be applied if local protocols permit. In many localities, application requires an order from a physician. (p. 583)

69. (D) A fractured femur is best immobilized with a traction splint. (p. 585)

70. (A) Before immobilizing a fractured knee, assess for distal PMS function. If there is no pulse, you may need to manipulate the extremity. (p. 585)

71. (B) The best method for immobilizing a suspected ankle fracture is a pillow splint. (p. 586)

72. (B) A sprain is an injury in which ligaments are torn. (p. 572)

73. (C) Definitive care for open extremity injuries is not provided in the prehospital setting. All other choices are true. (p. 572)

74. (D) Muscle is attached to bone by tendons. (p. 567)

75. (B) A partial-thickness burn involves the epidermis and dermis. (pp. 545, 547)

76. (A) The entire back of an adult patient's right upper extremity is 4.5% (the entire arm is 9, so half is 4.5%) and her entire chest (which is 9%) is therefore 9 + 4.5 = 13.5%. (pp. 548–549)

77. (C) A moderate burn involves superficial burns covering more than 50% of the body surface. (p. 550)

78. (A) Partial-thickness burns cause swelling and blistering. (pp. 545, 547)

79. (D) A patient suffering chemical burns to the skin caused by dry lime should be treated by first brushing away the lime. Also, if you look up the chemical, you would note it should not be mixed with water or phenol. (pp. 551, 553)

80. (D) Acid burns to the eyes should be flooded with water for at least 20 minutes. (p. 553)

81. (A) A method for estimating the extent of a burn is the rule of nines. (p. 548)

82. (A) The number-one priority for all EMS personnel at a collision scene is wearing the appropriate protective clothing. The unsafe act that contributes most to collision scene injuries is failure to wear protective gear during rescue operations. (p. 721)

83. (A) When arriving at the scene of a collision, the first thing an EMT-B should do is evaluate hazards and calculate the need for additional support. (p. 720)

84. (D) The EMT-B cannot be responsible for protecting the patient from injuries sustained by not wearing a seatbelt. The EMT-B is responsible for protecting the patient from broken glass from the wrecked car, sharp metal in the wrecked car, and the environment. (p. 722)

85. (D) It is not your responsibility to describe extrication procedures to the bystanders; doing so could take too much valuable time. At the scene of an auto collision, the EMT-B should try to keep the patient's safety in mind, inform the patient of the unique aspects of the extrication, and keep his/her own personal safety in mind. (p. 722)

86. (C) A vehicle involved in a collision that is determined to be a simple access will not require equipment to get to the patient. (p. 731)

87. (C) When applying a short spine board, the EMT-B should never apply a chin strap to the patient. (p. 630)

88. **(D)** Do not pull the patient out the side windows. To assist with patient access, the EMT-B should initially try opening each car door, roll down windows, and ask the patient to unlock the doors. (p. 731)

89. **(A)** Requirements for speed of removal dictates the specific technique used for spinal immobilization of a patient at a collision scene. (p. 720)

90. **(D)** The steps should be 1) sizing up the situation, 2) stabilizing the vehicle, 3) gaining the access, 4) disentangling the patient. (p. 719)

91. **(D)** The number of ambulances in the region is not a consideration unless this is an MCI. Considerations for size-up of a collision include potential hazards, need for additional EMS units, and the number of patients involved. (p. 720)

92. **(C)** To minimize injuries at a collision, EMT-Bs should wear highly visible clothing so they do not get hit by a car while attending to their patient. Use the proper tools for the task and do not deactivate the safety guards on tools or you will be injured. It is not always feasible to wait until the police arrive on the scene. (pp. 721–722)

93. **(B)** The vehicle's catalytic converter can be a source of ignition at a collision because it is often over 1,200°F. (p. 727)

94. **(A)** The three-step process of disentanglement described in the text includes creating exitways by displacing doors and roof posts, disentangling occupants by displacing front end, and gaining access by disposing of the roof. Opening the trunk and disconnecting the battery cable are not priority tasks. (pp. 731–732)

95. **(B)** If a vehicle's electrical system must be disrupted, disconnect the ground cable from the battery. (p. 727)

96. **(D)** When positioning flares, use a formula that includes the stopping distance for the posted speed plus the margin of safety. (pp. 722, 724)

97. **(C)** Once the vehicle has been stabilized, the second part of an extrication procedure for patient rescue is to displace doors and roof posts. The first part is to dispose of the roof. (p. 732)

98. **(A)** The Emergency Medical Dispatcher (EMD) has told you the exact location of a collision, how many and what kinds of vehicles are involved, and any known hazards. Other information that would be helpful from the EMD concerning this collision would be how many persons are injured. (p. 694)

99. **(C)** The EMD does not need to ask the person's name. All other questions are pertinent. (p. 694)

100. **(A)** When operating a siren, be aware that the continuous sound of a siren could worsen a patient's condition. All motorists will not hear and honor your signal. If you use the siren continuously, there should be a valid reason for doing so. The noise from the siren can damage your ears over a period of time. (pp. 696–697)

101. **(D)** Factors that affect an ambulance's response to a scene include day of the week, time of the day, and detours. Danger zones usually cannot be planned for. (p. 698)

102. **(B)** If a patient develops cardiac arrest during transport, have the operator of the ambulance stop the ambulance so you can begin defibrillation. Also alert the hospital about the arrest. (p. 703)

103. **(C)** When transferring a nonemergency patient to the emergency department personnel, you should check to see what is to be done with the patient. (p. 703)

104. **(C)** The last step when transferring a patient is to obtain your release, which usually takes the form of a thank-you for the information provided. (p. 703)

105. **(C)** At the hospital, as soon as you are free from patient care activities, you should prepare the prehospital care report. (p. 705)

106. **(D)** Suction catheters, contaminated dressings, and blood-soaked linens are considered biohazards; unopened gauze bandages are not. (p. 705)

107. **(D)** Completeness and operability of equipment is not always ensured in the EMS/hospital equipment exchange program. Always quickly inspect it; if you find parts are broken or incomplete, notify someone in authority so the device can be repaired or replaced. (pp. 705, 707)

108. **(D)** Vigorous cleaning of the ambulance while parked at the hospital is prevented or restricted by time, equipment, and space. There is, however, no law against it. (p. 705)

109. **(A)** While en route to your quarters, radio dispatch that you are returning. (p. 707)

110. **(D)** You should air the ambulance en route to quarters. When you return to quarters, replenish oxygen cylinders, clean the interior of the ambulance, and prepare yourself for service. (pp. 707, 711)

111. **(D)** Antivenin solution is not routinely carried in an ambulance as it needs to be refrigerated, is expensive, and is rarely used. A poison-control kit should include paper cups, activated charcoal, and drinking water. (p. 691)

112. **(C)** The fixed suction system is not part of the first-in kit. All other answer choices are correct. (p. 689)

113. **(A)** The first thing to inspect on the ambulance when the engine is off is the body of the vehicle. (p. 692)

114. **(B)** Rescue tools should always be examined for rust and dirt. (p. 694)

115. **(B)** Along with physical and mental fitness, ambulance operators should be able to perform under stress. (p. 695)

116. **(D)** When driving an ambulance, you should realize that there are no state laws that grant the absolute right of way. (p. 696)

117. **(B)** The headlights of an ambulance should be turned on whenever the vehicle is on the road so it can easily be seen. (p. 697)

118. **(D)** To assume that there is no electrical hazard would be very dangerous. When a car collides with a utility pole, the EMT-B should assume obviously dead wires could be energized at any moment, that severed conductors may be energizing every wire, and wires may be charged at the highest voltage present. (p. 725)

119. **(B)** The easiest way to break tempered window glass is with a spring-loaded center punch. (p. 731)

120. **(D)** Airway passages do swell when a child has airway disease. All other signs listed are indications of a respiratory disease. (p. 669)

121. **(C)** The soft spot on top of an infant's head is called the fontanelle. (p. 664)

122. **(B)** Small children are referred to as abdominal breathers because they use their diaphragm for breathing. (p. 664)

123. **(C)** A child's compensating mechanism for shock fails at approximately 30% blood loss. (p. 668)

124. **(D)** In cases of sudden death syndrome, the EMT-B should provide resuscitation and transport to the hospital. (p. 676)

125. **(C)** Injuries to the center of the back and upper arms might lead you to consider child abuse. Multiple skinned knees and sprained ankles are common in children. (pp. 679–680)

126. **(A)** A child who is hypoxic will have a slowed heart rate. (p. 666)

127. **(D)** Artificial ventilations for an infant or child under 8 years of age should be provided at a rate of 20 per minute. (p. 666)

128. **(B)** If you suspect respiratory distress in a conscious toddler, you should not insert anything in the patient's mouth. This could set off spasms along the upper airway that will totally obstruct the airway. (p. 669)

129. **(C)** Children usually get lead poisoning from eating paint chips. (p. 674)

130. **(C)** Common causes of shock in children include infection, trauma, blood loss, and dehydration. (p. 668)

131. **(C)** A sunken fontanelle may indicate dehydration. (p. 664)

132. **(A)** Flowing oxygen over the face of a small child so it will be inhaled is referred to as the blow-by technique. (p. 666)

133. **(B)** A complication of a rapidly rising temperature in a child is often a seizure. (p. 672)

134. **(D)** A group of viral illnesses that cause inflammation of the larynx, trachea, and bronchi is called croup. (p. 670)

135. **(C)** A child ages three to six is referred to as a preschooler. (p. 663)

136. **(D)** The strong, white, fibrous material covering the bones is called the periosteum. (p. 565)

137. **(C)** The coming apart of a joint is referred to as a dislocation. (p. 572)

138. **(B)** Overstretching or overexertion of a muscle is called a strain. (p. 572)

139. **(B)** Proper splinting of a closed fracture is designed to prevent closed injuries from becoming open ones. (p. 574)

140. **(B)** Any force strong enough to fracture the pelvis also can cause injury to the spine. (p. 583)

141. **(D)** The Sager is a unipolar splint. Examples of bipolar traction splints include Hare, Fernotrac, and half-ring. (p. 576)

142. **(C)** The indications for a traction splint are painful, swollen, deformed mid-thigh with no joint or lower leg injury. (pp. 576, 582)

143. **(C)** The Hazardous Materials Technician actually plugs, patches, or stops the release of a hazardous material. First Responder Awareness rescuers are trained only to recognize the problem and initiate a response from the proper organizations. First Responder Operations rescuers are trained to initially respond to releases or potential releases of hazardous materials in order to protect people, property, and the environment. The most advanced level of training is for the Hazardous Materials Specialist; this level rescuer is expected to have advanced knowledge and skills and to command and support activities at the incident site. (p. 742)

144. **(C)** The "safe zone" should be established on the same level as and upwind from the hazardous materials accident site. This positioning prevents flowing liquids or burning gases from spreading into the "safe zone." (pp. 743–744)

145. **(B)** A resource that must be maintained at the work site by the employer and that must be available to all employees working with hazardous materials is called the *Material Safety Data Sheet*. This sheet generally name the substance, its physical properties, fire and explosion hazard information, health hazard information, and emergency first-aid treatment. (p. 745)

146. **(B)** EMS personal at a hazmat incident are responsible for caring for the injured and monitoring and rehabilitating the hazmat team members. (p. 748)

147. **(D)** When a patient is categorized as Priority 1 at an MCI, this means the patient has treatable life-threatening illness or injuries. (pp. 755–756)

148. **(A)** The MCI officer responsible for communicating with each treatment sector to determine the number and priority of the patients in that sector is called the staging officer. (p. 759)

149. **(C)** A Priority 2 patient at an MCI would be color-coded yellow. Priority 1 patients would be red, Priority 3 would be green, and Priority 4, black or gray. (pp. 755–756)

150. **(C)** Patients at an MCI who are assessed to have minor injuries are categorized as Priority 3. See answer #149. (pp. 755–756)

Chapter 35: Advanced Airway Management

MATCH TERMINOLOGY/DEFINITIONS

▶ **Part A**

1. **(M)** Alveoli—microscopic sacs of the lungs where exchange of carbon dioxide and oxygen takes place

2. **(K)** Bronchi—two large sets of branches that come off the trachea and enter the lungs (There are right and left mainstem bronchi.)

3. **(A)** Carina—fork at the lower end of the trachea where the two mainstem bronchi branch

4. **(J)** Cricoid cartilage—ring-shaped structure that circles the trachea at the lower portion of the larynx

5. **(O)** EIDD—esophageal intubation detector device that may be used to detect incorrect placement (or to verify correct placement) of the endotracheal tube

6. **(C)** Endotracheal tube—tube designed to be inserted into the trachea; oxygen, medication, or a suction catheter can be directed into the trachea through an endotracheal tube.

7. **(I)** Epiglottis—leaf-shaped structure that acts as a covering to the opening of the trachea and that prevents food and foreign matter from entering it

8. **(G)** Esophagus—tube that leads from the pharynx to the stomach

9. **(F)** Glottic opening—opening to the trachea

10. **(H)** Hyperventilate—to provide ventilations at a higher rate to compensate for oxygen not delivered during intubation or suctioning

11. **(D)** Hypopharynx—area directly above the openings of both the trachea and the esophagus

12. **(E)** Hypoxia—inadequate oxygenation, or oxygen starvation

13. **(B)** Intubation—insertion of a tube

14. **(N)** Laryngoscope—illuminating instrument that is inserted into the pharynx to permit visualization of the pharynx and larynx

15. **(L)** Larynx—voice box

▶ **Part B**

1. **(E)** Mainstem bronchi—either of the two (right or left) large sets of branches that come off the trachea and enter the lungs

2. **(G)** Nasogastric tube (NG tube)—tube designed to be passed through the nose, nasopharynx, and esophagus. It is used to relieve distention of the stomach in an infant or child patient.

3. **(H)** Nasopharynx—area directly posterior to the nose

4. **(I)** Oropharynx—area directly posterior to the mouth

5. **(A)** Orotracheal intubation—placement of an endotracheal tube through the mouth and into the trachea

6. **(J)** Sellick's maneuver—pressure applied to the cricoid cartilage to suppress vomiting and bring the vocal cords into view; also called cricoid pressure

7. **(D)** Stylet—long, thin, flexible metal probe

8. **(B)** Trachea—"windpipe"; the structure that connects the pharynx to the lungs

9. **(F)** Vallecula—groove-like structure anterior to the epiglottis

10. **(C)** Vocal cords—two thin folds of tissue within the larynx that vibrate as air passes between them, producing sounds

MULTIPLE-CHOICE REVIEW

1. **(C)** The area directly above the openings of both the trachea and the esophagus is called the hypopharynx. (p. 765)

2. **(B)** The groove-like structure anterior to the epiglottis is called the vallecula. The carina is the location where the trachea bifurcates into the right and left mainstem bronchi. (p. 765)

3. **(B)** Food is more apt to be aspirated into the right mainstem bronchus rather than the left mainstem bronchus because the right splits off the carina at less of an angle than the left. (p. 765)

4. **(A)** The brain's center for respiratory control is located in the brainstem. The cerebellum controls fine-motor coordination, and the cerebrum contains the centers of higher cognitive abilities. The pons functions as a bridge between the cerebrum and cerebellum. (p. 765)

5. **(C)** The endotracheal tube is primarily intended to be inserted into the trachea and functions to provide direct access to the trachea. This allows positive pressure ventilation without the hazards of aspiration. Medication administration and suctioning are also possible via the tube, although these are not the primary functions of the tube. (p. 769)

6. **(A)** Orotracheal intubation allows direct ventilation of the lungs, bypassing the entire upper airway. (p. 769)

7. **(C)** When placing the endotracheal tube, the EMT-B uses direct visualization. Rapid-sequence, blind, and surgical techniques are performed by paramedics. (p. 769)

8. **(D)** Orotracheal intubation provides complete control of the airway and minimizes the risk of aspiration. It also

provides for better oxygen delivery and allows for deeper suctioning of the airway. (p. 769)

9. **(C)** During orotracheal intubation attempts, the heart rate may decrease, not increase, due to vagal nerve stimulation. Monitor the patient's heart rate closely. Complications of orotracheal intubation include hypoxia from prolonged attempts, soft-tissue trauma to the lips, gums, or airway structures, and gagging and vomiting. (p. 769)

10. **(B)** When the endotracheal tube is advanced too deeply, right-mainstem intubation commonly occurs. (p. 770)

11. **(C)** The most serious complication of endotracheal intubation is unrecognized esophageal intubation, which will rapidly result in death. Mainstem bronchus intubation, bradycardia, and airway trauma are also potential complications. (p. 770)

12. **(A)** The EMT-B should reassess the location of the endotracheal tube each time the patient is moved to prevent complications from accidental extubation. The tube can easily be displaced just enough to remove it from the trachea. Be sure to reassess the tube position after each move. (p. 770)

13. **(C)** Most adult patients can be intubated using a size 2 or 3 straight blade or size 3 curved blade. (p. 771)

14. **(C)** The straight blade is designed so that the tip of the blade is placed under the epiglottis. (p. 771)

15. **(D)** The curved blade is designed so the tip of the blade is placed into the vallecula. (p. 771)

16. **(A)** The cuff at the distal end of the endotracheal tube usually seals with 8 to 10 cc of air. Infant tubes are cuffless. (p. 771)

17. **(C)** When using an endotracheal tube on an infant or child less than eight years of age, do not expect to see a cuff on the tube. In these pediatric patients, the cricoid cartilage serves as a "cuff." (p. 771)

18. **(B)** No matter what the internal diameter of the endotracheal tube, it has a standard 15-millimeter adapter so the bag-valve mask can easily be attached. Infant and child tubes are cuffless, therefore, they do not have an inflation valve or pilot balloon. (p. 771)

19. **(C)** It is generally accepted that the average size adult male should receive either an 8.0 or 8.5 mm tube. (p. 771)

20. **(C)** In an adult, the properly placed tube will have the 22 cm mark at the teeth. (p. 771)

21. **(D)** Once the lubricated stylet is inserted, the endotracheal tube should be shaped like a hockey stick. This facilitates tube placement. (p. 772)

22. **(D)** Prior to securing an endotracheal tube, insert an oral airway as a bite block, listen to both lungs, and listen over the epigastrium. Do not suction down the tube until it is properly taped into place or you may accidentally extubate the patient. (p. 773)

23. **(C)** Endotracheal tube length is dependent upon the tube diameter; the tube length during placement is unimportant. Items that should be checked prior to an intubation attempt include the laryngoscope light bulb, cuff on the tube, and the shape formed by the stylet in the tube. (p. 777)

24. **(C)** The laryngoscope is designed to be held in the left hand. Do not use it as a fulcrum as you may break the patient's teeth. (p. 777)

25. **(A)** The Sellick's maneuver is designed to help reduce vomiting by indirectly compressing the esophagus. In addition, it often brings the vocal cords into view. (p. 777)

26. **(B)** The correct order for verifying tube placement by auscultation for the presence of breath sounds is first the epigastrium, then left, then right chest apex. (p. 778)

27. **(C)** If the breath sounds are diminished or absent on the left but present on the right, it is likely the tube has advanced into the right mainstem bronchus. (p. 778)

28. **(B)** The EMT-B should make no more than <u>two</u> attempts at orotracheal intubation. If both attempts fail, insert an oral airway, continue to ventilate the patient with high-concentration oxygen via bag-valve mask, and aggressively suction the airway. (p. 779)

29. **(D)** The narrowest portion of the infant's or small child's airway is the cricoid ring. The proper sizing of the uncuffed tube is critical to ensure an appropriate seal of the ET tube. (p. 780)

30. **(B)** A #1 straight blade is preferred for use in infants and small children. (p. 780)

31. **(C)** A nasogastric tube (NG) is commonly used in an infant or child patient to decompress the stomach and proximal bowel. (p. 782)

32. **(B)** When you are unable to adequately ventilate the child or infant patient due to distention of the stomach, you should consider the use of a nasogastric tube. (p. 782)

33. **(D)** The major contraindication for an NG tube placement would be head or major facial trauma due to the potential of placing the tube directly into the brain. (p. 782)

34. **(A)** The NG tube should be measured from the tip of the nose around the ear to below the xiphoid process. (p. 782)

35. **(D)** Do not hook the NG tube up to the suction unit. Once the NG tube is passed gently downward along the nasal floor, the EMT-B should confirm tube placement by aspirating stomach contents, secure the tube in place with tape, and confirm placement by auscultating the epigastrium while injecting 10–20 cc of air. (p. 783)

COMPLETE THE FOLLOWING

1. The four indications for when to perform orotracheal intubation include: (p. 773)
   - inability to ventilate the apneic patient
   - to protect the airway of a patient without a gag reflex or cough
   - to protect the airway of a patient unresponsive to any painful stimuli
   - cardiac arrest

2. The six complications of deep suctioning that can be avoided by hyperventilation include: (p. 786)
   - cardiac dysrhythmias
   - hypoxia
   - coughing
   - damage to the lining (mucosa) of the airway
   - spasm of the bronchioles if catheter extends past the carina
   - spasm of the vocal cords during orotracheal suctioning

VIRTUAL STREET SCENES

1. Be prepared to extubate the patient, assuring that you have suction available at the patient's side.

2. Yes. The patient is critical, and ALS would be helpful.

3. Remove the tube, and reintubate the patient.

4. Yes. The tube needs to be placed with the patient's head and neck manually stabilized in an in-line position. You also should consider a straight blade.

ALS-Assist Skills

MATCH TERMINOLOGY/DEFINITIONS

1. **(G)** Cricoid pressure—gently pressing the thumb and index finger just to either side of the medial throat and over the cricoid cartilage to bring the patient's vocal cords into view

2. **(C)** Drip chamber—chamber from which the drops of IV fluid flow

3. **(E)** ECG—measurement of the electrical activity of the heart on a graph

4. **(B)** Flow regulator—stop cock located below the drip chamber that can be pushed up or down to start, stop, or control the flow rate

5. **(F)** Infiltration—when an IV needle has either punctured a vein and exited the other side or has pulled out of the vein and the fluid is flowing into the surrounding tissues instead of into the vein

6. **(H)** IV—intravenous line inserted into a vein so that blood, fluids, or medications can be administered directly into a patient's circulation

7. **(D)** Macro drip—drip chamber used when a higher flow of fluid is needed (for a multi-trauma victim in shock, for example)

8. **(A)** Mini drip—drip chamber used when minimal flow of fluid is needed (with children, for example)

9. **(I)** Needle port—opening below the flow regulator on an IV set into which medication is injected

MULTIPLE-CHOICE REVIEW

1. **(C)** The "gold standard" of airway care is the endotracheal tube because it can be inserted directly into the trachea, forming an open pathway for air, oxygen, or medications to be blown into the lungs. (p. 794)

2. **(D)** Typical patients who need an endotracheal tube inserted include patients in pulmonary or cardiopulmonary arrest, patients in need of airway control, and those in respiratory failure due to overdose (or fluid in the lungs, asthma, asphyxia, or allergic reaction). A patient with full-thickness burns to the extremities would not need such assistance unless his level of responsiveness diminished. (p. 794)

3. **(A)** Prior to an intubation attempt, you may be asked to hyperventilate the patient. During the attempt, you may be asked to press on the neck to help bring the vocal cords into view. (p. 794)

4. **(A)** You do not shock a patient during an intubation attempt. During the intubation attempt, you may be asked to stand by and be prepared to begin ventilations, to gently press on the sides of the cricoid cartilage, and maintain neck stabilization. (pp. 795–796)

5. **(B)** Once the endotracheal tube is inserted in the trachea and the cuff is inflated, the paramedic should confirm placement by first using an esophageal intubation detector and then auscultating. See answer #6. (pp. 794–795)

6. **(D)** We do not listen over the lower abdomen. After inserting the tube, the intubator should listen with his stethoscope over the left lung, the right lung, and the epigastrium to confirm placement. Once the intubator assures the proper placement, then the ET tube is taped into place using an oral airway as a bite block. (pp. 794–795)

7. **(A)** If during the movement of the patient the ET tube is moved, you should notify the paramedic, who will immediately recheck placement. If the tube is pushed in, it will most likely enter the right mainstem bronchus, preventing oxygen from entering the patient's left lung. If the tube is pulled out, it can easily slip into the esophagus and send all the ventilations directly to the stomach, denying the patient oxygen. This is a fatal complication if it goes unnoticed before the tube is anchored in place. (p. 795)

8. **(B)** If you are ventilating a breathing patient with a BVM, you should time your ventilations with the patient's respiratory efforts. Do not decrease the oxygen concentration. (p. 795)

9. **(C)** If, when ventilating, you feel a sudden change in the resistance, this could be caused by air escaping through a hole in the lungs and filling the space around the lungs, which is called a tension pneumothorax. (p. 795)

10. **(B)** When ventilating a patient in cardiac arrest with a BVM, with each defibrillation attempt you should remove the bag from the tube. If you do not do this, the weight of the unsupported bag may accidentally displace the tube. (p. 795)

11. **(B)** It is important to note the mental status changes of patients who are intubated because they may wake up and bite on the tube, or they may attempt to pull out the tube. (p. 795)

12. **(A)** After the paramedic injects some medication down the tube, if you are assigned to ventilations, you may be asked to hyperventilate the patient to increase the rate at which medication enters the bloodstream through the respiratory system. (p. 795)

13. **(C)** If the patient has a suspected cervical-spine injury, your role will be to maintain in-line spinal stabilization throughout the procedure. (p. 795)

14. **(C)** A standard procedure used to alert EMS personnel to life-threatening heart rhythm disturbances is the ECG. (p. 796)

15. **(D)** Interpreting the ECG is the responsibility of personnel with additional training in its interpretation. The EMT-B should know how to turn on the ECG monitor and change the battery, change the roll of paper, and record an ECG strip. (p. 796)

16. **(B)** When assisting with an ECG, you should try to get in the habit of applying the leads to the electrode and then to the patient. If you apply the electrodes to the leads while they are on the patient, this creates some discomfort. (p. 796)

17. **(D)** When preparing the patient's skin for ECG electrodes, dry the area, remove oil, and shave the patient's skin. You may also apply an antiperspirant to the patient who is sweating. Do not apply alcohol to the skin as it could burn the patient if defibrillation is necessary. (p. 796)

18. **(D)** In the most common electrode configuration, the red electrode is placed on the left lower chest. White is right, and red is ribs. (p. 796)

19. **(B)** In the most common electrode configuration, the green or black electrode is placed under the center of the left clavicle. (p. 796)

20. **(D)** A mini drip IV administration set produces 60 drops for every cc. (p. 797)

21. **(A)** A macro drip IV administration set produces 10 to 15 drops for every cc. (p. 797)

22. **(D)** When inspecting an IV fluid bag, always check for expiration date, clarity of the fluid, and leaks in the bag. (pp. 797–798)

23. **(A)** When removing the protective covering from the port of the fluid bag and the protective covering from the spiked end of the tubing, be very careful to maintain sterility. If these parts touch the ground, they must <u>not</u> be used. (p. 798)

24. **(B)** The IV line is flushed prior to using it on a patient because it prevents introducing an air embolism into the patient's vein. (p. 798)

25. **(C)** The patient's blood pressure has nothing to do with the IV flow rate. Interruptions in the flow of an IV can be caused by a closed flow regulator, a constricting band left on the patient's arm, and kinked tubing. (pp. 798–799)

COMPLETE THE FOLLOWING

1. You may be asked to carry out four steps in the process of applying electrodes: (p. 796)
   - Turn on the ECG monitor.
   - Plug in the monitoring cables or "leads."
   - Attach the monitoring cables to the electrodes.
   - Apply the electrodes to the patient's body.

Stress in EMS

MATCH TERMINOLOGY/DEFINITIONS

1. **(I)** Acceptance—during this phase of grief, the dying person comes to peace with impending death

2. **(F)** Alarm reaction—first stage of the body's response to stress in which the sympathetic nervous system increases its activity in what is known as the "fight or flight" syndrome

3. **(B)** Cortisol—hormone that influences your metabolism and your immune response

4. **(C)** Critical incident—any situation that triggers a strong emotional response

5. **(E)** Cumulative stress reaction—reaction that is a result of prolonged recurring stressors in our work or private lives

6. **(H)** Debriefing—formal, highly structured process employed to assist individuals who are experiencing acute stress reactions; it includes six phases: fact, thought, reaction, symptom, teaching, and re-entry.

7. **(G)** Defusing—shorter and less structured form of debriefing usually led by a peer support member

8. **(D)** Delayed stress reaction—posttraumatic stress disorder, which may occur at any time, days to years, following a critical incident; also called PTSD

9. **(J)** Grief—emotional reaction to a loss that includes the process of recovery and adjustment to the loss

10. **(A)** Stress—state of physical and/or psychological arousal to a stimulus

MULTIPLE-CHOICE REVIEW

1. **(B)** You cannot always predict stressors or avoid them. Stressors that you are exposed to as an EMT-B may be the result of environmental factors, your dealings with other people, and your self-image or performance expectations. (p. 800)

2. **(A)** The three stages of the general adaptation syndrome as described by Dr. Hans Selye include the alarm reaction, resistance, and exhaustion. The other answer choices (acceptance, denial, and bargaining) are stages of grief. (p. 800)

3. **(C)** Cortisol, which influences your metabolism and immune response under stress, is produced by the endocrine system. (p. 800)

4. **(C)** The stress triad, which occurs late in the exhaustion phase, involves enlargement of the adrenal glands, wasting of the lymph nodes, and bleeding gastric ulcers. People in the third stage tend to have heart attacks, not cancer. (pp. 800–801)

5. **(B)** Another term for burnout is cumulative stress reaction, which occurs as a result of prolonged recurring stressors in our work or private lives. PTSD (posttraumatic stress disorder, also know as delayed stress reaction) is usually based on a delayed reaction to one critical incident. (p. 801)

6. **(D)** If a sign or symptom of acute stress reaction is not too severe or long-lasting (such as overeating for 24 hours), it may be uncomfortable, but not dangerous and does not require intervention. However, any sign or symptom that indicates an acute medical or psychological problem does require intervention. (p. 801)

7. **(D)** Boredom and apathy are early signs of cumulative stress reaction. Late signs include headaches and stomach ailments, sleep disturbances, and loss of emotional control. (p. 801)

8. **(B)** The ultimate key to preventing or managing cumulative stress lies in seeking balance in one's life. It will not be necessary to replace EMS with another career if you keep stress in check. Drugs and alcohol do not solve problems; they only contribute to them in the long run. (p. 802)

9. **(D)** Investigation of job-related stress reveals that oftentimes it is not the job itself that is the stressor, but rather organizational and functional factors. The leader's use of sensible, humane management practices can help relieve job-related stress. (p. 803)

10. **(C)** The phases of grief generally follow this order: denial and isolation, anger, bargaining, depression, and acceptance. (pp. 803–804)

COMPLETE THE FOLLOWING

1. Signs and symptoms associated with an acute stress reaction that require intervention may include: (p. 801)
   - acute medical problems (such as chest pain, difficulty breathing, or abnormal heart rhythms)
   - acute psychological problems (such as uncontrollable crying, inappropriate behavior, or a disruption in normal rational thinking)

2. The six phases of a CISD are: (p. 802)
   - fact
   - thought
   - reaction
   - symptom
   - teaching
   - re-entry

Basic Cardiac Life Support Review

MATCH TERMINOLOGY/DEFINITIONS

1. **(G)** Biological death—when brain cells die

2. **(K)** Brachial pulse—pulse measured by feeling the major artery of the arm; the absence of this pulse is used as a sign, in infants, that heartbeat has stopped and CPR should begin.

3. **(L)** Cardiopulmonary resuscitation—actions you take to revive a person—or at least temporarily prevent biological death—by keeping the person's heart and lungs working

4. **(D)** Carotid pulse—pulse felt between the groove of the Adam's apple and the muscles located along the side of the neck

5. **(C)** Clinical death—when breathing and heartbeat stop

6. **(E)** 50:50 rule—requirement that the amount of time you spend compressing the patient's chest should be the same as the time spent for release

7. **(F)** Gastric distention—bulging of the stomach that may be caused by forcing air into the patient's stomach during rescue breathing

8. **(J)** Head-tilt, chin-lift maneuver—maneuver that provides for maximum opening of the airway

9. **(B)** Heimlich maneuver—manual thrusts to the abdomen used to dislodge an airway obstruction

10. **(M)** Jaw-thrust maneuver—maneuver used to open the airway of a patient with a suspected spine injury

11. **(N)** Line of lividity—red or purple skin discoloration that occurs when gravity causes the blood to sink to the lowest parts of the body and collect there

12. **(O)** Recovery position—lying the patient on the side to allow for drainage from the mouth and to prevent the tongue from falling backward

13. **(A)** Rescue breathing—providing artificial ventilations to a person who has stopped breathing or whose breathing is inadequate

14. **(I)** Substernal notch—general term for area of the lower border of the sternum

15. **(H)** Xiphoid process—short triangular piece of cartilage (tough, elastic gristle) that extends from the bottom of the sternum

1. **(B)** When a patient's breathing and heartbeat stop, the brain cells will begin to die after 4 to 6 minutes. Heart, liver, and kidney cells begin to die after about one hour. (p. 817)

2. **(D)** Once clinical death occurs, brain cells begin to die within 4 to 6 minutes. However, it usually takes 10 minutes for biological death to occur. (p. 817)

3. **(C)** In the ABC method of cardiopulmonary resuscitation, the "A" stands for airway. (p. 817)

4. **(C)** In the ABC method of cardiopulmonary resuscitation, the "C" stands for circulation. (p. 817)

5. **(D)** To determine if an adult or child is pulseless, the EMT-B should check for a pulse at the carotid artery. (p. 818)

6. **(A)** To determine pulselessness in an infant, the EMT-B should use the brachial artery. This is because the carotid pulse is difficult to determine in an infant. (p. 818)

7. **(B)** If you are alone, after determining unresponsiveness in the adult, the next thing you should do before starting CPR is to activate EMS. (p. 818)

8. **(C)** When an unconscious patient's head flexes forward, the tongue could cause an airway obstruction. (p. 818)

9. **(C)** One of the best ways way to relieve an airway obstruction due to the positioning of the patient's tongue is the head-tilt, chin-lift maneuver. The jaw-thrust maneuver is used on a trauma patient. (p. 818)

10. **(C)** The head-tilt, chin-lift maneuver should not be used on a diving accident victim due to the potential for cervical-spine injury. (p. 818)

11. **(A)** The recommended maneuver for opening the airway of a patient with possible cervical-spine injury is the jaw-thrust maneuver. (p. 819)

12. **(B)** After opening the airway in a patient who requires rescue breathing, the EMT-B should inflate the patient's lung with two slow breaths. (pp. 819–820)

13. **(C)** Initial ventilations did not result in chest rise. Your next step is to perform airway clearance techniques. (pp. 819–820)

14. **(B)** A common problem in the resuscitation of infants and children caused by improper head position or too quick ventilations is gastric distention. (p. 820)

15. **(B)** In adult rescue breathing, the EMT-B provides 10–12 breaths every minute. (p. 820)

16. **(A)** Infants should be ventilated at the rate of one breath every 3 seconds (60 seconds ÷ 20 breaths per minute = 3 seconds). (p. 820)

17. **(C)** When a patient has a distended abdomen due to air being forced into the stomach, the EMT-B should be prepared to suction should the patient vomit. Do not decrease the oxygen concentration; pressing on the abdomen would produce vomiting. (p. 822)

18. **(A)** The recovery position is used because it protects the airway and allows for drainage from the mouth. It also prevents the tongue from blocking the airway. (p. 822)

19. **(C)** When delivering chest compressions during CPR, avoid using a stabbing motion to deliver compressions. Use a rhythmic 50% compression–50% relaxation motion. (p. 826)

20. **(D)** The CPR compression point is located on the lower half of the sternum, centered between the nipples (p. 824)

21. **(B)** Before beginning artificial ventilation, assess the patient's breathing for no more than 10 seconds. (p. 825)

22. **(D)** For an adult, the one-rescuer compression-to-ventilations ratio is 15 : 2. (p. 826)

23. **(C)** The adult CPR compression rate in one-rescuer CPR is 100 times a minute. (p. 826)

24. **(C)** The adult CPR compression rate in two-rescuer CPR is 80–100 times a minute. (p. 826)

25. **(B)** In two-rescuer CPR, the ratio of compressions to ventilations is 15 : 2. (p. 826)

26. **(C)** When performing CPR on an adult, the sternum is depressed $1^1/_2$ to 2 inches. (p. 826)

27. **(B)** When performing CPR on an infant, the sternum is depressed $^1/_2$ to 1 inch; in children 1 to $1^1/_2$ inches; in adults $1^1/_2$ to 2 inches. (p. 826)

28. **(B)** When performing CPR on a child, the sternum is compressed $^1/_2$ to 1 inches. (p. 826)

29. **(D)** The compression rate when performing CPR on an infant is at least 100 times a minute. (p. 826)

30. **(C)** When opening the airway of an infant, use a slight head-tilt. Full hyperextension of the neck can cause the airway to close. (p. 829)

31. **(B)** With effective CPR, the patient's pupils may constrict. Dilation occurs when the patient is hypoxic. (p. 829)

32. **(D)** CPR compressions are delivered to children with the heel of one hand. The fingertips are used to deliver compressions for infants. (p. 827)

33. **(A)** With the exceptions of endotracheal intubation or defibrillation, CPR should not be interrupted for more than a few seconds. (p. 829)

34. **(B)** If you are treating a patient with a partial airway obstruction, poor air exchange, and gray skin, you should treat the patient for a complete airway obstruction. (p. 830)

35. **(B)** Complete airway obstruction in a conscious patient is indicated by an inability to speak. Crowing, gurgling, and snoring are all sounds of partial airway obstruction. (p. 830)

36. **(C)** When you have recognized complete airway obstruction in a conscious adult patient, you should deliver a series of five Heimlich maneuvers. Only unconscious patients are placed in a supine position when ventilations are attempted. (p. 832)

37. **(D)** To deliver abdominal thrusts to an unconscious patient, place the patient in the supine position. (p. 832)

38. **(D)** You are treating an unresponsive adult patient with a complete airway obstruction. You have been unsuccessful in your attempts to ventilate the patient. You should continue with abdominal thrusts, finger sweeps, and reattempt ventilations. (p. 832)

39. **(C)** When treating an 8-month pregnant female who has a complete airway obstruction, the EMT-B should use chest thrusts. (p. 832)

40. **(B)** If a patient has a partial airway obstruction and is able to speak and cough forcefully, you should carefully watch the patient. Do not interfere with the patient's attempts to expel the foreign body. However be prepared to provide

help if the partial airway obstruction becomes a complete obstruction. (p. 834)

41. **(C)** A major difference between the adult and child obstructed airway procedure is blind finger sweeps are not used with children. Chest thrusts and back blows are used on infants. (p. 834)

42. **(B)** While you are trying to clear an obstructed airway in an adult, the patient loses consciousness. You open the airway, perform finger sweeps, and attempt to ventilate. If this fails, retilt the head and again attempt to ventilate. (p. 833)

43. **(B)** You have been unsuccessful in initially ventilating an unconscious infant. You reposition the head and attempt to ventilate again but are unsuccessful. Your next step is to perform back blows and chest thrusts. (p. 833)

44. **(D)** Signs of choking in an infant are lack of a strong cry, ineffective cough, agitation, wheezing, blue color, and breathing difficulty. (pp. 835)

45. **(C)** To correct a complete airway obstruction in an infant, position the patient in the head down position (see Scan BCLS-10). This allows gravity to aid removal and fluids to drain. (p. 835)

COMPLETE THE FOLLOWING

1. The special circumstances in which the EMT-B should not initiate CPR even though the patient is pulseless include: (pp. 829–830)
   - A line of lividity
   - Decomposition
   - Mortal injury
   - Rigor mortis
   - Stillbirth

2. Situations in which the EMT-B may stop CPR include: (p. 830)
   - Spontaneous circulation occurs (then provide rescue breathing as needed)
   - Spontaneous circulation and breathing occur
   - Another trained rescuer can take over for you
   - You turn care of the patient over to a person with a higher level of training
   - Upon order of Medical Director or patient's physician
   - If you become physically exhausted (e.g., backcountry rescue)